INSULIN TREATMENT IN PSYCHIATRY

INSULIN TREATMENT IN PSYCHIATRY

PROCEEDINGS OF THE INTERNATIONAL CONFERENCE
ON THE INSULIN TREATMENT IN PSYCHIATRY
HELD AT THE NEW YORK ACADEMY OF MEDICINE
OCTOBER 24 TO 25, 1958

Edited by:

MAX RINKEL, M.D.

(Boston, Massachusetts)

and

HAROLD E. HIMWICH, M.D.

(Galesburg, Illinois)

PHILOSOPHICAL LIBRARY

New York

Printed in the United States of America

In Memory of
Manfred Sakel's Contribution to Psychiatry.

INTRODUCTION

On October 24 and 25, 1958, an International Conference on the Insulin Treatment in Psychiatry was held at the New York Academy of Medicine under the joint chairmanship of Harold E. Himwich, Galesburg, Illinois; Max Rinkel, Boston, Massachusetts; and Andrew K. Bernath, New York City, New York. This conference was sponsored by Dr. D. Ewen Cameron, Montreal, Canada; Dr. Jacques S. Gottlieb, Detroit, Michigan; Dr. S. Bernard Wortis, New York City, New York; and the Manfred Sakel Foundation.

This volume includes the papers presented at this International Conference and also the ensuing discussion which raised many more questions that demand investigation. A glance at the list of authors and panel members will show that the most distinguished proponents and opponents of the insulin shock treatment were well represented.

It was the purpose of this conference to assess the value of insulin treatment of psychoses, to provide a global view of the use of such treatment, to learn about its failures as well as its successes, and to compare its results with those of other therapies.

It may seem that insulin therapy in schizophrenia is so thoroughly established that there is little reason for reassessment at this time, 30 years after Sakel inaugurated this method of treatment. Yet in a general review of the literature we find such comments as: "After 20 years of research with insulin treatment in schizophrenia the published evidence is inconclusive and contradictory," and the author adds that, "Insulin treatment in schizophrenia continues to pose a major challenge to research."

A really provocative paper was by Ackner, who published one of the most thoroughly and logically controlled pieces of research in this field, although limited to a comparison of barbiturates and insulin coma and with only a six-month follow-up. We shall quote only the last sentence of his summary: "No conclusion can be drawn about the therapeutic value of the coma regime, but the results suggest that insulin is not the specific therapeutic agent."

A number of authors positively stated, in the recent literature, that there is no difference in the outcome between schizophrenics treated with insulin coma and those with chlorpromazine. Other authors recently reported that oral and intravenous glucose alone produced the same results as insulin therapy.

Probably the most devastating attack on insulin therapy was published by Bourne, based on a review of literature and considerable imagination. In his conclusion he makes the following statements: "Recent trends in the psychiatric literature reveal that disillusion with the insulin coma treatment of schizophrenia has steadily spread in the past four years. Since the method has no rationale, and since even its empirical basis now cannot withstand critical inspection, it is of interest to know why it gained almost unanimous acceptance. Probably three circumstances are at the bottom of it. The first is that a movement for the reform of mental hospitals and for their conversion from inactively custodial asylums to therapeutic centers was bound to grow in the last 20 years. The second is that such a movement would inevitably have promoted treatment methods that involved optimistic and individual attention to psychotic persons. The third is that in the early 'thirties when all this began, schizophrenics were considered inherently inaccessible to psychotherapy, since Freud adumbrated that they were incapable of forming a transference relationship. . . . The psychiatrist in training probably suffers most damage. Juniors are often posted to the insulin unit so that, at its foundations, their knowledge of schizophrenia requires no preoccupation with its subtle psychology and no experience of psychotherapy. Even the proper use of ECT is impeded because it is learnt as a casual procedure, administered sporadically and without system, as an adjuvant to the insulin ritual."

One experiment (Whitehorn et al) tends to confirm this speculation in that it compares two groups of psychiatrists, one psychotherapeutically effective, the other not effective. Only in the second group the results of treatment were enhanced by insulin treatment. This experiment lends emphasis to the frequent observation that insulin therapy is often used as a last resort when other methods have failed.

Bowes cites the following objections to the insulin coma therapy: It is merely an adjuvant to group psychotherapy, a messy form of treatment, expensive, time-consuming, somewhat dangerous, and emotionally upsetting to the staff. However, Patton of the same hospital expresses a different opinion which reads as follows: "Some patients [with drug therapy] seem to reach a degree of improvement short of readiness for discharge, but then stagnate for weeks in a quiet, contented seclusive state. In the ataractic-push group, I have yet to find a method to break up this stagnation. With insulin coma therapy, the patient could usually be stimulated to further improvement by discussion or interpretation of his actions or his semi-stuporous remarks, at the time of awakening from comas. Analytically oriented interpretations flowed freely on such occasions. It may be that insulin coma therapy is the treatment of choice for the quiet withdrawn patient, lacking gross physical evidence of tension. . . . On insulin coma therapy, conflict material, brought vividly into consciousness each morning, may result in desensitization, so there is less need for psychotic defenses and recovery ensues."

Sakel, in his posthumously published book *Schizophrenia,* met some of these objections by his statement: "The perfunctory application of the treatment will of course achieve results but this will be confined to cases that are relatively simple and the doctor will draw the conclusion that the difficult cases simply have not responded to the treatment. Favorable response to a perfunctory application which unfortunately is too widely used now, seems to indicate that the therapeutic scope of the treatment is much wider than I originally anticipated. But this only shows how much greater a percentage of cures could be achieved if the treatment were applied on the minutely regulated and adaptable lines laid down above."

In 1937, Poetzl, writing in the *Wiener Klinischen Wochenschrift*, stated, on the basis of his experience, that "Sakel's method of insulin shock is the first one I have seen that has achieved real success in the attempt to secure the reversal of the schizophrenic process."

In 1958, Hoff, in his introduction to Sakel's book on schizophrenia, makes the following statements: "Unfortunately, even today the therapeutic benefits of insulin shock treatment, which have been attested to by Dr. Sakel and his collaborators all over the world, are denied many patients merely because their physicians have failed to appreciate the significance of Dr. Sakel's detailed instructions for administering treatment. . . . Despite the development of new somatic methods of treatment of mental disorder, due largely to the stimulus provided by Dr. Sakel's innovation, the basic concepts of insulin shock therapy of schizophrenia have remained almost unchanged. It is an eloquent testimony to the genius of its discoverer that throughout the period since its inception the administrators of the Psychiatric Clinic of Vienna have not deemed it necessary to deviate from the classical procedure of insulin therapy, as outlined by Dr. Sakel, in any essential."

The following pages present the views of the contributors and discussants on the present status of "The Insulin Treatment in Psychiatry." These views and the evidence on which they are based demonstrate that insulin therapy is not outmoded and is still essential in psychiatry.

Max Rinkel, M.D., and Harold E. Himwich, M.D.
Editors

x

Officers
of the International Conference on the Insulin Treatment
in Psychiatry

Honorary President: Professor Otto Poetzl—Vienna, Austria

Chairmen

Harold E. Himwich, M.D.—Galesburg, Illinois

Max Rinkel, M.D.—Boston, Massachusetts

Andrew K. Bernath, M.D.—New York City, New York

.

SPONSORS

D. Ewen Cameron, M.D.
Professor of Psychiatry and Chairman of Department, McGill University; Psychiatrist-in-Chief, Royal Victoria Hospital; Director, Allan Memorial Institute of Psychiatry, Montreal, Canada.

Jacques S. Gottlieb, M.D.
Director, Lafayette Clinic; Professor in Psychiatry, Wayne State University, Detroit, Michigan.

S. Bernard Wortis, M.D.
Professor of Psychiatry and Neurology, New York University, College of Medicine, New York City, New York.

Manfred Sakel Foundation
17 East 63rd Street
New York City, New York

PLANNING COMMITTEE FOR
THE MANFRED SAKEL FOUNDATION

Dr. Bela Schick
Mr. Richard De Rochemont
Mr. Emerson Foote
Mr. George Hammond
Mr. Philip Liebmann
Mr. J. P. McEvoy*
Mr. Irving Sartorius
Mrs. Louis S. Gimbel, Jr., Chairman

*Deceased

MEMBERS OF THE PANEL

RALPH W. GERARD, M.D.—Director of Laboratories, Mental Health Research Institute, University of Michigan, Ann Arbor, Michigan.

JACQUES S. GOTTLIEB, M.D.—Director, Lafayette Clinic; Professor in Psychiatry, Wayne State University, Detroit, Michigan.

ALEXANDER GRALNICK, M.D.—Director, High Point Hospital, Port Chester, New York.

MILTON GREENBLATT, M.D.—Assistant Superintendent, Massachusetts Mental Health Center, Boston, Massachusetts; Assistant Professor of Psychiatry, Harvard Medical School.

PAUL H. HOCH, M.D.—Commissioner of Mental Hygiene, State of New York, Albany, New York; Professor of Clinical Psychiatry, College of Physicians and Surgeons, Columbia University, New York, New York.

HANS HOFF, M.D.—Professor, Vorstand der Psychiatrisch-Neurologische Klinik der Universität Wien, Vienna, Austria.

LOTHAR B. KALINOWSKY, M.D.—Research Associate in Psychiatry, College of Physicians and Surgeons, Columbia University, New York, New York; Psychiatric Research, New York State Psychiatric Institute and Hospital, New York, New York.

NATHAN S. KLINE, M.D.—Director of Research, Rockland State Hospital, Orangeburg, New York.

JAMES MANN, M.D.—Director of Psychiatry, Boston State Hospital, Boston, Massachusetts.

A. C. PACHECO E SILVA, M.D.—Professor of Clinical Psychiatry, University of São Paulo, Brazil.

FEDERICO SAL Y ROSAS, M.D.—Chief Physician, Home for Women of the Victor Larco Herrera Hospital, Lima, Perú.

WILLIAM SARGANT, M.D.—Physician in Charge, Department of Psychological Medicine, St. Thomas' Hospital, London, England.

GERALD J. SARWER-FONER, M.D.—Director of Psychiatric

Research, Consultant in Psychiatry, Queen Mary Veterans Hospital, Montreal, Quebec, Canada.

RAYMOND W. WAGGONER, M.D.—Director & Chairman, Department of Psychiatry, University of Michigan, University Hospital, Ann Arbor, Michigan.

HAROLD G. WOLFF, M.D.—Department of Neurology, Payne Whitney Psychiatric Clinic; The New York Hospital, New York, New York.

JOSEPH WORTIS, M.D.—Director, Division of Pediatric Psychiatry, The Jewish Hospital of Brooklyn, Brooklyn, New York.

CONTRIBUTORS

ARNOLD, O. H., M.D.
Privatdozent, Psychiatrisch-Neurologische Klinik der Universität Wien, Vienna, Austria.

BENNETT, IVAN F., M.D.
Clinical Investigator, Lilly Laboratory for Clinical Research, Indianapolis, Indiana.

BERNATH, ANDREW K., M.D.
Clinical Assistant in Psychiatry, New York University; Staff Psychiatrist, Bellevue Hospital Center Psychiatric Division.

BERMANN, GREGORIO, M.D.
Formerly Professor of Psychiatry, University of Cordoba, Argentina.

BOGOCH, SAMUEL, Ph.D., M.D.
Director, Neurochemical Research Laboratory and Senior Psychiatrist, Massachusetts Mental Health Center (Boston Psychopathic Hospital); Department of Psychiatry, Harvard Medical School, Boston, Massachusetts.

BOWMAN, KARL M., M.D.
Former President of the American Psychiatric Association; Professor Emeritus, Department of Psychiatry, University of California Medical Center, San Francisco, California.

DELGADO, HONORIO, M.D.
Professor, Universidad Mayor De San Marcos, Facultad De Medicina, Catedra De Psiquiatria, Lima, Peru.

DUSSIK, KARL T., M.D.
Physician in Charge, Insulin Therapy Research and Teaching Unit, Metropolitan State Hospital, Waltham, Massachusetts; Clinical Instructor in Psychiatry, Tufts

University, School of Medicine.

HIMWICH, WILLIAMINA, Ph.D.

Thudichum Psychiatric Research Laboratory, Galesburg State Research Hospital, Galesburg, Illinois.

HOCH, PAUL H., M.D.

Commissioner of Mental Hygiene, State of New York; Professor, New York State Psychiatric Institute, New York City, New York.

HOFF, HANS, M.D.

Professor, Vorstand der Psychiatrisch-Neurologische Klinik der Universität Wien, Vienna, Austria.

PACHECO E SILVA, A. C., M.D.

Professor of Clinical Psychiatry, University of Sao Paulo, Brazil.

SAL Y ROSAS, FEDERICO, M.D.

Chief Physician, Home for Women of the Victor Larco Herrera Hospital, Lima, Peru.

SARGANT, WILLIAM, F.R.C.P.

Physician in Charge, Department of Psychological Medicine, St. Thomas' Hospital, London, England.

SAWYER, CHARLES H., Ph.D.

Professor of Anatomy, University of California School of Medicine at Los Angeles and Veterans Administration Hospital, Long Beach, California.

WEISS, DANIEL M., M.D.

Assistant Chief, Closed Ward Section; Administrative Assistant to the Chief, Psychiatry and Neurology Service, Veterans Administration Hospital, Boston, Massachusetts; Senior Clinical Instructor, Tufts College Medical School.

WORTIS, JOSEPH, M.D.

Division of Pediatric Psychiatry, The Jewish Hospital of Brooklyn, Brooklyn, New York.

Messages

Professor OTTO POETZL, M.D., of Vienna, Austria, the
honorary president of this conference, the first to recognize
the potential value of insulin treatment in schizophrenia
and the one who encouraged Manfred Sakel in his experiments, sent the following message:

I welcome you here this evening on this most mem-
orable occasion although I regret that I cannot do so in
person. It would have given me the greatest pleasure to
be present at this International Conference on the Insulin Treatment in Psychiatry, which commemorates the
discovery made, thirty years ago, by my friend and col-
league, Manfred Sakel. In his spirit—that of a great
scientist and humanitarian—you have the opportunity
provided by this meeting to expand the search for the
imbalances in the basic life processes, adding to our
knowledge of curing and helping the men and women
who suffer from mental illness. My greetings and con-
gratulations to the men of science and the lay people
who have made this International Conference a reality!

Another message came from Professor HONORIO DELGADO,
of Lima, Peru, which reads as follows:

I am pleased to extend my best wishes to the International Conference on the Insulin Treatment in Psychiatry as their meetings realize a successful completion
which results from its excellent organization. I am sorry
that reasons beyond my control prevent me from being

present. However, I join my colleagues in Peru in expressing my personal esteem to the memory of Manfred Sakel and my admiration for the progress of psychiatry in the United States.

Other messages, conveying best wishes, have been received from: Dr. Wilfred Bloomberg, Commissioner of Mental Health of the State of Connecticut; Professor Max Müller, Director of the Psychiatric Clinic, Bern, Switzerland; and Dr. Seymour S. Kety, of the National Institute of Mental Health.

GREETINGS

S. Bernard Wortis, M.D.

Read by Dr. Morris Herman

Dr. S. Bernard Wortis, who is one of the sponsors of this meeting, has asked me to substitute for him. He is away on a teaching mission in Israel, Iran, and Australia, and he regrets his inability to be here with you in person.

Greetings should be warm but brief, so that the business of the meeting can proceed without undue delay. Greetings to all the members of the conference, particularly to the committee that worked so hard to make this conference possible and to the chairmen who will mold the material into a cohesive whole.

It is now almost a year since the death of Dr. Manfred Sakel, the discoverer of the hypoglycemic insulin treatment of schizophrenia. It was in Bellevue Hospital, when Dr. Karl Bowman was director, that Dr. Sakel did some of the earliest work in insulin therapy in this country. The results of the treatment appeared miraculous then, and led to a wave of enthusiasm and great optimism. Time has tempered this reaction. But the wave of interest in the physiological processes relevant to schizophrenia and all mental processes has persisted and even grown. It can truly be said that Sakel's discovery marked the fruitful beginning of the biochemical approach to mental disease.

Now we have come to a point where stock taking is appropriate. We pause to take breath so that we can advance with greater speed and greater certainty. The participants of this conference will survey and make available pertinent data which will undoubtedly be a framework for future advances in the field.

D. Ewen Cameron, M.D.

Mr. Chairman, Ladies and Gentlemen:

May I say how delighted I am that this large and representative meeting has been drawn together. It has long seemed to me that not only those of us who have been actively engaged in the development of this first of the effective therapies of schizophrenia but also those of us who represent other fields of work in psychiatry should gather together in testimonial to this pivotal advance in the treatment of the mentally sick.

The impact of insulin treatment of schizophrenia can, of course, be readily demonstrated in statistical form and has appeared in this manner in countless publications. But it is most sharply perceived, and may be related most readily, in terms of personal experience.

It was in March 1936 that the research staff of the Worcester State Hospital, of which I was a member, first began to explore the use of this treatment. It was an exciting and, in some ways, a disturbing adventure insofar that we had never had an opportunity to see the treatment carried out beforehand, and could discover no other place in the country which at that time had started its use. After we had been working for some months, however, Dr. Sakel, accompanied by Dr. Joseph Wortis, visited the hospital and we learned a great deal more about the management of the treatment.

Nonetheless, during those first few months I gained an indelible impression of the resolution, the fortitude and the vision which are required to press forward into a totally new field and, at the meeting, held in Boston, of the Society of Neurology and Psychiatry I had the pleasure of testifying to these qualities in Dr. Sakel, whom I introduced.

Later, there followed a gathering of the Clinical Directors of the New York State Hospitals at Wingdale, where Dr. Sakel put on a brief course of instruction, and the insulin coma treatment for schizophrenia was launched in this country. For the next two years at Worcester, Mass., most intensive studies were carried out by all sections of the research department upon the insulin treatment.

The spread of this form of treatment across the country was enormously rapid and for several years to come was the primary topic of interest at the annual meetings of the American Psychiatric Association.

The introduction of insulin hypoglycemia for schizophrenia gave an immense stimulus to the therapy of schizophrenia, and I should like to stress the fact that, whatever may be the fate of the insulin coma treatment itself, there is no doubt that after Dr. Sakel's introduction of this method of treatment the therapy of the schizophrenic patient was enormously accelerated and the whole future of individuals suffering from this condition was materially changed.

From the 1930's onward there have appeared, one after another, new therapeutic approaches to the condition, and we have, above all things, changed our attitude towards schizophrenia, so that we no longer take it as something hopeless, we no longer approach it in the Kraepelinian sense: in the sense of an inevitable dementia.

From the very first months of this therapy in this country, men turned with new interest to studying the earliest possible manifestations of schizophrenia, since it was early asserted, and correctly so, that the sooner in its development the condition was treated, the more hopeful the results. Men turned, also, to the study of the best possible circumstances under which the treatment could be given. Some men, it is true, attempted to put the treatment on a mass-production basis; and one heard of immense, long wards, lined on the one side with men and on the other with women, undergoing this treatment. But the most inquiring and enterprising soon realized that the circumstances under which the treatment was carried out, the circumstances of care and solicitude, were of the utmost importance.

Dr. Sakel gave further impetus to that by his insistence that the physician should remain in the closest possible contact with the patient through the development of his coma and should seek to follow, even into the depths of the coma, the slightest possible changes in the patient's expression, his restlessness and, in a word, should look for the most delicate indications of the status of the patient, seeking to interrupt him when his total condition, and not merely his physiological condition, seemed most favourable.

Following upon this, there soon branched out a widening interest in the dynamics of the schizophrenic patient; and there sprang up, in natural relation to this, the development of the "total push" method, which has been modified into our current highly organized rehabilitation programs for the schizophrenic patient.

It was early recognized, also, that profound comas which produced serious, temporary memory defects might be of particular value in the treatment of specially recalcitrant cases. And there has moved from this a growing interest in the use of amnesia, produced by whatever means, as a method of treatment of deeply established aberrations of human behavior.

We may also claim, quite reasonably, that our early studies of the most favourable circumstances under which insulin could be carried out started us on a train of thought now expressing itself in our spreading knowledge of the nature of the therapeutic community and of the psychotherapeutic organization of the ward—and, indeed, of the hospital as a whole.

Impetus was given in still other directions. First among these should be mentioned the problem of relapse. To meet these, carefully contrived follow-up services have been developed in many centers. It is true that these follow-up services are concerned more with offering psychotherapeutic facilities, or facilities for electroshock. Nonetheless, the problems of relapse, the causes and their prevention, received much support from the tremendously widespread use of the insulin treatment of schizophrenia.

Finally, I would refer to the speculation which this treatment engendered, at least in some of us, with regard to the nature of the reparative process in schizophrenia. The old working model of repair of a wound, which was almost implicit in the thinking of most of us in earlier years, has given place to much more sophisticated ideas concerning recovery. We now see recovery as perhaps occurring on the basis of more than one system, among these systems being the interesting concept of the short-circuiting of damaged areas.

In a word, then, there has been an immense shift in our whole approach to the problem of schizophrenia. Our attitude now is one of determination, of the utilization of all possible therapeutic resources. It is an approach, above all things, of hope and of the expectation of success, and this shift in attitude is justified. Today, schizophrenia is no longer the formidable thing that it was prior to the introduction of the insulin treatment. Tomorrow is bright with hope. With success leading to confidence, and confidence to further success, the early future promises final victory over this long-dreaded and desperate disease.

For the starting up of this great, long, gathering train of events, we must be profoundly indebted to Dr. Manfred Sakel.

JACQUES S. GOTTLIEB, M.D.

I would first like to express my appreciation, and I am sure the appreciation of all of you, to the Manfred Sakel Foundation for making possible this International Conference on the Insulin Treatment in Psychiatry. Certainly, too, we are indebted to Dr. Harold E. Himwich, Dr. Max Rinkel and Dr. Andrew K. Bernath for bringing together a most distinguished and sophisticated panel of physicians and investigators who have been concerned with the evaluation of insulin coma therapy, its manifestations and its mechanisms of action. To them I bring my sincerest greetings, for I anticipate that through their efforts those of us in the audience will gain much from this endeavor.

It was in 1927, as all of you know, that Manfred Sakel first announced his method for treating morphine addiction through the use of insulin in sub-coma amounts. It was only a short time thereafter when he applied this technique to patients with schizophrenia that some began to improve and gradually the method of insulin coma therapy developed. For 25 years the value of insulin coma therapy in the treatment of the patient with schizophrenia has been debated. It is my sincere hope that at this meeting an authoritative statement of the value of insulin coma therapy will be forthcoming. I am also in hopes that some of the important mechanisms by which insulin affects the organism will be described.

Irrespective of the final judgment of the value of insulin in the treatment of the psychiatric patient, the impetus given to psychiatric research, particularly the biological aspects of psychiatric research, by the method introduced by Sakel cannot be denied. I well remember the tremendous enthusiasm of the late 1930's for the application of insulin coma treatment to psychiatric patients. I am also familiar with the disappointments and the gradual, general decline that has occurred in the use of this technique throughout this country. The rejection of the technique, however, has not led to the rejection of other avenues of research. Rather, the fact that such a daring procedure was possible and that in some way it may have an important bearing upon the pathophysiology of mental disorder has stimulated innumerable others to seek other pathophysiologic mechanisms in their patients.

Of course, it is true that during this intervening 25 years there has been great growth in the science of biochemistry. No longer need this science be considered a study of static mechanisms, for it now lends itself very well to the study of the dynamic aspects of the organism's function. Moreover the new biochemical techniques which have become available as the result of the application of some of the findings in the physical sciences has opened a much broader field of study even to including the very essentials of life itself. This is not to deny the significance or importance of the psychological and social factors in the genesis of psychiatric disorders, rather it is to make more meaningful the effects of these experiences in producing the response tendencies of the organism.

The research horizons in psychiatry are broadening rapidly. Not too long ago it was only possible for us to study the behavioral effects of the environmental forces, both physical and social, as they impinged upon the organism. Much was learned as the organism's responses could be studied in both objective and subjective terms. This horizon is subject now to considerable expansion for not only is it possible to add to our study a definition of the biological limitations of the organism but also to explore the physiologic and chemical mechanisms by which the organism functions. In this way research has truly become dynamic and holistic. In this way we may really develop a unitary theory of man; a theory of man in health and disease. Much broader vistas are therefore before us than was possible 25 years ago, yet a significant spark was lit at that time which may have more meaning through the impetus to research that it gave than its direct evaluation as viewed by us today and tomorrow at this meeting.

I greet all of you with the hope that educational profit and research urge will be ours.

ACKNOWLEDGMENTS

The editors take this opportunity to express their gratitude to Mrs. Louis S. Gimbel, Jr., Chairman of the Planning Committee of the Manfred Sakel Foundation, for her most outstanding and enthusiastic assistance and continuous inspiration, and to the New York Academy of Medicine for its hospitality.

We also wish to thank the sponsors for their interest and cooperation, inaugurating this important conference, and all the authors and participants who made it possible.

We owe appreciation to Mr. Charles R. Atwell, Miss Barbara A. O'Connell, and Mrs. Rose Morse for their untiring editorial assistance. The speedy publication of the proceedings of the conference also deserves special mention of the Publisher, The Philosophical Library.

CONTENTS

PART ONE
HISTORICAL CONTRIBUTIONS

1 History of the Organic Treatment
 of Schizophrenia   3
 Hans Hoff
2 The History of Insulin Shock Treatment   19
 Joseph Wortis

PART TWO
PHYSIOCHEMICAL RESEARCH

3 Hormonal and Other Blood Changes Occurring
 During Insulin Hypoglycemia Treatment   45
 Ivan F. Bennett
4 Biochemical Changes in the Brain Occurring
 During Insulin Hypoglycemia   85
 Williamina A. Himwich
5 Electroencephalographic Changes in the Brain
 During Insulin Hypoglycemia   106
 Charles H. Sawyer
 Discussion   126
6 Summary   138
 Harold E. Himwich

PART THREE

CLINICAL RESEARCH AND FOLLOW-UP STUDIES

7   Insulin Treatment in England and Its Relation to
        Other Physical Therapies   145
    William Sargant
8   The Sakel Method in the Argentine   159
    Gregorio Bermann
    Discussion   164
9   Trends in Insulin Treatment in Psychiatry   172
    Karl M. Bowman
10 Insulin Therapy As Compared to
        Drug Treatment in Psychiatry   181
    Paul H. Hoch
    Discussion   187
11 Results and Efficacy of Insulin Shock Therapy   199
    O. H. Arnold
    Discussion   222
12 Indications of Insulin Therapy   231
    A. C. Pacheco e Silva
13 Notes on the Application of the Sakel Method in
        Mental Patients in Perú   240
    Federico Sal y Rosas
    Discussion   251
14 Insulin Therapy of Schizophrenia in Perú—
        Our Twenty Years of Experience   253
    Honorio Delgado
15 Modification of Anxiety Subsequent to
        Insulin-Induced Mild Hypoglycemia   266
    Andrew K. Bernath
    Discussion   292
16 Insulin Coma Therapy in a
        Veterans Administration Hospital   298
    Daniel M. Weiss
17 The Place of Sakel's Insulin Coma Therapy in
        An Active Treatment Unit of Today   316
    Karl Theo. Dussik
    Discussion   332

18 Neuraminic Acid in the Cerebrospinal Fluid of
        Schizophrenic Patients   343
    Samuel Bogoch
    Discussion   358
19 Summary   360
    Max Rinkel

                    PART FOUR
                    APPENDIX

    Appendix   375
    Index   382

Part One

HISTORICAL CONTRIBUTIONS

Chapter 1

HISTORY OF THE ORGANIC TREATMENT OF SCHIZOPHRENIA

HANS HOFF

Schizophrenia and epilepsy belong to the first psychotic manifestations recognized by man. The old Egyptians described epilepsy long ago and suggested surgical treatment. Schizophrenia too was recognized as a disease of the mind with organic changes in the brain, with the thought that the cause was a particularly disturbed combination of the supposed gas and blood in the ventricles.

Earliest Organic Treatments

The treatment of psychoses started in the latter part of the Middle Ages, with the belief that the disease was caused by the devil who had taken possession of the mentally afflicted or by miraculous influences of a divine nature. It is interesting to know that the old Egyptians, later followed by the Greeks, combined a kind of organic treatment with the magic influence of gods. The patients were brought to the temples for this purpose. The desire to treat such patients caused a great deal of economic competition among physicians on different islands in the Aegean sea. In the temples, patients were put into some kind of sleep mostly induced by alcoholic drinks. The sleep treatment lasted for days, or even weeks. It was assumed that God Eskulap would appear in some disguised form and expel the evil spirits, during sleep. Also, attempts were made to treat some organic changes in the supposed relation between fluid and gas in the ventricles of the brain. It is quite interesting to note that during those days the importance of dreams already played a part, and mental diseases were thought to be of organic origin.

Period of Mystic Religious Ideas

The Middle Ages brought about a change in concept. Religious and mystical origins were given prominence in the development of mental disease. The patients were either thought of as saints or as persons possessed by the devil. The treatment consisted of either putting such patients into prisons and dungeons or attempting to drive the devil out of them through religious ceremonies. It is possible that some kind of psychotherapy was attempted during that time while the idea of treatment by belief seems to have been one of the fundamentals of this religious period of psychiatry.

The period of liberal thinking brought a change in the attitude of physicians and laymen with regard to psychiatry and especially to schizophrenia. There was a time when pathological-anatomists tried to find an organic basis for diseases of all kinds. The structures of the body became the focus of research and soon there was a descriptive pathological anatomy of almost all diseases, with the exception of some diseases of the brain. The first such reports were about the discoveries of the brain pathology in general paresis and in senile dementia, which seemed to be in accordance with the general line of the organic basis of the mental disorder. These discoveries brought a trend toward organic and biological treatment of such diseases. The period of mere social improvement and mere symptomatic treatment in psychiatry seemed to be over. The first man to break through the ignorance and inactivity in treating mental disorders was Wagner-Jauregg with his malaria treatment of general paresis. This enormous success in our position towards mental diseases and the optimistic view in psychiatric treatment soon led, however, to a phase of disappointment.

Development of the Concept of Schizophrenia

The excellent work of German and Swiss psychiatrists had already provided a good description of entities regarded as mental diseases, and one of the greatest achievements has been the description of dementia praecox. At first the idea prevailed that these diseases must be 1) produced by the same cause, 2) must take the same course and 3) lead to the same final stage. None of these points was present in the first description of dementia praecox; neither did they have the same cause, nor did they follow the same course, and also the end was different in each case. The description of the different forms of the disease was such an outstanding one that the idea of dementia praecox became accepted in psychiatry. Soon objections concerning the name of the disease arose. Not only was dementia absent in most patients, but it also became evident that the disease did not start in early stages of life in all cases. Therefore the name of schizophrenia was chosen by Eugen Bleuler. The dynamics of the disease itself became of interest. Stransky's excellent work showed that some intrapsychic ataxia played a very important part in the dynamics of schizophrenia. Berze thought there was a functional disequilibrium between the cortex and the big ganglia in the depth of the brain. The organic nature of this disease seemed further to be proved by the fact of its hereditary transmission. It was thought that the causes of the disturbances of the mind arose through heredity. Hereditary transmission seems to be an inevitable fate for those patients who are born under this unlucky star. Therefore, psychiatry began to make a sharp distinction between the organically based diseases, where the germs of intoxication seemed to play a great part, and the so-called functional disease, in which the hereditary factors seemed to be the main cause for the illness, although their pathological-anatomical causes could not be proved. Therefore it was an essential decision from the viewpoint of prognosis to distinguish between the so-called confusional states in which intoxication was supposed to play the most important part, and schizophrenia in which heredity was thought to be the cause. The first group meant a situation of danger to life, but if the patient was able to overcome this danger then the prognosis appeared to be good. Schizophrenia meant a bad prognosis. But there were border-line cases which had often showed long-lasting remissions. Were they to be labeled schizophrenic too? These doubts arose owing to the fact that the disease, as described by E. Bleuler, is not well defined and does not seem to correspond to the rules of the Kraepelinian concept.

During this period the interest of psychiatry changed from mere descriptive attitudes to psychodynamic concepts of mental disease. But the treatment of the so-called functional psychoses like schizophrenia or manic depressive psychosis still lay in the shadow of pessimism.

The Endocrine Period

Psychiatrists seemed to be fascinated by the endocrine changes of the patients suffering from schizophrenia in the final state of the disease. These endocrine disturbances caused visible changes in the bodies of our patients and in the expression of the function of the endocrine glands. Irregularity in menstruation, appearance of beards in women, obesity were some of the noticeable signs. At the same time changes in vascularization of hands and feet appeared. Therefore it seemed that treatment should be directed toward these visible changes. The period of endocrine treatment of schizophrenia began. First the function of the endocrine glands was enhanced by giving the patients pituitary glands, testicular and/or ovarian extracts, powders of dried thyroid glands. Subsequently it was thought that in patients suffering from schizophrenia there was lack of glandular function of the opposite sex and so the men received ovarian extracts whereas, to the women, testicular extracts were administered. Finally it was thought that not an underfunction of different glands, but rather dysfunction of one or several endocrine glands prevailed. Therefore, some patients were castrated and an extract of normal glands derived either from other human beings or from animals was implanted in their body. The disturbances of menstrual cycles in women concomitant with the appearance of homosexual trends in the course of schizophrenia, and also the appearance of rare remissions after some treatment of the above-mentioned types, added some impetus to the process. Pathological and anatomical findings in the endocrine glands in the final states of schizophrenia also supported the idea of this treatment.

If we look back at the "endocrine" period, we see that it was characterized by treatments with an approach lacking in scientific criteria, which was almost forced upon the medical profession by unhappy and desperate relatives of the patients. The findings of Kretschmer on the constitutional factor of schizophrenia did not alleviate the feeling of pessimism and hopelessness in the case of schizophrenic patients.

Early Shock Treatments

Already towards the end of the Middle Ages and the beginning of the new period an interest developed in attempting to treat schizophrenics by some form of shock. In Switzerland at this time schizophrenics were put into nets and lowered into lakes until they were almost drowned and then pulled out again. Sometimes short-lasting remissions were witnessed. In other countries patients were hit with chains and whips. Some of these patients died. But again there were some very impressive recoveries and remissions. This kind of primitive shock-treatment was considered to be of a magic nature. It was believed that the devil had possession of the human body and mind, and the only logical consequence of such ideas seemed to be the attempt to make the devil's stay in these strange places of residence as miserable as possible.

Malaria Treatment

The discovery of malaria fever as a cure gave rise to an attempt to obtain results similar to those in the malaria treatment of general paresis by nonspecific fever treatment. Again an interesting factor arose: sometimes after a very serious physical condition the patient improved. Schilder was one of the first who gave weight to the description of Cervantes of the dying Don Quixote. Don Quixote, the constitutional schizophrenic type, full of psychopathological ideas and adventures, had seen his own life clearly during the process of his death. Another example is a patient of Schilder who was suffering from schizophrenia for many years and who recovered while dying of tuberculosis.

Certain psychiatrists came up with the idea of the potential value of shock-treatments. Stransky described a schizophrenic patient who in a delusional state escaped from a mental asylum, then climbed an electric pole from which he was thrown to the ground. This left him in a serious physical condition for weeks, but also left him free of any psycho-pathological symptoms. In spite of the fact that this patient died due to consequences of his fall, a new development of treatment had been inaugurated.

Prolonged Sleep Treatment

Kläsi in Switzerland treated schizophrenic patients with sleeping cures. Patients were kept under sleeping drugs for weeks. The rationale of this treatment was not quite clear. It was thought possible that rest would cure the sick mind just as inactivity cures a sick lung. However, the treatment was fraught with danger. First of all, it was difficult to get the patients to fall asleep and then equally as difficult to wake them up because of the barbiturate drugs which were used during the cure. But this form of treatment showed some success.

Early Psychosurgery

A very ingenious form of treatment was attempted by Pötzl, but no further investigations followed his first attempt. Pötzl had described some people with lesions of the brain showing symptoms similar to schizophrenia. Of course they were not suffering from schizophrenia as a disease. He found a disturbance of a distinct system in the brain causing such specific symptoms and signs. He described this fiber system of the brain as consisting of thalamocortical and thalamo-commissural connections. He therefore made the attempt in some schizophrenics to change the pathological function of the brain system by causing injury to the thalamus itself. This came close to the starting point of one of the organic treatments of schizophrenia called psychosurgery.

In different countries the idea came up that schizophrenia had nothing to do with organic changes of the brain. These scientists accepted schizophrenia as nothing else but an alteration of behavior patterns caused by a disturbance of the relationship between an over-anxious mother and her child. This hereditary transmission must have the same foundation in a changed reaction of the whole brain or in parts of ganglion cells. Therefore, the idea of the biological treatment of schizophrenia was never completely abandoned. New research has been started again and again in the direction of the organic basis of the disease.

The First Sakel Treatments

In former investigations shock had been shown as a possible treatment in schizophrenia, but medicine had no way of controlling the danger of death caused by these treatments. During this time Sakel came to Vienna from Germany as a refugee. At the time Prof. Wagner-Jauregg had a young lady patient who was suffering from schizophrenia as a result of an unhappy love-affair. She already had marked signs of changes in her body, such as obesity, and also changes in female secondary sexual signs such as the growth of a beard. Wagner-Jauregg, weighing the psychological cause which appeared to be at the root of the disease, had made a good prognosis. He promised the parents that the child would be completely cured after a year of internment in a well known private institution. The cure consisted of symptomatic treatment by bromides and barbiturates, and psychotherapy, which helped to build the girl's personality. However, after a year of treatment, the patient, who had come from Poland, became even worse than at the time of her arrival. The mother told me that she planned to commit suicide together with her daughter. I went to Sakel, who had already tried insulin treatments successfully in some cases of drug-addiction, and in some restless schizophrenic patients. He suggested making an attempt with the use of a full insulin shock treatment, in the case of this unhappy girl. Not knowing what the results would be we started the treatment in a private institution, without any protection from the law. To our surprise, after the second shock the girl seemed very coherent and started to speak with her mother, a thing which she had refused to do during her last six months' stay. However, she had another relapse after a few days, but a few more shocks led to a complete recovery which she has maintained to this day.

The second patient, who came from Spain, confirmed our first impression. We informed Pötzl of the results of our therapeutic attempt and he offered Dr. Sakel all the facilities of the Psychiatric Department of the University of Vienna, for his investigations. Dr. Sakel, under the supervision of Prof. Pötzl, cooperated with Dr. Dussik and Dr. Palisa, and developed the standard insulin treatment which is used at the present time.

Sakel's and Pötzl's Theories

Dr. Sakel's working theory held that under the influence of the shock treatments, sick and defective cell connections in the brain would be separated. Sakel believed that such defective connections were caused by psychological influences on cells which, on the basis of hereditary factors, are prone to such defective connections. He believed that after the chemical separation the tendency of the organism to normality and to homeostasis would be greater than the abnormal psychological tendencies, and therefore after complete disruption normal connections would be established. He felt it would be necessary to destroy pathological connections again and again to interrupt the tendency towards defective connections permanently. Pötzl, who enthusiastically introduced this new treatment in his University Hospital, had a somewhat different opinion on the effect of the insulin shock treatment. He believed that in the hypoglycemic coma, malfunctioning ganglion cells would be destroyed. These cells, according to Pötzl, work like a "störsender" (jamming radio transmitter). The destruction of these cells makes it possible for the remaining cells to go on working, undisturbed in the normal pattern. Pötzl called this the "Mauserung" (moulting) of the brain.

Cardiazol (Metrazol) Shock Treatment

In 1934 Meduna introduced Cardiazol shock. Under the treatment with insulin, sometimes patients had epileptic fits. It is doubtful whether such a treatment alone is more successful than the hypoglycemic coma. Nevertheless, at the time the connection between epileptic fits and this treatment of schizophrenia was uncertain. Meduna had the idea that epileptics did not get schizophrenia, and therefore he wanted to make schizophrenics into epileptics, hoping in this way to cure schizophrenia. The supposed opposition between schizophrenia and epilepsy was completely wrong. We know quite a number of epileptics who developed schizophrenia. According to the Viennese School, the connection between schizophrenic and epileptic delirium is quite apparent. Nevertheless Meduna's contribution to the treatment of schizophrenia was the introduction of drugs which caused epileptic convulsions. Cardiazol treatment alone did prove to be more successful in catatonic attacks but was not effective in paranoid and hebephrenic forms of schizophrenia.

Electric Shock Treatment

The fact that epileptic fits had some effect on schizophrenia made Cerletti and Bini experiment with induction of epileptic fits by electrical currents, thus creating electric shock treatment. This method had some advantage over the Metrazol shock treatment. Patients in the beginning of the Metrazol injections had a terrible feeling of being destroyed, of "explosiveness" in the brain, while electric shock was too sudden in its effect to be perceived by the patient; therefore it caused less fear than Metrazol shock treatment. The standard treatment of 20 electric shocks was introduced in schizophrenia as a minimum. Kalinowsky propagated this treatment in parts of Europe and the United States. His introduction of the treatment showed clear judgment and he was free from excessive or overrated expectations. The Vienna School came to the conclusion that the electric shock treatment proved successful in catatonic cases, whereas its success was far less impressive in the cases of paranoid schizophrenia. Electric shock and insulin did not show the same positive results in hebephrenic forms of schizophrenia.

Arguments About Sakel's Treatments

Sakel's contribution had been quite clear. He showed that at the beginning of the treatment there was sometimes even an accentuation of the psychosis, while later on during the treatment the psychosis disappeared completely. It was possible to send a great number of schizophrenic patients home. The repercussions in the psychiatric world were enormous. The amount of resistance against the new form of treatment was strong. The argument ran the usual way. Sakel was accused of not being the first man who introduced this kind of treatment, although I do not know of any other man who worked so intensively in this line. Even the severity of schizophrenia was doubted. Of course there have been great difficulties in the nomenclature of schizophrenia. What is schizophrenia? There might be a difference of opinion in defining schizophrenia, between the United States and Europe. There is without any doubt a group of cases which show spontaneous remissions, especially in the first stage of the disease, but there is also an enormous group of schizophrenics populating our mental asylums. The relatives of the schizophrenic patients will tell us how severe this disease is. Finally, the success of insulin treatment in schizophrenia countered opposition from different places. Sakel made clear that the insulin treatment will only help during the first one and one-half years of the disease, and he also showed us that the technique of the insulin treatment is difficult because it includes some danger. Many tried to mitigate the shock by changing it completely in such a way that Sakel would have never accepted it. So-called incomplete shocks have been introduced in the therapy of schizophrenia. The time of a possible success had elapsed in many cases; quite useless treatments have been supplied and frequently one and one-half years have been allowed to pass without any insulin treatment. What ought to be done with these patients?

The Period of Psychosurgery

In 1953 Moniz operatively destroyed Areas 9, 10 and 11 (according to Brodman), following Pötzl's idea that the relationship in schizophrenia is pathologically disturbed. As a consequence of this operation degeneration of the dorsomedial nucleus of the thalamus appeared. In some patients, hallucinations and delusions disappeared, but many cases paid for this success by the loss of initiative, intelligence and judgment. It looked as if the function of the brain had descended to a lower level.

Spiegel and Wycis in this country tried another procedure by electrocoagulation of the dorsal medial nucleus of the thalamus, and they believe that they will have some success without having to make their patients pay so heavily with loss of intelligence, adaptation and judgment. These different methods of treatment, like the destruction of the nucleus amygdale, were combined in the so-called psychosurgery.

The Period of Psychotherapy

Psychiatry is always characterized by fashion. The period of psycho-surgery was followed by a reaction, where schizophrenia was not accepted as a mental disorder but more or less as a kind of abnormal behavior pattern in which hallucinations and delusions make some sense or are a reaction of the individual to his abnormal behavior. The period of psychotherapy in schizophrenia started. Success was experienced in a few cases. The treatment lasted long and the mental asylums all over the world are crowded once more with patients suffering from schizophrenia who were untreated. Insulin treatment was applied less in the world, but the new kind of psychotherapy supported by occupational therapy and activities could not even show any definite success. Patients suffering from schizophrenia showed better adaptation but cure of the disease was rare and almost limited to pseudoneurotic forms of schizophrenia described so well by Hoch. Of course some of the patients improved remarkably well with insulin treatment, while as many others had relapses.

Tranquilizers and Neuroleptics

The discovery of tranquilizers and neuroleptics developed a new hope concerning the treatment of schizophrenia. Psychiatry seemed to become a pharmacological problem, which made it possible to keep the patient in a long lasting sleep, even in hibernation. Success has been claimed in many quarters, in the treatment of young as well as elderly patients. According to our own experience, tranquilizers and neuroleptics can only improve symptoms but have no influence whatsoever on the disease itself. The psychiatric diseases consist of reactions of the healthy part of the individual to the disease, and again the reaction to his surroundings and his home environment. If we improve the symptoms we also improve the patient's relationships, which only means improving the condition of the patient without really being able to treat the disease. A perfectly achieved adaptation is naturally not a cure. Psycho-pharmacological methods proved to be a great success in the case of schizophrenic patients by *advancing* the personality and the human relationships of our patients. But all these are not a direct cure for schizophrenic patients. INSULIN TREATMENT IS THE ONLY SUCCESSFUL BIOLOGICAL TREATMENT OF OUR TIME. A great number of our patients treated with insulin shocks showed signs of relapses; therefore the Viennese School to which Dr. Sakel belonged tried to treat the patient in a multi-factorial way.

The Organic Nature of Schizophrenia

We are in full agreement with Sakel and believe in the organic nucleus of schizophrenics invested by heredity. The proof of the organic nature of schizophrenia consists of:

1. *Hereditary factors:* Mono-ovarial twins show a concordance of schizophrenic reaction in 92% according to recent investigations. Even twins of this kind who grow up and receive education separately from the very first day of their birth, often show schizophrenic reactions of similar type. These similarities have been studied extensively and carefully by Hartmann. Based on his observations we believe that the tendency to schizophrenia is inherited whereas the psychic content and the complexes of those patients are not.

2. *Constitution:* Statistic correlation of schizophrenia with the asthenic type is secure while the correlation between this type and introversion is not completely statistically secured.

3. *Pathologic-anatomical findings:* Papez and other authors believed that form and frequency of destruction of ganglion cells is of a specific nature in schizophrenia. In involvement of the ganglion cells of the 3rd and the 5th layer of the cortex, changes of the cells in the dorso-medial nucleus of the thalamus appeared almost in every brain of all long lasting schizophrenic states. They were naturally not present in the cases of patients who died in the early stages of schizophrenia.

4. *Examinations of spinal fluid, of blood and of the reaction of blood vessels,* have shown a greater number of abnormalities in the field of metabolic changes, as well as vegetative reactions, and also in the field of hormones. The frequency of these abnormalities is, according to statistical findings, much higher than in an average normal personality. Of course, we also have to consider secondary changes caused by disorganized life, hospitalization and the pressure of emotional changes.

5. *Modern biochemical examinations revealed under stress,* disturbances of phosphorus metabolism. Other investigations of a biochemic nature and enzyme studies reported by Richter, Elkes, Himwich along with a few others, at the symposium in Strasbourg, showed no typical schizophrenic reaction.

Our own examinations revealed in all cases of schizophrenic patients a disturbance of incorporation of administered pyruvic acid. It shows itself in an abnormal reaction to organic and inorganic phosphates. These changes may be caused by 2 factors:

a) *Mutations of the genes.* The inclination to such disturbances is always present in the organism. It reveals itself, however, only by an over-optimal loading with pyruvic acid and then leads to a disturbance of the incorporation of this substance in the carbohydrate metabolism.

b) The disturbance may be caused by an anomaly of transamination, again caused by the mutation of the genes.

6. *The similarity of some of the symptoms* and signs of schizophrenia with pathologically well defined symptoms of patients with brain injuries is remarkable. We must believe that in schizophrenia some part of the brain is in a state of dysfunction.

Insulin Treatment of Paranoid Schizophrenia—

Method of Choice

We are of the opinion that *insulin treatment is the standard method of choice for paranoid schizophrenia.* We may enhance this treatment by introducing electric or Cardiazol (Metrazol) shock treatment during the cure. We believe that this kind of treatment must be amplified by psychotherapy which can be started during the last stage of insulin treatment. We believe also that the relatives have to be taken under treatment to learn to understand the problems which schizophrenia elicits in patients already marked by heredity. We believe that occupational therapy, activity, expressions and music therapy, have a place in restoring the self-confidence and self-esteem of our patients. We also believe that social workers, too, have their place in this treatment, by helping the patient to find his right position in life. But we think that the insulin treatment is the paramount treatment of paranoid schizophrenia at present. In catatonic states electric shock should be used first. If afterwards symptoms still remain, insulin shock should be started. We think that only in the case of hebephrenic patients, treatment with neuroleptics has been proved to be more successful than the insulin treatment. Of course, in these cases the cure consists of maximal adaptation and not complete elimination of the disease itself.

Sakel Method—A Milestone in Modern Psychiatry

What great changes have taken place since Sakel's discoveries! Psychiatry had already received a method of active therapy through the psychodynamic approach of Freud, and the introduction of malaria treatment of general paresis. Psychiatry today possesses the most active therapy of any branch of medicine. More than 80% of the patients who have been in mental asylums are returning to their families. The population of the mental asylums is changing. The so called capitamortua of the old schizophrenic types are disappearing. Therefore we can help schizophrenic patients, and we are more interested in the personality, not because of curiosity, but because of its being the center of medical research and human activity. I think Sakel has really created a milestone in the development of modern psychiatry.

Chapter 2

THE HISTORY OF INSULIN SHOCK TREATMENT

JOSEPH WORTIS, M.D.

Manfred Sakel was not the first to use insulin in the treatment of psychoses. Soon after the successful isolation of insulin in 1922, Cowie, Parsons, and Raphael (1923 and 1924) tried a combination of 2 to 10 units of insulin with glucose in cases of depression, with favorable effects on the sugar curves, but without other signs of clinical improvement in the patients. Targowla and Lamache in 1926, and Puca in 1927 successfully used daily doses of up to 45 units combined with glucose to improve the appetite and nutrition of several psychotic subjects. Targowla and Lamache noted the disappearance in the course of treatment of the motor symptoms of a subject with catatonic stupor; Puca even remarked that one of his cases recovered completely after a month of treatment, but none of them followed the lead.

Miskolczy of the Budapest University Clinic (1927) had good results in promoting the nutrition of psychotic subjects with 30 units a day. Becker (1928) recommended single doses as high as 100 units to make patients eat. Haack (1929) confirmed his good results and reported some curious experiences:

A catatonic patient had been refusing nourishment for three years. For ten months she lay continually in bed in a rigid attitude, was completely mute and had to be tube fed daily. On March 4, 1929, she was given 30 units of insulin. Half an hour later she asked for food and ate without further help. An hour and a half later she opened her eyes, sat up in bed, talked to the nurse, and asked if she could get up. She remained accessible for two days and then relapsed into her previous stupor. On March 8 she was given 30 units, on March 9 another 30 units, and later 40 units again without effect. On March 10 she was given 60 units at midday. At 3 P.M. she opened her eyes and spoke, but would not eat. At 5:55 P.M. she went into hypoglycemic shock, with cyanosis, respiratory distress and irregular pulse. She was quickly aroused with intravenous glucose. The patient thereupon opened her eyes, sat up and expectorated. She began to speak, at first confusedly, and then more and more intelligibly, said that she had pain in her chest that she might have inherited from her father, and that she wanted some milk with a lot of sugar in it right away. She ordered some meat and plenty of bread for herself for the following day, and then said that she felt terrible after the injection and thought she would die. The patient remained active and friendly for the next two days and ate with appetite. She then became apathetic again but up to the time of the report (three weeks later) continued to eat without help.

Insulin was now being more widely used to combat malnutrition and anorexia in psychotics, and such mental improvement as occurred was only incidentally noted. Paul Schmidt in 1928 was the first to deliberately use insulin for its therapeutic effect on the psychosis as such. He administered 60 to 80 units of insulin a day with good effect; stuporous patients grew active, agitated patients grew calm, and his results on the whole were positive. But this author, like those preceding him, always combined the insulin injection with carbohydrate administration and warned against the danger of hypoglycemia.

In America, Appel, Farr, and Marshall (1928 and 1929) gave 31 psychotic subjects up to 70 units of insulin a day in divided doses, followed by carbohydrate administration, with similar results. They permitted mild hypoglycemia to develop but quickly interrupted incipient coma. They concluded that insulin was good for malnutrition in psychotic subjects. Moreover, they reported that 7 of the 31 patients showed mental improvement. A patient with dementia praecox, for example, who had been uncooperative for a year, became agreeable and cooperative, and a depressed patient with profound somatic delusions and chronic vomiting, lost many of her delusions, stopped vomiting, and began to joke, laugh and play games. But they wrote, "The effect of the treatment on the mental status is difficult of appraisal," and like Targowla, Lamache, Schmidt, and Puca before them, they did not follow the lead.

In the following years a long series of favorable reports on the use of insulin for malnutrition in psychotics appeared. Jaschke (1929), using doses up to 40 units a day for malnutrition, reported marked mental improvement in one case after insulin treatment. Rosenthal and Beyer (1929), using similar doses, reported beneficial effect on the mental state of 11 out of 20 psychotic subjects, mostly cases of depression, and Gallinek (1929), using somewhat larger doses, reported slightly better results with over 20 subjects.

Roberti (1930) claimed excellent results with a 45-day course of insulin treatment with doses up to 30 units. He reported three full remissions in as many cases of paranoia, and felt that the treatment promoted recovery in five cases of confusional toxic psychoses. Results in three cases of schizophrenia were negative. Stanesco (1930) successfully used small amounts of insulin (15 units a day) as an accessory in a combined treatment of a case of catatonic stupor. Slotopolsky (1931) in an elaborate paper on the use of insulin for psychotics who were unwilling to eat, stated for the first time that a hypoglycemia reaction was sometimes desirable. But the author was thinking mainly of his patients' appetite, and added that severe hypoglycemic reactions or hypoglycemic coma should be avoided at all costs. He therefore concluded that the single dose should never exceed 30 units, and that hypoglycemia should never be permitted to last longer than two hours. The author also incidentally reported that insulin had a definite and protracted sedative effect on disturbed patients, and that the patient sometimes actually "awakened" from his psychosis. "This may be of therapeutic value," he said, but he did not follow the lead. Gründler (1931) also successfully used insulin for intractable anorexia in psychotics. Küppers and Strehl (1933) in a careful report of 35 cases confirmed all these results. They used single doses of 20 to 50 units and sometimes waited as long as four hours to see if patients would eat spontaneously. In six cases of schizophrenia they observed the disappearance of symptoms of catatonic stupor, in two cases for a protracted period. One case died of complications following hypoglycemic shock (apparently because insufficient intravenous sugar was administered). The authors were inclined to question the therapeutic importance of the hypoglycemia as such, and warned against marked hypoglycemic reactions.

Steck (1931) at first used insulin to promote the appetite of psychotics and later (1932) reported the beneficial effect of insulin (10 units four times a day) on disturbed patients. He noted particular improvement in a few cases following symptoms of shock, and emphasized the significance of both the hypoglycemia as such and the associated increase in parasympathetic tone. This author claimed priority for the introduction of insulin in the treatment of catatonic excitement, but as we have seen, his observations were reported after the appearance of the papers of Paul Schmidt (1928) and Slotopolsky (1931) where similar observations are recorded.

In the U.S.S.R., Mebel (1932) reported similar results. In France E. Jacob and Pierre Doussinet (1933) reported marked improvement or complete cure in a series of psychotic patients with ketosis who were subjected to intensive insulin treatment. Amounts up to 160 units a day were used, but always in combination with sugar, and the authors warned against hypoglycemic coma.

Charlotte Munn (1935) of Rockland State Hospital in New York used 20 to 30 units of insulin a day followed by carbohydrates in the treatment of a series of psychotic subjects. The "possibility of the occurrence of hypoglycemia or insulin shock," she wrote, "was an ever present worry." But she remarked, in reporting one female case of schizophrenia, "It is of interest that during moderately severe insulin shock the catatonia entirely disappeared and she talked freely and moved about easily for an hour or so." She noted mental improvement in a number of her fourteen subjects, during or following treatment, but was not disposed to attribute it to the insulin.

Sharp and Bahr (1934), using 30 units a day in divided cases, noted mental improvement in one out of their five psychotic subjects and did not regard their result as encouraging. Parfitt (1936) found insulin a useful accessory to the somnifen (diethylamine salts of diethyl and allylisopropyl barbituric acid) sleep treatment of psychoses. Bennett and Semrad (1936) treated malnutrition in 25 psychotic subjects with doses of 5 to 15 units of insulin, t.i.d., followed by carbohydrates. "At times," they noted, "striking improvement in behavior, mentation and return of normal affective tone came coincidentally with the weight gain," but they were not sure that the insulin treatment was responsible.

The preceding account of the literature will serve to show that there was from the beginning considerable agreement among the various workers that insulin is a valuable aid in the treatment of malnutrition in psychotics. The point of special interest for us, however, is the surprising frequency of the reports of mental improvement in association with insulin treatment. Almost all of the reports contain some incidental comment on this effect. At least three of the workers already mentioned—Haack in Germany (1929),

Steck in Switzerland (1932) and Munn in America (1935)—actually noted and reported particular improvement following insulin shock; but none of them followed the lead. A fourth report, by Torp, of striking improvement in a schizophrenic subject following an unintentional insulin shock is recorded in the Norwegian *Magasin for Laegevidenskapen* for July 1932, and will be found in translation on page 38 of the Wilson report. Sakel was, however, the first to introduce hypoglycemic shock as a therapeutic principle, the first to devise a relatively safe procedure for managing hypoglycemic shock, and the first to elaborate a successful method of treatment on that basis. Starting from altogether different premises (and without knowledge of these other reports) Sakel was led to his discovery through quite different channels.

It should be kept in mind that Sakel, following his graduation from The University of Vienna in 1925, worked for the next succeeding years in the field of internal medicine. During the years 1927 to 1933 he was chief physician in the Lichterfelder Hospital in Berlin. This was a private psychiatric hospital where abstinence cures for morphinism were frequently administered. Struck by the resemblance between the stormy withdrawal symptoms and hyperthyroidism, Sakel began to use insulin as a vagotonic antagonist to the sympathotonic overactivity he observed during the abstinence cures, finding to his surprise that hypoglycemic insulin shock was especially helpful to his patients. After some crude animal experimentation in his kitchen he was convinced that insulin shock was not the dangerous calamity it was supposed to be and could be a valuable tool in the treatment of excitement. He proceeded to apply it systematically in the management of other types of psychiatric excitement, including schizophrenia, with good results. Though he courted great risks with this bold experimentation, with typical confidence in his own observations he felt he was on the road to great discoveries, and returned to Vienna to work as a volunteer assistant on the University psychiatric service to develop his work and to interest Professor Pötzl. The tactic succeeded and Pötzl, though schooled in the thoroughly skeptical tradition of Central European psychiatry, became convinced that the treatment was effective, and sponsored Sakel's work throughout the stormy period of claims and counter-claims and sharp attack that followed. "The first treated cases that I saw," wrote Pötzl, "convinced me that this method of treatment outclassed any other presently available." The initial report of results was made at a meeting of the Viennese Medical Society in November 1933, and a brief account of the presentation published soon after in the *Wiener medizinische Wochenschrift*. Three weeks later a vigorous and lengthy attack on the proposed treatment by Professor Josef Berze appeared in the same journal. Berze criticized it for its lack of rationale, its faulty scientific documentation, its dangers and its very questionable results. Besides, he said, it wasn't really new. "This treatment must be rejected," he concluded. Other similar attacks were not long delayed.

Sakel's first results on a large series of cases were reported in the *Wiener medizinische Wochenschrift* for 1934-35. The first detailed account of the results of hypoglycemic treatment of a large series of schizophrenic subjects was made in 1936 by Dussik and Sakel. In 58 cases in which the first marked mental change occurred less than six months prior to treatment, they found that 70.7 per cent of the cases responded with full remission, and a further 17.3 per cent with good social remission and capacity for work, making a total of 78 per cent of positive results. Of the remaining cases of longer duration, 47.8 per cent responded with good social remissions, and 19.6 per cent with full remission. It should be remarked, however, that relatively few of these cases were of more than a few years' duration.

A second large series of 111 cases treated by Sakel's method was reported by Max Müller of Munsingen, Switzerland in September 1936.

At Paris in November 1936 Müller reported a total of 136

cases treated. In cases of less than 6 months' duration, he had 89.8 per cent of full or good remissions of which 73 per cent were full remissions. In cases of six to eighteen months' duration he had 82 per cent full or good remissions of which 50 per cent were full remissions, and in cases of more than a year and a half duration he had 45 per cent of full or good remissions of which only 0.5 per cent were full remissions. There was one fatality.

This confirmatory work was particularly impressive, not only because of the reputability of its author, but also because it was based on the combined statistics of 11 Swiss hospitals, all using a uniform and standard technique. Müller's own cases comprised about half of the total number but all the physicians had been trained by Müller, who had in turn received his training from the Viennese school.

I was fortunately able to observe Sakel's treatment in Vienna in 1934, reported on it at a staff meeting at the Phipps Clinic in March 1935 and called attention to the work in the *Journal of Nervous and Mental Disease* for February 1936. Early in 1936 several workers in this country undertook treatment of schizophrenics according to Sakel's method. By September 1936 work was already under way in at least three American hospitals, though Cameron and Hoskins should be credited with having started the first actual treatment in this country. Glueck's enthusiastic account of his observations in Vienna and Munsingen, published on September 26th, 1936, stimulated further widespread interest in this country. Thanks to the energetic support of Dr. Karl Bowman, then director of Bellevue Psychiatric Hospital, on November 12, 1936, several cases under treatment at Bellevue were presented at the New York Society for Clinical Psychiatry. Steinfeld reported favorable results of treatment in three out of four cases in the *Journal of the American Medical Association* for January 9, 1937. At a symposium at the New York Academy of Medicine on January 12, 1937, Cameron reported ameliorative changes in most of his group of fifteen chronic cases, Glueck reported improvement in most of his twelve cases, and we reported three full remissions and beneficial effects in other cases in a series of 13 cases at Bellevue which had already been treated at that time.

What followed thereafter is history. Although the scientific literature has been preponderantly positive up to the present time, it was nevertheless soon realized that the cures were not permanent. Patients relapsed over the years and a ten year follow-up shows no great difference between those who had the advantages of the treatment and those who did not. Though this might be construed as proof of its inefficacy, those who work with the treatment realize that these remarkable remissions, often lasting for years, are a major accomplishment, a scientific breakthrough of great interest and importance. A year or two after introduction of insulin shock treatment to this country, Meduna's convulsive treatment became a formidable rival, followed later by lobotomy, and most recently by the new drug treatments which initiated a broad new approach to the therapy of the psychoses. Figure 1 gives some idea of the interest in these new treatments as reflected in the number of scientific publications in the world's literature on each subject over the years.

Sakel's contribution to psychiatry can be viewed in two ways: he was the first to successfully develop a treatment for schizophrenia, the hypoglycemic insulin shock treatment, which has proved its value and maintained its usefulness up to the present day. But he was also the first successful proponent of a physiological approach to the treatment of psychoses, a contribution which goes far beyond his discovery of a new treatment, a treatment which he well knew would be superseded in time by better treatments to come. In fact it was his advocacy of a physiological approach which led to the sharpest opposition, especially in this country, and it was his victory in this struggle which marked his greatest success and paved the way for great new developments thereafter. Although it was only 25 years ago that

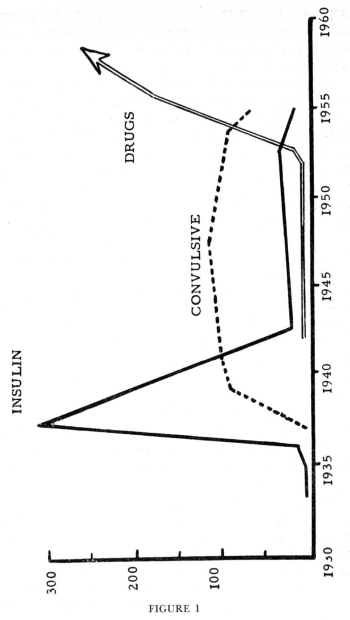

FIGURE 1

The number of articles published each year in the world's medical literature on insulin, convulsive and drug treatment of psychoses.

his new treatment was first proposed, so much has changed since then that it will be helpful to reconstruct the memories of that time and see Sakel's contribution in historical perspective. In the years when Sakel was developing his treatment, European psychiatry was still largely dominated by Kraepelinian views and Kraepelin regarded dementia praecox as an organic disease that would sooner or later yield to medical treatment. Bumke, in the 1929 edition of his textbook, which can be regarded as fairly representative of Central European thinking at that time, declared (p. 684):

> I am convinced that every attempt to reduce dementia praecox to psychological terms will become superfluous as soon as we discover the organic basis for these disorders. Nobody doubts this any more: not only the physical but even the psychological symptoms are in all probability based on organic or toxic factors. . . .

But in this country the revolt against Kraepelinian concepts was far advanced. Adolf Meyer, the dean of American psychiatrists and the leading influence in that period (see Vol. 5, *Proc. Assn. for Research in Nervous and Mental Disease*, p. 14, 1929), while advocating a broad and rather diffuse formulation of "reaction types" based on a multiplicity of factors, spoke of "the possibility of dynamic factors which may enter at several of the integrated levels" . . . a view which in practice led to a very insistent emphasis on psychology. Dr. McFie Campbell, a pupil of Meyer's, in developing Meyer's concept at the same meeting, was challenged by Dr. Morton Prince, who rose from the audience to say, "Dr. Campbell, I have obtained the impression that you interpret schizophrenia (dementia praecox) entirely in terms of psychological reaction or interest of the individual. Do I understand you to hold that this process is primary . . .?" Dr. Campbell answered in some noncommittal fashion, but the aura of psychological interest and emphasis remained.

Actually Adolf Meyer and his school did not like the organic emphasis and were disturbed by the advent of Sakel's pharmacological treatment. A number of leading American psychiatrists who did not wish to publicly voice their principled objections to this approach, privately discouraged it. Though Adolf Meyer agreed to participate in the special insulin treatment evening in this New York Academy of Medicine on January 12, 1937, the first large meeting of its kind, he wrote to me a few days earlier:

> There are two extremes in the attempts to play the savior role in psychiatry: work at the root—which is evidently *not* insulin work—and importations which have next to nothing specific to do with psychiatry but exploit the patient and resources through and for imported interests; and this is the case of insulin. I am always sorry to see the latter get on the top. Whenever it does, my interest wanes. I have allowed the paresis problem to pass into the domain of the lues department because paresis is a "dirty" experiment of nature without localizing or any other control being possible. I am willing to leave it to the spirochaetist. And with insulin we deal with even more of an importation apt to divert the attention completely from the illness by absorbing the attention in the direction of something pharmaceutical. I am not belittling the interest and the experiment, but I hope you understand me fully. It is too easy for non-psychiatrists to assume a dominant position and to become more or less antipsychiatric in the field. Therapy by the way of experimental pathology, along lines which have nothing to do with the disease process except as a starter and in the role of medical dominance acceptable to the patient and relatives and the profession will always have to prove itself. As soon as it becomes dominant by diverting the attention from what after all is the crux of it all, viz., the therapy at the root and in terms of life, it should only hold itself if success justifies the always dis-

turbing disruption and usurpations by some narrow technician.

I naturally shall not inject this note into the discussion of January 12. The meeting will anyhow be one in partibus infidelibus, i.e., governed by non-psychiatric interests and all I can expect to do is not to stir up the problem of psychiatry, but to balance what is sound in the work.

Not long afterwards, when public interest in these new approaches began to seem dangerously high, the Public Education Committee of the American Psychiatric Association issued this warning:

The widespread publicity, including radio dramatization of the so-called "insulin shock" treatment for schizophrenia for dementia praecox has resulted in many inquiries being directed to the Committee on Public Education of the American Psychiatric Association, as to the curability of dementia praecox by this form of treatment in particular.

The impression that there never has been and is now no treatment for dementia praecox, except through insulin therapy, is entirely erroneous. While dementia praecox has a less favorable outlook than many other forms of mental illness, much has been done and there are many forms of therapy, each promising something. It is hoped, and may prove to be a fact, that the so-called insulin shock treatment for dementia praecox will find a useful place among the forms of treatment, but its exact value has yet to be determined, and it can be stated definitely that it is not a specific, nor by any means a cure for all cases of dementia praecox.

It would be a source of regret should insulin shock treatment be a means of holding out a false hope to the families of tens of thousands of sufferers from dementia praecox, when this hope most certainly cannot be widely realized with present day knowledge of insulin therapy. It is, however, at the present time receiving careful study in the New York and Massachusetts state hospital systems, Bellevue Hospital, New York, and other scientific centers, but it should not be undertaken except by those adequately trained to meet the dangers connected with the treatment.

Objections came from other sources too, for this was a treatment that was developed not in the cloistered halls of our medical academies, and not documented with refined scientific or statistical data. Quite the contrary. One very distinguished neuropsychiatrist wrote, "Such a naive mixture of physics, chemistry, physiology and circumlocution has rarely appeared in a medical journal. It is scientific hypothesis degenerating to mixed metaphor!" But a year later the same author wrote, "The general consensus appears to be that [the procedure] constitutes a distinct contribution to the treatment of schizophrenia. . . ." And there the matter rested.

This period had its amusing aspects too. In some hospitals where a group would start insulin treatment in the face of the (understandable) critical skepticism of colleagues, as the treatment began to prove its value new groups on the staff would back the new convulsive treatment and you would get factions of insulinists and metrazolites. The same thing happened with some private hospitals which got off to a late start on the insulin work, and then began to specialize in convulsive treatment.

Sakel was sometimes bitter about the advent of convulsive therapy. Actually the first deliberate use of convulsive reactions for purposes of psychiatric treatment was Sakel's contribution, since he observed and reported the beneficial effect of insulin convulsions, and even tried to provoke them. It is unfortunate that Sakel was never given due credit for this. On the other hand Sakel was unduly alarmed by the convulsions, overestimated their dangers and never developed a systematic treatment out of them. This was Meduna's contribution, for which he must be fully credited. Both treatments together represented important new advances and helped open up a whole new area of psychiatric interest.

I would like to conclude on a personal note: it was a real pleasure to look over my old files to review this material. It was a wonderful period, full of excitement, with an atmosphere of great events surrounding it. Something really new and good was coming into psychiatry. There were difficulties, obstacles, debates and conflict, but the fights were good fights because big principles were involved and what was at stake was an aspect of human welfare. Moreover it was good to be on the winning side, for time has vindicated Sakel and his associates. What more could one ask? But medicine moves on: New issues and fresh problems arise, some of them merely new forms of the old struggle, because as Remy de Gourmont once said, *Il y a encore des gens qui rougissent d'avoir un corps.*

Bibliography of Some of the Early Literature

Anderson, C. L'Insulinthérapie dans la démence précoce. Extrait des Compt.-Rendus du Congrès des Med. Aliénistes et Neurologistes de France et des Pays de langue française. Brussels, July 1935. *Ann. Med.-Psych.*, 2:312, 1935.

v. Angyal, L. Uber die motorischen und tonischen Erscheinungen des Insulinschocks. Beiträge zur Physiologie und Pathologie des menschlichen Stirnhirns bei der Insulinbehandlung Schizophrener. *Zeit. Neur.*, 157:35, 1937.

v. Angyal, L., and Sakel, M. Insulinbehandlung des Pubertätsirreseins. *Orv. Hetil.*, 80:359, 386, 1936. (Hungarian.)

Appel, K. E., Farr, C. B. and Marshall, H. K. Insulin in

undernourished psychotic patients. *J.A.M.A.*, 90:1788, 1928; also: *Arch. Neur. Psych.*, 21:149, 1929.

Baranowski, L., Borysowicz, J., Marzynski, M., Ossendowski, A., Paradowski, J., and Witek, St. (Insulin method of treatment of schizophrenia.) *Rocz. psych.*, 25:161, 1935. (Polish.)

Bauer, M. E. Essais de traitement des affections schizophréniques par la méthode de Sakel. *Ann. Med. Psych.*, 94 T. II. 682, 1936.

Becker. Insulin bei nahrungverweigernden Geisteskranken. *Psychiat.-Neurol. Woch.*, 30:547, 1928.

Benedek, L. *Insulin-Schock-Wirkung auf die Wahrnehmung.* Berlin: Verlag Karger, 1935.

Bennett, A. E., and Semrad, E. V. Value of insulin treatment in undernourished psychiatric patients. *Am. J. Psych.*, 92:1425, 1936.

Berglas, B., and Susic, Z. Uber die Hypoglykämie-schockbehandlung der Schizophrenie. *Psychiat.-Neurol. Woch.*, 38:599, 1936.

Bersot, M. H. Le syndrome neurologique du choc insulinique. Soc. Méd.-Psycholog. Séance du 23 Nov. 1936. *Ann. Méd. Psych.*, 94:665, 1936.

Berze, J. Die Insulin-schock-Behandlung der Schizophrenie. *Wien. Med. Woch.*, 83:1365, 1933.

Borysowicz, J., and Marzynski, M. (Further remarks on the treatment of schizophrenia with large doses of insulin.) *Rocz. Psych.*, 28:70, 1936. (Polish with French abstract.)

Borysowicz, J., Paradowski, J., Rose, J., Witek, St., and Zalewski, W. (Insulin treatment of schizophrenia.) *Rocz. Psych.*, 28:26, 1936. (Polish with French abstract.)

v. Braunmühl, A. Die Insulinschockbehandlung der Schizophrenie. *Münch. Med. Woch.*, 84:8, 1937.

Bresler, J. Insulin in der Psychiatrie. *Psychiat.-Neurol. Woch.*, 39:14, 1937.

Bumke, O. *Lehrbuch der Geisteskrankheiten* Munich, Bergmann Verlag, 1929.

Bychowski, G., Kaczynski, M., Konopka, C., and Szczytt, K. (Experiences with the hypoglycemic shock method of treatment of psychoses.) *Rocz. Psych.*, 28:105, 1936. (Polish with French abstract.)

Bychowski, G. (Psychoanalysis and the induced hypoglycemic state.) *Rocz. Psych.*, 28:165, 1936.

Campbell, C. M. On the definition or delimitation of the schizophrenic type of reaction. *Proc. Assoc. Res. Nerv. Ment. Dis.*, 5:16, 1925.

Claude, H., and Rubenovitch, P. Traitement de la schizophrénie par le choc insulinique. Soc. Méd. Psycholog. Séance du 23 Nov. 1936. *Ann. Méd. Psych.*, 94:676, 1936.

Cobb, S. Review of Neuropsychiatry for 1937. *Arch. Int. Med.*, 60:1098, 1937.

Cobb, S. Review of Neuropsychiatry for 1938. *Arch. Int. Med.*, 62:883, 1938.

Cowie, D., Parsons, J. P., and Raphael, T. Preliminary report: insulin and the mental state of depression. *J. Mich. State. Med. Soc.*, 22:383, 1923.

Cowie, D., Parsons, J. P., and Raphael, T. Insulin and mental depression. *Arch. Neur. Psych.*, 12:522, 1924.

Dameshek, W., Myerson, A., and Stephenson, C. Insulin hypoglycemia: mechanism of neurologic symptoms. *Arch. Neur. Psych.*, 33:1, 1935.

De Châtel, A., and Palisa, C. Das Elektrokardiogramm im schweren hypoglykämischen Schock. *Klin. Woch.*, 14:1784, 1935.

Ederle, W. Schizophrenienbehandlung durch hypoglykämischen Schock. Report at the meeting of the Med. Gesellschaft at Giessen. *Münch. Med. Woch.*, 83:120, 1936.

Ederle, W. Remarks at 2. Jahresversammlung der Gesellschaft Deutscher Neurologen. u. Psychiater. *Der Nervenarzt.*, 9:629, 1936.

Feissly, R. Traitement insulinique des états de denutrition chez les sujets non diabétiques. *La Presse Med.*, 34:196, 1926.

Franke, G. Zur Frage der Epileptiformen Anfallsbereitschaft im Insulinschock. *Psychiat.-Neurol. Woch.*, 39:63, 1937.

Friedlaender, K. Insulinschock-Behandlung der Schizophrenie. *Psychiat.-Neurol. Woch.*, 38:520, 1936.

Frostig, J., Kister, J., Manasson, A., and Matecki, W. (Experimental study of the insulin treatment of schizophrenia.) *Rocz. Psych.*, 28:136, 1936. (Polish with French abstract.)

Gallinek, A. Erfahrungen mit Insulin in der Psychiatrie. *Arch. f. Psychiatr.*, 88:19, 1929.

Geller, W. Erfahrungen mit der Insulinbehandlung der Schizophrenie nach Sakel. *Psychiat.-Neurol. Woch.*, 38:628, 1936.

Georgi, F. Humoralpathologische Bemerkungen zur Insulinschocktherapie bei Schizophrenen. *Schweiz. Med. Woch.*, 66:935, 1936.

Giauni, G. Modificazioni elettrocardiografiche negli squilibri glicemici. *Clin. med. ital.*, 67:309, 1936.

Glueck, B. The hypoglycemic state in the treatment of schizophrenia. *J.A.M.A.*, 107:1029, 1936.

Glueck, B. The Induced hypoglycemic state in the treatment of the psychoses. *New York State J. Med.*, 36:1473, 1936.

Grimaldi, L. and Tomasino, A. Terapia de shock insulinico nella schizofrenia. *Schizofrenia*, 4:127, 1935.

Gross, M. Insuline et Schizophrénie. *Schweiz. Med. Woch.*, 66:689, 1936.

Grundler, W. Über Anwendung von Insulin bei hartnäckiger Nahrungsverweigerung. *Psychiat.-Neurol. Woch.*, 33:157, 1931.

Guiraud, P., and Nodet, C. H. Principes et technique de l'insulinothérapie. Soc. Méd.-Psychologique. Séance du 23 Nov. 1936. *Ann. Méd.-Psych.*, 94:670, 1936.

Haack, H. Insulin bei nahrungsverweigernden Geisteskranken. *Psychiat.-Neurol. Woch.*, 31:195, 1929.

Hadorn, W. Das Herz im Insulinchock. *Schweiz. Med. Woch.*, 66:936, 1936.

Hirschmann, J. Über Insulinbehandlung bei Schizophrenie. *Psychiat.-Neurol. Woch.*, 39:13, 1937.

Hoagland, H., Rubin, M. A., and Cameron, D. E. Electroencephalogram of schizophrenics during insulin treatments. *Am. J. Psych.*, 94:183, 1937.

Hoff, H. Hypoglykamie-Schockbehandlung von Psychosen. *Wien. Klin. Woch.*, 49:917, 1936.

Hutter, A. Nieuwe Behandelung von Dementia Praecox? *Nederl. Tijdschr. Geneesk.*, 80:2320, 1936.

Jacob, E., and Doussinet, P. Traitement insulinique d'un groupe de cetoses en pathologie mentale. *Bull. gén. de thérap.*, 184:12, 1933.

Jaschke, D. Die Behandlung der Nahrungsverweigerung mit Insulin. *Psychiat.-Neurol. Woch.*, 31:545, 1929.

Journal of the A.M.A. Editorial; Hypoglycemic Shock Treatment of Schizophrenia, 107:1720, 1936.

Kronfeld, A. Personal communication to Dr. Manfred Sakel. Dated Feb. 17, 1937.

Kronfeld, A. and Sternfeld, E. (On the treatment of schizophrenia with insulin shock.) Publication of the Gannushkin Institute, 1936.

Kronfeld, A., and Sternfeld, E. Paper read at the All-Soviet Psychiatric and Neurol. Congress. Dec. 1936. Congress Report.

Kubo: quoted by Wilson (see below), P. 52.

Kuppers, K. Remarks at 2. Jahresversammlung der Gesellschaft Deutscher Neurologen u. Psychiater. *Der Nervenarzt*, 9:629, 1936.

Kuppers, K., and Strehl. Insulin bei Nahrungsverweigerung. *Psychiat.-Neurol. Woch.*, 35:337, 1933.

Lancet: Leading Article: Insulin in Schizophrenia. 1:1418, 1936. Leading Article: Insulin in Schizophrenia. 2:750, 1936.

Langfeldt, G. Die Insulin-schok-behandlung der Schizophrenie. *Psychiat.-Neurol., Woch.*, 38:483, 1936.

Langfeldt, G. Effect of large doses of insulin in schizophrenia, *Nord, Med. Tidsckrift.* 12:1833, 1936.

Lehmann-Facius. Remarks at 2. Jahresversammlung der Gesellschaft Deutscher Neurologen u. Psychiater. *Der Nervenarzt.*, 9:629, 1936.

Lichter, C., and Lichter, N. *Le Traitement de la schizophrénie par de fortes doses d'insuline.* Vol. Jubilaire en l'honneur du Prof. Dr. C. Parhon. Publié par la Société Roumaine de Neurologie, Psychiat., Psycholog., et Endocrin. p. 281, 1934.

Maier, H. W. Remarks at the Congrés des Médecins Aliénistes et Neurologistes de France et des Pays de Langue Française. Session 40. Basel, Zurich, Berne, and Neufchâtel. July 20-25, 1936. *L'Encéphale,* 31:294, 1936.

Mauz. Remarks at 2. Jahresversammlung der Gesell. Deutscher Neurolog. u. Psych. *Der Nervenartz,* 9:629, 1936.

Mebel, M. Versuch einer Anwendung des Insulins in psychiatrischer Praxis. *Sovet. Psichonevr.,* 8:41, 1932. (Russian with German summary.)

Meyer, A. Evolution of the Dementia Praecox Concept. Proc. Assoc. Res. Nerv. Ment. Dis., 5:3, 1925.

Mira, E. El metodo de Sakel para el tratemiento de la esquizofrenia. *Rev. Med. de Barcelona,* 24:529, 1935.

Miskolczy, D. Insulinmastkur bei Nerven u. Geisteskranken. *Psychiat.-Neurol. Woch.,* 29:34, 1927.

Müller, Max: Le traitement de la schizophrénie par l'insuline. Société Médico-Psychologique, Seance du 23 Nov. 1936. *Ann. Med.-Psych.,* 94:649, 1936.

Müller, M. Die Insulinschocktherapie der Schizophrenie. *Der Nervenarzt.,* 9:569, 1936.

Müller, M. Die Insulinschockbehandlung der Schizophrenie. *Schweiz. Med. Woch.,* 66:929, 1936.

Munn, C. Insulin in catatonic stupor. *Arch. Neur. Psych.,* 34:262, 1935.

v. Pap, Z. Erfahrungen mit der Insulinschoktherapie bei Schizophrenen. *Monatsch. f. Psychiatrie u. Neurologie,* 94:318, 1937.

Parfitt, D. N. Treatment of psychoses by prolonged narcosis

(using somnifene, barbital derivatives, with and without insulin). *Lancet*, 1:424, 1936.

Pisk, G. Über ein "Zeitraffer" phänomen nach Insulinkoma. *Zeit. f. d. ges. Neur. u. Psych.*, 156:777, 1936.

Pötzl, O. Introduction to Sakel's *Neue Behandlungsmethode der Schizophrenie*. Vienna and Leipzig; Verlag Moritz Perles, 1935.

Pötzl, O. Remarks at the Viennese Gesellschaft der Aerzte. Nov. 1933. *Wien. Klin. Woch.*, 46:1372, 1933.

Puca, A. La insulino-terapia nei malati di mente. *Rass. Studi. Psichiat.*, 16:461, 1927.

Roberti, C. E. La terapie insulinica nelle malattie mentali. Nota preventiva. *Rass. Studi Psichiat.*, 19:628, 1930.

Rose, J. (Blood sugar curves in the course of insulin treatment of schizophrenia.) *Rocz. Psych.*, 25:178, 1935, and *Warszaw Czas. Iek.*, 12:555, 1935.

Rosenthal, C. and Beyer. Insulinbehandlung psychischer Erkrankungen. *Arch. f. Psychiatr.*, 88:504, 1929.

Rutkowski, A. (Results of the insulin therapy of schizophrenia at the Psychiatric University Clinic of Wilna.) *Rocz. Psych.*, 28:94, 1936.

Sakel, M. Neue Behandlung der Morphinsucht. *Zeit. Neur.*, 143:506, 1933.

Sakel, M. Theorie der Sucht. *Zeit. Neur.*, 129:1930.

Sakel, M. *Neue Behandlungsmethode der Schizophrenie*. Vienna: Verlag Moritz Perles, 1935.

Sakel, M. Zur Methodik der Hypoglykamiebehandlung von Psychosen. *Wien. Klin. Woch.*, 49:1278, 1936.

Sakel, M. Neue Behandlungsart Schizophrenser u. verwirrter Erregter. In the Proceedings of the Gesellschaft der Aerzte in Vienna. *Wien. Klin. Woch.*, 46:1372, 1933.

Sakel, M. Neue Behandlung der Morphinsucht, *Deutsch. Med. Woch.*, 42:1777, 1930.

Schmid, H. Zur Histopathologie der Sakelschen Hypoglykämiebehandlung der Schizophrenie. *Schweiz. Med. Woch.*, 66:960, 1936.

Schmid, M. H. L'histopathologie du choc insulinique. Soc. Méd.-Psychologique. Séance du 23 Nov. 1936. *Ann. Méd.-Psych.*, 94:658, 1936.

Schmidt, Paul. Über Organtherapie und Insulinbehandlung bei endogenen Geistesstörungen. *Klin. Woch.*, 7:839, 1928.

Sharp, W. L., and Bahr, M. A. Results of insulin therapy in mental patients. *J. Indiana M.A.*, 27:210, 1934.

Slotopolsky, B. Insulin bei nahrungsverweigernden Geisteskranken. *Zeit. Neur. Psych.*, 136:367, 1931.

Stanesco, J. Psychothérapie analytique associée à différents agents endocriniens et médicamenteux (insuline, etc.) dans la thérapeutique de la schizophrénie (syndrome catatonique). *Semaine d. hôp. de Paris*, 6:378, 1930.

Steck, H. Insulinwirkung bei psychotischen Erregungzuständen. *Schweiz. Med. Woch.*, 14:748, 1932.

Steck, H. Remarks at the Congrès des Médecins aliénistes et Neurologistes de France et des Pays de langue Française. 40 Session, 1936. *L'Encéphale*, 31:294, 1936.

Steinfeld, J. Insulin Shock Therapy in Schizophrenia (with subsequent Progress notes). *J.A.M.A.*, 108:91, 1937.

Strecker, H. Insulin in Schizophrenia (A letter). *Lancet*, 1:1498, 1936.

Strecker, H. Die Insulinbehandlung der Schizophrenie. *Münch. Med. Woch.*, 83:649, 1936.

Targowla, R., and Lamache, A. Le Traitement par l'insuline des états d'anorexie de sitiophobie et de dénutrition dans les troubles psychonévropathiques. *Prat. Méd. Franc.*, 5:452, 1926.

Targowla, R. La cure d'insuline dans les états neuro-psychopathiques. *Gaz. Méd. de France*, 2:47, 1930.

Targowla, R., and Lamache, A. L'insuline dans les états d'anorexie, de sitiophobie, et de dénutrition chez les psychopathes. *La Presse Méd.*, 34:1285, 1926.

Teenstra, P. E. M. Die Behandlung schizophrener Psychosen mit Insulinschocks. *Nederl. Tijdschr. Geneesk.*, 80:17, 1936.

Torp, H. Psykioke og nevrologiske forandringer efter hypo-glykemisk koma hos en schizofren. *Norsk Magasin for Laegevidenskapen*, 93:760, 1932.

Traczynski, J. (Hematological studies of patients undergoing insulin treatment.) *Rocz. Psych.*, 28:157, 1936.

Weygandt, W. Über aktive Schizophreniebehandlung. *Psychiat.-Neurol. Woch.*, 37:608, 619, 1935.

Wilson, I. A study of hypoglycemic shock treatment in schizophrenia. Board of Control, H. M. Stationery Office, London, 1936.

Wortis, J. Sakel's 'Neue Behandlungsmethode der Schizophrenie.' (A review.) *J. Nerv. Ment. Dis.*, 83:215, 1936.

Wortis, J. Bradycardia with Hypoglycemia (A letter). *J.A.M.A.*, 106:2089, 1936.

Wortis, J. On the response of schizophrenic subjects to hypoglycemic insulin shock. *J. Nerv. Ment. Dis.*, 84:497, 1936.

Wortis, J. Cases illustrating the treatment of schizophrenia by insulin shock. Proceedings of the N. Y. Society for Clinical Psychiatry. Nov. 12, 1936. *J. Nerv. Ment. Dis.*, 85:446, 1937.

Wortis, J. and Roberts, J. Insulin shock treatment in the psychoses. *Am. J. Nursing*, 37:494, 1937.

Wortis, J. Common acne and insulin hypoglycemia. *J.A.M.A.*, 108:971, 1937.

Part Two

PHYSIOCHEMICAL

RESEARCH

Chapter 3

HORMONAL AND OTHER BLOOD CHANGES OCCURRING DURING INSULIN HYPOGLYCEMIA TREATMENT

Ivan F. Bennett

Introduction

A neuroendocrine basis for the effectiveness of insulin-induced hypoglycemia in the treatment of psychiatric conditions was consistently defended by Sakel. He believed in the existence of psychotically functioning nerve cells which, because of their hyperactivity, were more sensitive to the hypoglycemic-blockade than the normal ones. Deprived of carbohydrate these aberrant cells were forced into hibernation and reverted to normal functioning. The use of an endogenous substance such as insulin was a natural method leading to superior and more permanent results. Its parasympathetic activity neutralized the excessive sympathetic stimulation of the nervous system seen as psychotic symptoms. With the restoration of normal autonomic homeostasis the patient regained his normal state.[1]

In a discussion of hormonal and blood changes one should include a review of studies involving the autonomic system as reflected in the Mecholyl or Funkenstein Test and changes in carbohydrate metabolism including those seen with the Glucose and Insulin Tolerance Tests. Following a discussion of insulin sensitivity a fitting transition can then be made from this to a consideration of the role played by the contra-insulin hormones, notably growth hormone, the 11,17-oxycorticosteroids acting through ACTH and, of course, adrenaline.

I. *Autonomic Nervous System Variables*

In 1943 Gold, using 15 mg. mecholyl chloride before and after insulin shock therapy in thirty-three catatonic patients, noted 66 percent of the group exhibited improved sympathetic activity following therapy. This was seen in an increased rate of recovery from the lowered systolic pressure, a reduction in the time required for it to return to its baseline or to rise above its original level. In this group 75 percent showed clinical improvement.[2] Using nine schizophrenic patients with twelve controls, Shurley and Morris measured the response of the autonomic nervous system to the Insulin Tolerance, Adrenaline, and Mecholyl Tests, prior to and following the termination of therapy. The schizophrenic patients showed a decreased response as compared to the controls before insulin. Following the course of treatment there was an increase in sympathetic activity. Those with the greater response again showed a more satisfactory clinical state.[3] Funkenstein *et al.* cite one case of a patient with a pretreatment epinephrine-precipitable anxiety whose clinical improvement was accompanied by the elimination of this type of anxiety.[4] Such an effect was confirmed by Alexander who believes that epinephrine-precipitable anxiety is a favorable prognostic sign for successful therapy, especially when that therapy is insulin shock.[5] Because of the influence of extraneous factors influencing blood pressure Vanderkamp *et al.* used a number of variables to predict improvement in insulin shock therapy. In addition to blood pressure, these included pulse rate, sweating, salivating, flushing, pupillary changes, and global reactivity. They were separately rated on a 5-point scale and graded from no change to marked responsiveness. In the seventy-five patients evaluated before and after treatment, the pulse rate deviation variable was found to have a significantly greater predictive power than the Funkenstein Test index of systolic blood pressure groupings. Maximum correlations occurred at the 7-minute observation period following mecholyl injection, pulse rate deviations correlating .63 and systolic blood pressure deviations −.34 with insulin improvement.[6]

In the Funkenstein phenomenon Gellhorn finds evidence for a group of schizophrenic patients characterized by a hyporeactive sympathetic hypothalamus who benefit from the increased sympathetic activity initiated by insulin shock. The clinical improvement is mirrored in a normal sympathetic reactivity.[7] In addition, however, he emphasizes the role of anoxia from hypoglycemia raising blood pressure. The resulting increase in impulses from the chemoreceptors potentiates the augmented sympathetic impulses.[8] Alexander's opinion is that there is a balanced stimulation during insulin shock therapy of both divisions of the autonomic nervous system at different shock levels. Therefore the treatment reduces excessive reactions to both cholinergic and adrenergic stimuli.[9]

II. Effect on Carbohydrate Metabolism

The fall in blood glucose following insulin administration is, of course, the most characteristic finding. Since this may be due to either an increased rate of glucose removal or to a decreased rate of glucose replacement, the process is a complicated one. The fall in serum potassium and inorganic phosphate[10a, 10b, 11] is due to their movement with the glucose from the extracellular fluid into the cell. Others, though, have found no change in the potassium level.[12, 13] The increased gluconeogenesis from protein due to release of adrenocortical hormones explains the lowered amino acid blood level.[14] Increased serum protein and sodium with decrease in the serum chloride have been attributed to the hemoconcentration and marked sweating during shock therapy.[10a, 10b] These investigators also noticed a decrease in bicarbonate which was statistically significant and they believed this is linked with the failure to utilize oxygen. The effects on acid-base, electrolyte, and water balance are secondary to those on carbohydrate, fat and protein metabolism.[15] Or, in other words, the effect of insulin on these blood constituents is secondary to the increase in the metabolism of glucose.

a. Effect on the Glucose Tolerance Test

After discovering that insulin, in doses producing hypoglycemia, in diabetic patients gradually diminishes carbohydrate tolerance and aggravates the diabetes, Maher and Somogyi noted a similar effect when 20 units of insulin daily were given to nondiabetic, tuberculous patients for over six months as an appetite stimulant. This was also observed in schizophrenic subjects undergoing insulin shock therapy.[16] It was reasoned that the prolonged compensatory hyperglycemia potentiated the decrease in the carbohydrate tolerance. Looney and Cameron, determining the glucose tolerance curve before and after insulin shock therapy in seven patients, likewise found a decrease following therapy. They concluded that the adrenaline response slowed down the formation of liver glycogen and so prevented the removal of blood sugar.[17] On the other hand, Proctor *et al.* reported that the clinical improvement following insulin therapy was accompanied by an increase in the glucose tolerance phenomenon,[18] while Borenz and his group, using the IV glucose tolerance test, showed no change before and after treatment.[19] While they mention preparation of patients by weeks of an adequate carbohydrate diet, Olsen and Neutzel, in normal subjects, could find no variation in response to the test dose of insulin when a high or low carbohydrate diet or a low caloric diet were successfully given.[20]

In Pfister's series of 104 normal subjects and 184 schizophrenic patients, oral ingestion of levulose (100 Gm.) resulted in a steep, brief rise and a gradual fall in the normal group. The acute schizophrenic patients showed a rapid rise with values above normal and a relatively slow fall, while the chronic members exhibited a slow rise which often failed to reach the maximum in the 2-hour period. The delayed response was attributed to a defective autonomic apparatus.[21]

A reduced glucose tolerance, though, is seen when the sampling is broadened to include nonschizophrenic patients. On this basis, Freeman *et al.* concluded that the test is related to emotional tension and is not specific for the psychoses.[22] Furthermore, Hinkle and Wolf, studying the effects of stressful life situations on the blood glucose level, observed that, if the subject is newly exposed to a stressful situation, the glucose tolerance curve is usually flatter than normal. But, if he has been exposed for some time to stress and is then given glucose, the glucose tolerance curve is higher and more prolonged than it is in the absence of stress.[23]

While reports are contradictory it would appear that changes in the clinical state following insulin therapy can be accompanied by improvement in the glucose tolerance.

b. Effect on the Insulin Tolerance Test

Pfister administered 0.2 units of insulin/kilogram of body weight to normal and schizophrenic subjects and compared the insulin tolerance curves. The normal response was a fall 20 to 30 percent below the fasting level of blood sugar in the first half hour and a return to the original level after the first hour. The schizophrenic group had a slow and delayed response. The chronic members were unable to make an adequate compensation as shown by a feeble and delayed rise.[21] While Borenz *et al.* noted a greater rigidity of response to both the glucose and insulin tolerance tests, they were unable to detect any significant changes following insulin shock therapy.[19] In the group of 16 schizophrenic patients given test doses of insulin by Harris, some showed a normal response, and others, either an increased or decreased sensitivity. Three of the patients showed a greater drop in blood sugar after insulin shock treatment, which he found contrary to the experience of Banting *et al.* who observed increase in insulin resistance following insulin shock treatment in one schizophrenic patient. Harris found no correlation between the tests and subsequent dose of insulin required to produce coma. A decrease in insulin resistance was not necessarily accompanied by clinical change.[24]

Nadeau and Rouleau used a glucose-insulin tolerance test on four insulin-resistive patients who had shown flat insulin tolerance curves. Following this procedure they found an unexpected sensitivity towards insulin and hypoglycemia. This was interpreted as being due to the temporary inactivation of insulin antagonists produced by the initial hyperglycemia. During this phase, both exogenous and endogenous insulin act without inhibition inducing an effective level of hypoglycemia. The administration of glucose before insulin in the management of insulin-resistant patients undergoing shock therapy was proposed.[25] They also could see no consistent correlation between response to the insulin tolerance test and the dose necessary to induce coma.

Both the glucose tolerance and the insulin tolerance tests can show changes following insulin shock therapy. Such changes though are so unpredictable that they cannot be used as prognosticators of therapeutic result.

III. *Insulin Resistance*

When one recalls a depancreatized man requires only 35 to 50 units of insulin daily to control the resulting diabetes[26] and the requirement for some diabetics of 500 to 5000 units of insulin daily in the presence of acute infections,[27] the variation in dose required to produce coma in schizophrenia does not seem so extreme.

Von Braunmühl believed a patient requiring 300 units of insulin for the production of coma showed "absolute resistance."[28] This has been commonly accepted, possibly because the dose limit for sensitivity in diabetes has been set at 200 units of insulin for control.[26] However, the problem is not peculiar to these two groups.

Olsen and Neutzel, using 1/40 unit of crystalline insulin/ kilogram of body weight intravenously, have observed insulin resistance in those with collagen, neoplastic, hepatic and infectious diseases, as well as in certain endocrine disorders. They see these as non-specific stresses to which the body responds by an increase in adrenocortical activity.[20] As evidence they cite the study of Conn *et al.* in which the administration of ACTH to normal subjects in diabetic-producing amounts resulted in an increased resistance to endogenous insulin. The mean percent fall from fasting values of blood sugar in the acutely ill patients was 12.3 percent after thirty minutes and in the chronically severely ill group, 17.4 percent. The normal control was 39.0 percent. Mansour and Hewitt, though, found no direct correlation between adrenocortical activity and insulin sensitivity when adult rats were exposed to cold stress. After one day there was increased adrenocortical activity without change in blood sugar or insulin sensitivity. Hyperglycemia and hypersensitivity to insulin appeared after six days of exposure while adrenocortical activity remained high. This persisted after nine days even though by then the adrenocortical activity had returned to normal levels. It was postulated that blood sugar changes were produced by adrenaline and other mechanisms.[29]

The author in a special study of 113 schizophrenic patients receiving insulin coma therapy has observed 15 who required over 1500 units of insulin for induction of coma. The average time for the initial coma was 13 days and the average dose required was 2000 units. There was no sex difference. In those who developed coma on less than 1500 units daily, the 71 males had their first coma on the sixth day with an average dose of 900 units, and the 27 females on the same day with an average dose of 750 units. Maintenance dose for continuation of one hour of coma was 700 units in the insulin-resistant group of 13 males and 150 units in the insulin-normal group. The females required 900 units and 50 units respectively for maintenance. The Bond and Shurley technique of insulin dosage adjustment was used.[30] The daily dose was increased rapidly by geometric progression, starting with 50 units on the first day, 100, 200, 400, and 800 on successive days and then by 200-unit increments until coma was attained. Patients were kept in treatment for 3 hours daily, 5 days a week for 12 weeks. Three of the insulin-resistant patients were given over 2000 units daily for 45 or more days without evidence of the development of insulin sensitivity.

Some of the theories proposed to explain resistance to insulin have a direct bearing upon metabolic changes occurring during insulin shock therapy.

a. The Role of Insulin

The insulin content of blood from 27 schizophrenic patients and 10 normal controls was assayed in the hypophysectomized-adrenomedullated rat by Gellhorn and associates. In the absence of emotional excitement, both groups showed the same amount of insulin in the blood. The insulin content of the blood from schizophrenic patients was greatly increased under emotional excitement. In 21 of the

27 cases, while there was no evidence of blood sugar change in their own blood, there was a marked fall in the blood sugar of the test animal so severe as to produce coma. In the remaining 6 an increase in blood sugar level was shown, indicating an adrenaline increase. A hypoglycemic response in the rat was seen, though no coma. While the normal subjects showed a slight rise in their blood sugar during excitement, the blood samples produced no hypoglycemic response in the test animal. It was concluded that the two groups do not differ with regard to insulin secretion in periods of rest, but that with emotional excitement there is an increased insulin secretion in the patient group without a concomitant rise in the adrenaline level. The psychotic group was considered to respond to stress with excessive vagoinsulin activity whereas the normal subjects showed a predominance of sympatheticoadrenal activity.[31]

This would explain the observation of Scheflen and Reiner who noted patients sensitive to insulin shock therapy had deep, quiet, and slowly terminated comas characterized by parasympathetic predominance. Refractory patients experienced light, active comas often terminating spontaneously and characterized by sympathetic predominance. In their group of 100 patients, the insulin-sensitive patients after treatment displayed passivity, withdrawal, asthenia, listlessness, and easy fatigability, while the refractory ones showed marked anxiety, paranoid dread, aggressiveness and resistiveness.[32]

Psychophysiologic resistance was also studied by Patterson using 27 patients who received group psychotherapy with the insulin shock treatment. Attitude toward treatment was related to the amount of insulin required for coma, total coma time, number of adverse reactions, and length of treatment required. The patients were divided into four groups with characteristic attitudes. Those who considered the therapy as a last ditch type of treatment responded very poorly during the therapy. They showed a high physiological resistance, as determined by the criteria above, and a low rate of discharge (14.2 percent). Patients in the second group accepted insulin as genuine treatment, or even as the treatment of choice in their case. They showed low physical resistance to insulin and a high rate of discharge (100 percent). Those in the third group expressed no attitude toward the treatment and showed a low physical resistance to insulin coma. There was no attitude and there was no change, the discharge rate being 33.3 percent. The fourth group initially felt insulin therapy was hopeless but during the course of treatment they became more optimistic. This was accompanied by a striking change in lowered physical resistance to insulin and a subsequent improvement. Discharge rate was 88.9 percent. It was reasoned that the initial attitude gave them a psychophysiological handicap which could not be compensated for.[33]

It has been shown that blood insulin levels do vary with stress and that there may be a psychophysiological relationship altering the individual's response to insulin during shock therapy. The importance of establishing baselines not only in regard to blood sugar levels but in terms of the patient's level of apprehension or anticipation previous to a test or therapy should be emphasized.

b. Hyperglycemic Factors

Meduna, Gerty, and Urse reported that blood samples from 60 percent of their schizophrenic patients showed an anti-insulin effect when tested in rabbits. This was seen as a decrease in the drop in the blood sugar and a more rapid return of the blood sugar to original levels as compared with blood from normal persons.[34] Later Meduna and Vaichulis isolated a hyperglycemic factor from the urine of a particular group of schizophrenic patients (oneirophrenics). This group showed an abnormal carbohydrate metabolism characterized by a resistance to insulin, a pseudo-diabetic reaction to the Exton-Rose test, and a protracted sugar-tolerance curve during the intravenous glucose tolerance test.[35] They were said to have a good prognosis for remission, either spontaneous or following shock therapy. Harris had some patients whose serum had this anti-insulin effect, but others showed little or no such activity.[24] Goldner and Ricketts could find no evidence of an anti-insulin factor in the blood of schizophrenic patients.[36] They mentioned that Kraines had not only extreme variations from person to person, but different results with the blood of the same patient examined from day to day. Morgan and Pilgrim though did find such a factor in the urine of schizophrenic individuals and not in the urine of normal subjects.[37]

Harris mentioned that DeWesselow and Griffiths in 1936 found an anti-insulin substance in the blood of diabetic patients.[24] Using the isolated rat diaphragm Marsh and Haugaard found that serum from both normal and diabetic subjects contained significant amounts of such material but that serum from insulin-resistant individuals contained excessive quantities.[38] These substances rapidly inactivated some or all of the insulin added to the preparation and glucose had no effect on the reaction. A hyperglycemic factor from normal human urine which contained urinary amylase, derived probably from blood serum amylase, was extracted by Moya and Hoffman. It was believed that blood serum amylase might influence the storage of liver glycogen.[39]

There is then evidence for a hyperglycemic factor in serum and urine which is present in normal humans. Those showing insulin resistance have a higher concentration. It is possible that this may apply to some schizophrenic individuals showing resistance to insulin shock therapy.

c. Insulin Antibodies

Lerman has demonstrated the presence of substances in the blood of insulin-resistant diabetic patients which protect animals against the hypoglycemic effects of insulin and which show the characteristics of various antibodies. His clinical material suggests that the return of normal insulin sensitivity is dependent upon the disappearance of these immune bodies and he cites other examples of similar fluctuations in antibody titer. He recommends the treatment of insulin resistance by repeated insulin injections to bring about a desensitization.[40] Confirmation of a desensitization reaction was shown experimentally by Corwin who gave nondiabetic dogs 1 unit of insulin/kilogram of body weight intravenously every two hours until convulsions occurred. The amount of insulin required to produce convulsions progressively decreased for three days. After the third day, the amount became stabilized in each animal and in all of the 26 dogs tested. The blood sugar levels, the rapidity of the development of hypoglycemia and the depth of the hypoglycemia were similar on subsequent days.[41] The administration of large doses of intravenous insulin (400 units/kilogram of body weight) in rabbits was found by Naatanen to produce less shock and less hypoglycemia than small doses (10 units/kilogram of body weight). Repeated large doses though produced severe reactions. It was concluded that a pituitary factor was responsible for the initial resistance but that this was exhausted by continual administration of the large dose.[42] Here, too, there was an increase in insulin sensitivity with repeated insulin shock.

Berson and Yalow differentiate serum anti-insulin factors as being insulin antibodies and insulin antagonists demonstrable in the absence of a history of exogenous insulin administration. Insulinase is most representative of the second group and is responsible for half of the circulating insulin being degraded in thirty-five minutes in vivo.[43] In a previous paper Berson et al. administered insulin-I[131] intravenously to diabetic and schizophrenic subjects. The latter were insulin shock patients. Plasma or serum samples were obtained from normal subjects and, after the addition of insulin-I[131], these were also evaluated by paper and starch block electrophoresis. Binding of insulin-I[131] was never observed in the absence of previous insulin therapy, but was always present in those who had received insulin treatment for three months or longer. Two schizophrenic patients who had been receiving insulin shock therapy for six weeks and three and one-half months, respectively, showed the presence of such binding. Two others receiving therapy for three and one-half weeks and eight weeks, respectively, showed no binding. The binding of the insulin-I^{131} to gamma globulin prevents it from passing rapidly through the capillary wall and the insulin is not utilized. Insulin resistance results. Such a binding globulin fulfills the criteria for an antibody and is an insulin-transporting rather than a precipitating one. As with hydrocortisone and several of the anterior pituitary hormones, the rate of inactivation of insulin is a constant one extending over a wide range of hormone concentrations far exceeding physiological limits. One subject is cited who, while receiving 640 units of regular insulin subcutaneously, had the same rate of disappearance as the controls. They emphasize that while this pattern of rapid hormone inactivation is wasteful, it does allow for high concentrations in response to physiological demands or stress without the penalty of prolongation of effect after the need has passed.[44] Sudden breaking through of insulin resistance with a severe reaction could be explained as due to the release of the "trapped" insulin by dissociation of the insulin-globulin complex. Such a binding theory could also explain the ineffectiveness of large intravenous doses of insulin after massive intramuscular doses have failed. Horvath and Friedman, for example, found that doses of 120 units intravenously produced no greater effects than did those of 30 units.[45]

The presence of insulin resistance secondary to antibodies need not be suspected only if high doses of insulin are required. Arquilla and Stavitsky have shown antibodies to insulin in diabetic patients requiring between 120 and 1000 units of insulin daily.[46]

Insulin being a poor antibody producer, the rapidly developing resistance in the first two weeks of insulin shock therapy and the response to such treatment is probably to a large degree not associated with this but must be related to such insulin antagonists as the contra-insulin hormone.

IV. *Contra-insulin Hormones*

a. Adrenaline

It is well known that the insulin-induced hypoglycemia causes a release of adrenaline which, through hepatic glycogenolysis, produces an increase of liver glucose seen as hyperglycemia and so restoring the low blood sugar level. Other mechanisms may play a role, however, such as the inhibition of glucose utilization. Adrenaline may increase cellular hexosemonophosphate through phosphorylation of glycogen and so reduce glucose uptake.[47] Hökfelt found that injection of insulin in the cat depleted the adrenals of adrenaline but the noradrenaline content remained unchanged unless amounts sufficient to induce insulin shock were used.[48] Tietz and her co-workers in 1940 reported that within two hours following insulin administration to ten schizophrenic patients undergoing shock therapy, there was no change or only a slight rise or fall in blood adrenaline. There was a tendency toward an increase in most cases after three hours, and a more consistent rise was seen in all patients after four hours.[49] Weil-Malherbe and Bone, using the differential fluorometric method, followed the catechol amine level (adrenaline and noradrenaline) during insulin shock therapy. There was an unusually immediate and rapid drop after insulin with the lowest value half an hour after injection, occurring so soon it could not be attributed to hypoglycemia. The blood sugar continued to fall after blood adrenaline had stabilized at a lower level. The noradrenaline concentration remained unchanged. Disappearance of circulating adrenaline was believed due to its increased utilization in the liver because of the hypoglycemia.[50] A contradictory result reported by Holzbauer and Vogt, namely, elevation of adrenaline after intravenous insulin, was explained by Weil-Malherbe as due to difference in technique.[51] However, Millar, using the fluorometric estimation of adrenaline during insulin hypoglycemia, also reported an increased adrenaline level.[52] As additional evidence of the influence of insulin upon adrenaline metabolism, Von Euler and Luft found an increase in urinary excretion of adrenaline after intravenous insulin in normal subjects.[53]

The weight of evidence is that plasma adrenaline level increases following insulin administration. Adrenaline metabolism is accelerated from its secretion to its excretion.

b. Histamine

Intravenous histamine was used as a stress agent to evaluate the rapidity of ACTH response by Gray and Munson. A dosage level sufficient to cause marked difference between adrenal ascorbic acid concentration, comparing treated and control rates, was used. Within ten to fifteen seconds there was an increase in ACTH blood level. This was not shown with nicotine, tetraethyl ammonium chloride, or l-epinephrine. It was concluded that adrenaline does not play an essential part in the pituitary response to stress for the histamine test showed the pituitary was capable of responding in five to ten seconds.[54] Bliss et al. reported histamine decreases 17-hydroxycorticosteroid level but only when given in toxic amounts. When 5 I.U. of ACTH were given before the histamine, there was a normal response. It was surmised that histamine neither activates nor inhibits the pituitary adrenal cortex axis. Other adrenocortical activators such as bacterial pyrogen (Piromen), insulin, and the Antabuse-alcohol reaction did cause an increase in the 17-hydroxycorticosteroid level.[55]

A possible role of endogenous histamine, however, is shown in an interesting study done by Billig and Hesser in 1944. Blood samples from six patients receiving insulin shock therapy were bioassayed for histamine levels and a correlation was later made between the histamine level and the depth of coma. While the hypoglycemic reaction could not be correlated with the insulin dose or the blood sugar level, in four patients the peak of the histamine level did coincide with the greatest depth of coma. With insulin shock therapy there was up to a 789 percent increase (an average value of 0.353 micrograms/cc.) over the average preshock histamine level (0.045 micrograms/cc.) with an average level of 0.25 micrograms/cc. Since 90 percent of the histamine in the blood is carried in the white blood cells, especially the eosinophiles, the possibility of insulin increasing cellular and capillary permeability was considered. Evidence for this is the vascular damage seen in protracted insulin shock. They quote the observation of Heilbrunn and Liebert that the adrenaline level in deep coma is very low and mention is made of the antagonistic relationship between adrenaline and histamine.[56] Histamine is known to be an adrenaline antagonist and when administered to animals does stimulate the release of adrenaline. In toxic doses this results in an adrenaline-induced hyperglycemia.[56a] It is thus probable that the high histamine level during deep coma is a compensatory one.

c. The Thyroid

The effect of insulin shock therapy on thyroid function as determined by changes in serum protein-bound iodine, radioactive iodine uptake, basal metabolic rate and plasma cholesterol was studied over a two-year period by Bowman and his colleagues using seven patients. No significant changes were seen during treatment nor was there any positive correlation between improvement and such changes. This conclusion held for such other types of therapy as electroshock, combined shock, thyroid extract or psychotherapy.[57] The results were sustained when the number of patients studied was increased from twenty-five to forty-nine.[58] Emphasizing the wide frequency distribution of metabolic and endocrine functions in schizophrenia from subnormal through normal to the supranormal range, Batt *et al.* did show a difference in I^{131} uptake following effective insulin shock therapy. Their controls had the accepted normal range with the 24-hour I^{131} uptake falling between 25 and 50 percent of the injected dose.[59] Low thyroid activity is a bad prognostic sign if primary. If secondary to pituitary underfunction or if reciprocal to high adrenocortical activity, it may become normal with clinical improvement resulting. If it remains normal improvement is maintained, but if it becomes high the patient relapses. Normal thyroid activity is not influenced by insulin therapy, and when it does shift outside the normal range secondary to the stimulation of the anterior pituitary, prognosis is poor. High thyroid activity, if primary, is also a bad prognostic sign and is often aggravated during insulin therapy owing to additional anterior pituitary stimulation with increased secretion of the thyrotropic hormone. If the high thyroid activity is secondary to excessive anterior pituitary activity, with the additional stress of insulin therapy, the production of the thyrotropic hormone may become exhausted, leading to an improvement in the secondary hyperthyroidism. The return to normal thyroid activity is correlated then with clinical improvement.[60]

This clinical study confirms the evidence of others that the thyroid per se exerts only a minor influence on insulin response and emphasizes that changes in its metabolism only mirror alterations in that of the anterior pituitary.

d. The Stress Axis.

The most effective contra-insulin agents, ACTH and the growth hormone of the anterior pituitary and the adrenocortical steroids of the adrenal cortex, notably corticosterone, cortisone and hydrocortisone, will be considered together because of their close reciprocal activity in insulin metabolism.

(1) Eosinophile level

Best *et al.* consider the limits of normal for circulating eosinophiles to be from 70 to 450 eosinophils per cubic millimeter. They point out that day-to-day variation of the 8:00 a.m. count may be appreciable and that diurnal fluctuations, with an average midmorning fall of 20 percent below the 8:00 a.m. level and a night time peak 30 percent above it, are factors to be considered in the evaluation of eosinophile change. In general, eosinophilia is due to exogenous factors and eosinopenia to endogenous ones, notably adrenomedullary and adrenocortical hyperactivity.[61] A study of the effect of insulin hypoglycemia on the eosinophile and lymphocyte levels of eight schizophrenic patients was reported by Tsai *et al.* There was a uniform and significant decrease in both, the eosinopenia amounting to a 69 to 96 percent fall and the lymphocytopenia to a 38 to 70 percent fall. The maximal eosinopenia occurred 4 to 8 hours after insulin administration and 2 to 4 hours after the lowest blood glucose. The magnitude of the decrease had no relation to the number of previous insulin injections, dosage, nor to the clinical status following therapy. With the concurrent administration of glucose in two cases, the hypoglycemia was prevented and no significant eosinopenia or lymphocytopenia occurred. It was therefore concluded that adrenaline, not insulin, caused the adrenocortical activation in insulin-induced hypoglycemia.[62] In a study of eosinophile response to insulin in nine schizophrenic patients, Mann and Lehmann found the greatest drop in count was from 11:00 a.m. to 3:00 p.m., when the mean fall was 81.5 percent. They believed this reflected a "sugar stress" following heavy glucose administration at the termination of the insulin shock at 11:00 a.m. Of all the experiments those involving insulin shock therapy gave the most profound eosinopenia. Clinical improvement following therapy was usually accompanied or preceded by a rise in the eosinophile level.[63] In evaluating the role of somatic therapies, the eosinophile level was used as a measure of the function of the adrenal cortex by Alexander and Neander. Eosinophile counts were taken before therapy and every two weeks in a group of fifty-six patients. In 75 percent of the group that improved there was evidence of a decrease in adrenocortical function, as seen by an increase in the eosinophile count. They concluded the eosinophile count may give a clue to prognosis, based on the function of the adrenal cortex in response to the stress of a somatic therapy.[64] Freeman *et al.* reported a three-year follow-up study of patients who had developed an eosinophilia during insulin coma therapy and those who had developed a minimal eosinophilia response. Six of the seven who had shown an increase in eosinophiles improved during therapy, and four of the seven showed continued benefit of therapy three years later. Only one of the four who developed minimal eosinophilia improved during therapy and none was improved after three years.[65]

Insulin coma therapy was seen as an opportunity to study the effects of repeated acute stress upon the adrenocortical activity by Dohan and his group at the Coatesville (Pennsylvania) Veterans Administration Hospital.[66] The blood eosinophile count before, throughout, and after completion of a course of deep insulin shock therapy was studied in thirty-five patients. From Figure 1 it is evident that there is very little fall in eosinophile count by 10:00 a.m., three hours after the injection of insulin, and that the rate of fall between 10:00 a.m. and 1:00 p.m. is rapid and more or less the same throughout the course of insulin shock therapy, as indicated by the similarity of the slopes of the lines. The basal eosinophile count gradually rose during the first portion of the course of insulin therapy and tended to fall during the latter portion. These results are similar to those described by Mann and Lehmann.[63]

Figure 2 shows the course of the mean 7:00 a.m. (basal) eosinophile count on Monday and Friday before, during, and for two weeks after termination of insulin shock therapy.

Both the improved and the unimproved group showed a gradual rise in the mean Monday basal eosinophile count and the mean Friday basal eosinophile count in the early portion of therapy, falling slowly about halfway to the initial count during the latter weeks of treatment. The improved patients had a significantly higher basal eosinophile count (at $P < 0.05$ level) on Monday in the 4th, 6th, 8th, and 10th weeks of therapy. In addition, the mean basal eosinophile count in the improved group was higher than that in the

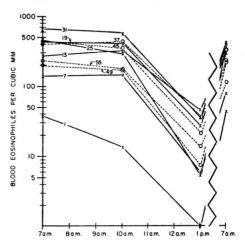

Fig. 1.—Blood eosinophile count at 7:00 a. m. on Monday and at intervals throughout the next 24 hours during the course of insulin shock therapy in a schizophrenic man.

This chart shows, on a semilogarithmic graph, the fall in eosinophiles found at the sixth hour (1:00 p. m.) after the injection of insulin, the insignificant fall three hours (10:00 a. m.) after the injection of insulin, and the rise to approximately the basal level or higher 24 hours after the injection of insulin. The slope of the lines between the 10:00 a. m. and 1:00 p. m. counts indicates that the percentage fall was approximately the same on the various Mondays. Also to be noted is the rise in the basal (7:00 a. m.) count, reaching a peak on the 31st day of insulin shock therapy, and the fall thereafter. The day of insulin shock therapy is indicated by the number on the line. The latter half of the course of insulin shock therapy is indicated by the dotted lines.

See note 66a.

unimproved group (P = 0.05) on both Mondays and Fridays. The difference between the mean of all basal counts and the initial Monday counts was also significantly greater in the improved group. There was no relationship, however, be-

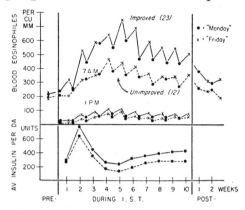

Fig. 2.—Course of the eosinophiles and insulin shock therapy (I. S. T.).

The chart shows the mean basal (7 : 00 a. m.) and six hours' postinsulin (1 : 00 p.m.) eosinophile counts on Monday and Friday throughout the course of insulin shock therapy, and the mean basal count two weeks thereafter for the improved (solid line) and the unimproved group (dashed line) of schizophrenic subjects. The mean basal count on Friday was consistently greater than the mean basal count on Monday throughout the course of I. S. T., but was not so before or after the course of I. S. T. The means of the 1 : 00 p. m. counts, post-therapy (not charted), were slightly lower than the respective means of the 7 : 00 a. m. counts for both the improved and the unimproved group. Counts before instituting therapy showed no significant difference of the 7 : 00 a. m. counts on Monday and Friday morning, and the 1 : 00 p. m. counts (not charted) were, in general, slightly lower than the 7 : 00 a. m. counts.

The lower section of the charts shows the mean insulin dose per day each week throughout the 10-week course of insulin shock therapy. Since only 12 of the 23 improved patients and 3 of the 12 unimproved patients had 12 weeks of I. S. T., the last 2 weeks of therapy in these patients are not charted. Figure 4 shows more clearly the relationship of the mean insulin dose per day each week to the mean of the basal eosinophile counts on Friday and Monday of each week.

See note 66a.

tween the degree of change in the basal eosinophile count and the level of improvement attained.

In both the improved and the unimproved group the same percentage of mean basal Friday count was higher than the mean basal Monday count throughout the course of insulin therapy. The greater incidence of the higher Friday counts is significant at the $P<0.001$ level. The variation in the Monday and Friday counts was suggestive of some decrease in adrenocortical activity during the weekdays when insulin shock was administered. Such variation did not occur before or after the course of insulin therapy and is not present in normal men.

The mean percent fall on Monday was greater than that on Friday for 19 of the 23 patients in the improved group and for 9 of the 12 patients in the unimproved group, or 28 out of 35 for both groups. This distribution is highly significant.

Fig. 3

—Relation of the mean daily insulin dose each week to the mean basal eosinophile count each week throughout the course of insulin shock therapy.

The data, when plotted on semilogarithmic graph, show a linear negative correlation. The position and slopes of the regression lines are significantly different. The possible significance of these relationships is considered in the discussion. The numbers by the symbols indicate the week of I. S. T. The first week is omitted, since the insulin dosage is primarily a routine matter until coma is produced. After induction of the first coma, the dose is manipulated (see "Methods") so as to produce coma with the minimum dose of insulin.

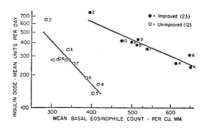

See note 66a.

Figure 3 illustrates the inverse relationship of the mean daily dose of insulin each week and the mean of the basal counts on Monday and Friday of each week for the improved and unimproved groups during the second to the tenth week of therapy, inclusive. The data, when plotted on a semilogarithmic graph, show a linear negative correlation. The position and slopes of the regression lines are significantly different.

(2) *The adrenocortical steroids*

In 1942 Tietz and Birnbaum measured an adrenaline-cortical compound (A-C substance) in twenty-nine patients receiving insulin therapy. In those that improved there was an increase in "A-C" levels which stabilized. In those that did not improve, there was a persistent low "A-C" level with great susceptibility to change with insulin shock therapy.[67] Bliss *et al.* took a one-day sample on eight schizophrenic patients during insulin shock therapy. Four of these were in the early stages of treatment and four had had over forty hours of coma. They noted no difference between the two groups as all the patients showed an increase in plasma 17-hydroxycorticosteroids. The increases after electroshock therapy, for example, were comparable to those following small amounts of corticotropin intravenously. Since much larger amounts of corticotropin have been given without clinical improvement, it was concluded that the increase in adrenocortical steroids following such shock therapies is coincidental and does not explain the therapeutic effectiveness of such treatments.[68]

Based on the relationship of changes in ketosteroid excretion rate and in thyroid function to the clinical outcome of insulin shock therapy, Batt *et al.* recognize four types of reaction. Type i: "standard" type: before treatment the ketosteroid excretion rate is very high, either in the upper normal range, or considerably above it at times. During insulin treatment, the ketosteroid excretion rate—sometimes after a short rise—goes down, falling to low levels or occasionally below the normal range. Mental improvement occurs at this time. Concomitant with these changes, thyroid function, low at first, increases but remains in the normal range. Type ii: "temporary improvement" type: these patients start as those above. When the ketosteroid excretion rate becomes low, some mental improvement is noted, and is still present when the ketosteroid excretion later tends to rise. Thyroid function, low at first, remains low or increases above the normal range. If the ketosteroids rise still further, the patient relapses. Type iii: "successful treatment" type: the ketosteroid excretion rate is initially low but increases into the normal range. Thyroid function either remains normal or becomes normal. Type iv: "unsuccessful treatment" type: ketosteroid excretion is below normal or is in the low normal range at the beginning. Thyroid function remains normal or moves to hypernormal range or where abnormally high remains so. They conclude that for improvement it is essential that the ketosteroid excretion rate and thyroid activity should both come into and remain in the normal range. If one of these values is found at the end of treatment to be outside the normal range a relapse can be predicted. Patients with high ketosteroid excretion rates show well-developed primary and secondary sexual characteristics. Prognosis for a favorable result from insulin coma therapy is more favorable in this group. Those with the ketosteroid excretion rate below the normal range are often sexually retarded, with an open inguinal canal as the most striking feature. They have had no schizophrenic patient with an open inguinal canal improve after insulin coma therapy.[59]

Marks *et al.* measured adrenocortical function before, during, and after a course of insulin coma therapy in a paranoid schizophrenic patient. The variables used were urinary 17-hydroxycorticosteroids, 17-ketosteroids, and circulating eosinophiles. Following the onset of insulin coma therapy, there was a moderate increase in daily urinary

17-hydroxycorticosteroid excretion, primarily from 7:00 a.m. to 3:00 p.m. A weekend drop, when insulin was not administered, was observed throughout the entire course, but was not noted during the pre-insulin control period. During the first six weeks, urinary 17-hydroxycorticosteroids varied between 9.5 and 15.5 mg./24 hours, whereas during the last half, the value ranged below 11 mg./24 hours. In contrast to the 17-hydroxycorticosteroids, urinary 17-ketosteroids were within the control range during therapy days and did not regularly decrease over the weekend. There was a progressive rise in eosinophiles with a peak level of 825 pr cu. mm. during the sixth week. Insulin coma, in contrast to major surgical operations, was seen as only a moderate adrenocortical stimulus.[69]

Dohan *et al.*, in addition to studying the eosinophile count, determined the changes in plasma 17-hydroxycorticosteroid concentrations and eosinophiles in three patients before, during and after insulin shock therapy.[66] During therapy, the mean rise in the plasma 17-hydroxycorticosteroid level from 7:00 a.m. to 10:00 a.m. was 8.3 gamma/100 ml. plasma. The mean fall from 7:00 a.m. to 10:00 a.m. prior to and after treatment was 3.7 gamma/100 ml. plasma. These values are significantly different ($P = 0.03$). The mean increase in the 11:30 a.m. specimen (from the 7:00 a.m. specimen) was 5.7 gamma during the therapy and the fall at 11:30 a.m. prior to and after treatment was 2.2 gamma (P approximately 0.1). These increases at 10:00 a.m. and 11:30 a.m. are comparable to the findings of Bliss and associates who demonstrated one hour following intravenous administration of 1 I.U. of corticotropin in fifteen to thirty seconds a mean rise in 17-hydroxycorticosteroids of 9.5 gamma/100 ml. of plasma and one hour later a mean value which was only 3.3 gamma above the initial values. Their percent fall in the eosinophiles, four hours after the intravenous injection of 1 I.U. of corticotropin was 67 percent. The mean fall of eosinophiles (7:00 a.m. to 1:00 p.m.) during insulin shock was 88 percent. The mean fall prior to and after therapy was 6 percent. This suggests the possibility that the 88 percent fall may be due to other factors than 17-hydroxycorticosteroids, such as adrenaline. It was concluded that the data could be interpreted as follows: (1) shock therapy decreased the basal secretion of hydrocortisone (and cortisone?), as indicated by the increase of the basal count on Friday but that this decrease in basal secretion is, in part, compensated for by the weekend rest, and that the compensation is not complete, as indicated by the gradual rise in basal eosinophile level; (2) that the ability to cause rapid release of hydrocortisone (and cortisone?) into the blood stream (in sufficient quantity to produce the approximately maximum depression of the eosinophiles for the time period measured) is not diminished by a course of insulin shock therapy, thus indicating that the productive capacity of the adrenal has not been completely inhibited; (3) that a change in rate of secretion due to the effects of repeated "stress" of both adrenocorticotropic hormone and of growth hormone may be the mechanism, in part, responsible for the inverse correlation of the mean basal eosinophile count each week and the mean daily dose of insulin given each week to produce coma; and (4) that a relationship may exist between the factors responsible for clinical improvement and the physiological mechanisms responsible for changes in the basal eosinophile count, since significant differences ($P = 0.05$) between the improved and the unimproved group have been demonstrated.

(3) *Growth hormone implications*

The data obtained above by Dohan and his associates supported the concept that with repeated severe stress there is a somewhat decreased basal secretion of adrenal cortex, possibly via partial inhibition of the hypothalamic-anterior pituitary-adrenal cortex axis. The inverse correlation of the basal level of the blood eosinophile count and the marked changes in the amount of insulin necessary to produce coma suggested the possibility that changes in the insulin resistance may be due to concomitant changes in the basal secretion of the anterior pituitary growth hormone and other anti-insulin factors. Two hypotheses were proposed to explain changes in "insulin sensitivity" during insulin shock therapy: (a) a smaller dose of insulin causes an approximately equal or greater fall in true blood glucose, or (b)

Fig. 4

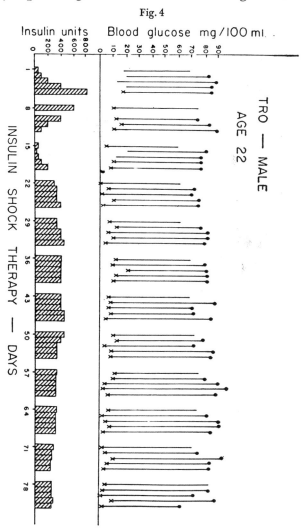

See note 66a.

the central nervous system is "sensitized" with development of stupor or coma at higher blood glucose concentrations. The following study by Bennett *et al.* supported the hypothesis that there was an enhancement of the blood-glu-

Fig. 5

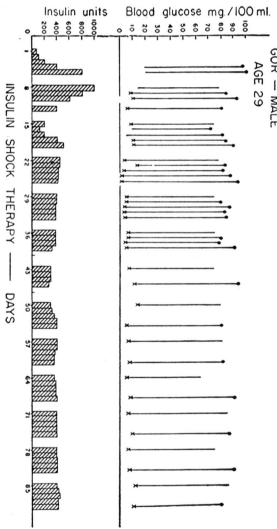

See note 66a.

cose-decreasing capacity of insulin.[70] True blood glucose concentrations were measured in three patients throughout the twelve-week course of insulin shock therapy; one with a constant dose of 400 units after the first three days, the other two with the insulin dosage adjusted according to the Bond and Shurley technique.[30] Glucose concentrations were measured every thirty minutes from 7:00 a.m. through 10:00

Fig. 6

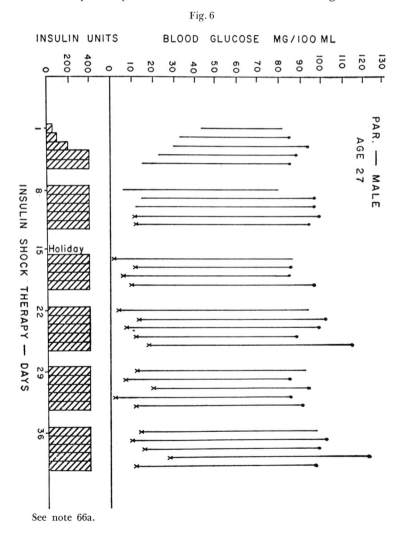

See note 66a.

a.m. In Figures 4, 5, and 6, the basal (7:00 a.m.) true blood glucose is indicated by a dot (·). The Monday 7:00 a.m. values omit the dot on the upper end of the lines. The cross (x) represents the blood glucose concentration of the first blood sample taken after the appearance of a reaction (stupor or coma). The lines without a cross on the lower end indicate the lowest blood glucose value (at thirty-minute intervals) on those days without a reaction. These charts show that the blood glucose concentrations shortly after the appearance of a reaction were, in 91 of 105 reactions, at the same level or below that associated with the

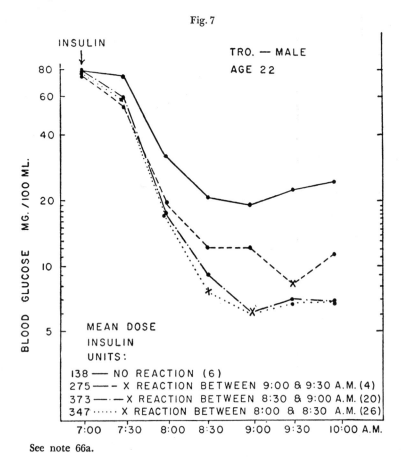

Fig. 7

INSULIN

TRO. — MALE
AGE 22

BLOOD GLUCOSE   MG. /100 ML.

MEAN DOSE
INSULIN
UNITS:
138 —— NO REACTION (6)
275 ——- X REACTION BETWEEN 9:00 & 9:30 A.M. (4)
373 —·— X REACTION BETWEEN 8:30 & 9:00 A.M. (20)
347 ······ X REACTION BETWEEN 8:00 & 8:30 A.M. (26)

7:00   7:30   8:00   8:30   9:00   9:30   10:00 A.M.

See note 66a.

initial reaction. The onset of reaction was associated in only fourteen instances with a glucose level higher than that at the time of the initial reaction. The charts also show that the pre-insulin glucose concentrations were, in general, lower on Mondays. Figure 7 shows the typical mean blood glucose values before and at half-hour intervals following insulin administration. The mean concentration associated with the appearance of an insulin reaction varied slightly, but it was lower than the mean lowest value found on non-reaction days. The rate of fall during the first one to one and one-half hours was about the same whether or not a reaction occurred on that day. But the concentration on non-reaction days did not reach the low levels associated with a reaction. In all three subjects there was a considerably higher proportion of early stupor or coma in the latter portion of the course of therapy. Figures 4 and 5 show that the differences in time of reaction were not due to the reactions occurring at a greater concentration in the latter period. It was shown by this study that these three subjects did not have an "increased sensitivity" of the central nervous system to the concentration of blood glucose. To produce a reaction, it was necessary for the blood glucose to fall to levels approximately equal to that present at the initial reaction, even though the dose of insulin necessary to produce these levels decreased considerably· In the third subject the dosage was maintained at 400 units daily. Change in "insulin sensitivity" was found to be due to changes in the response of blood glucose to insulin. It was suggested that recurrent stimulation of the contra-insulin hormones may result in a somewhat decreased basal production of these factors.

Summary

A neuroendocrine basis for the effectiveness of insulin hypoglycemic treatment was defended by Sakel. The use of an endogenous substance such as insulin to depress brain metabolism was seen as a natural method leading to superior and more permanent results. Since this therapy does have a beneficial effect, it was reasonable to seek an explanation for its effectiveness in areas involving insulin activity. Clinical observations and investigations of metabolic changes in the brain have furnished evidence of the tremendous effect on nervous tissue when the true blood sugar concentration falls to below 20 mg. percent. In our series the following correlations were seen: 81 of the 85 samples taken during deep coma showed a range from 0 to 10 mg. per 100 ml. and 65 of the 67 drawn during stupor showed less than 20 mg. per 100 ml. Of these 50 were below 10 mg. per 100 ml.[70]

The response of schizophrenic patients undergoing insulin therapy to tests involving the autonomic nervous system, carbohydrate metabolism, and insulin resistance are characteristic of patients with other disorders also associated with emotional tension or physiological stress. The inconsistent results are most probably explained by the lack of proper controls and baselines. Insufficient attention has been paid to such mental reactions towards the test or therapy as those of apprehension, anticipation or indifference. If this had been done, the changes in these variables would be more consistent and possibly of greater value. The question of insulin resistance (or sensitivity) refers to the changes in the individual's response to a given amount of insulin. This phenomenon is present not only in some cases of diabetes and schizophrenia but also in many other disorders. It can be explained as secondary, in some cases, to the development of insulin antibodies following prolonged insulin administration. Their effect on increased, continual, or decreased resistance has been thought as being due to the binding of the insulin which then cannot be utilized. In patients undergoing insulin therapy, however, the resistance is more likely the result of the contra-insulin hormones.

Basic endocrine relationships are upset by the administration of insulin far in excess of physiological needs. The influence on glucagon, prolactin, thyroid, and sex hormones is a minor and transitory one.[47] But there is a measurable effect on adrenaline metabolism and the 11, 17-oxycorticosteroids. The role of the anterior pituitary in releasing ACTH and growth hormone in response to insulin seems to be central in this problem of change in insulin resistance. With repeated administration of insulin, then, there is exhaustion of these antagonists and a corresponding decrease in their levels. During this phase the individual becomes insulin sensitive and smaller doses of insulin produce the same degree and duration of coma. The stress of insulin shock is not severe enough to inhibit totally the contra-insulin hormone group or to decompensate them entirely during the course of treatment. Clinical improvement often occurs if the excessive stimulation leads to normalization of the neuroendocrine system.

The gains from the use of insulin hypoglycemic therapy are that it is not only an effective form of treatment but it has also led to the development and testing of a hypothesis linking clinical improvement with physiological changes. In addition, it has made a unique contribution as a model of a controlled experimental situation involving repeated acute stress in the human.

Bibliography

1. Sakel, M. The classical Sakel Shock Treatment. A reappraisal. *J. Clin. & Exper. Psychopathol.*, 15:255, 1954.
2. Gold, L. Autonomic balance in patients treated with insulin shock as measured by mecholyl chloride. *A.M.A. Arch. Neurol. & Psychiat.*, 50:311, 1943.
3. Shurley, J. T., and Morris, H. M., Jr. Autonomic function in insulin coma therapy. *J. Nerv. & Ment. Dis.*, 114:532, 1951.
4. Funkenstein, D. H., Greenblatt, M., and Solomon, H. C. Autonomic changes paralleling psychologic changes

in mentally ill patients. *J. Nerv. & Ment. Dis.*, 114:1, 1951.

5. Alexander, L. Objective approaches to treatment in psychiatry. *Canad. Psychiat. Assoc. J.*, 2:77, 1957.

6. Vanderkamp, H., Norgan, A., Wilkinson, G. W., and Pearl, D. The mecholyl test as a predictor of improvement in insulin coma therapy. *Am. J. Psychiat.*, 114:365, 1957.

7. Gellhorn, E. *Physiological Foundations of Neurology and Psychiatry.* Minneapolis: The University of Minnesota Press, 1953.

8. Gellhorn, E. *Autonomic Imbalance and the Hypothalamus. Implications for Physiology, Medicine, Psychology, and Neuropsychiatry.* Minneapolis: The University of Minnesota Press, 1957.

9. Alexander, L. *Treatment of Mental Disorder.* Philadelphia: W. B. Saunders Company, 1953.

10a. Thorley, A. S., and Kay, W. W. Some biochemical aspects of hypoglycaemic coma (I). *Proc. Roy. Soc. Med.*, 44:969, 1951.

10b. Kay, W. W., and Thorley, A. S. Some biochemical aspects of hypoglycaemic coma (II). *Proc. Roy. Soc. Med.*, 44:973, 1951.

11. Harris, M. M., Blalock, J. R., and Horwitz, W. A. Metabolic studies during insulin hypoglycemia therapy of the psychoses. *A.M.A. Arch. Neurol. & Psychiat.*, 40:116, 1938.

12. Looney, J. M., Jellinek, E. M., and Dyer, C. G. Physiological studies in insulin treatment of acute schizophrenia. The blood minerals. *Endocrinology*, 25:282, 1939.

13. Gottfried, S. P., and Willner, H. H. Blood chemistry of schizophrenic patients before, during, and after insulin shock therapy: preliminary studies. *A.M.A. Arch. Neurol. & Psychiat.*, 62:808, 1949.

14. Harris, M. M., and Harris, R. S. Effect of insulin hypo-

glycemia and glucose on various amino acids in blood of mental patients. *Proc. Soc. Exper. Biol. & Med.*, 64:471, 1947.

15. Cantarow, A., and Schepartz, B. *Biochemistry* (2d ed.). Philadelphia: W. B. Saunders Company, 1957.

16. Maher, J. T., and Somogyi, M. Effect of insulin on carbohydrate tolerance of nondiabetic individuals. *Proc. Soc. Exper. Biol. & Med.*, 37:615, 1938.

17. Looney, J. M., and Cameron, D. E. Effect of prolonged insulin therapy on glucose tolerance in schizophrenic patients. *Proc. Soc. Exper. Biol. & Med.*, 37:253, 1937.

18. Proctor, L. D., Dewan, J. G., and McNeel, B. H. Variations in glucose tolerance observations in schizophrenics before and after shock treatment. *Am. J. Psychiat.*, 100:652, 1944.

19. Borenz, H. F., Schuster, D. B., and Downey, G. J. Effect of insulin shock therapy on glucose metabolism in schizophrenia. *J. Nerv. & Ment. Dis.*, 110:507, 1949.

20. Olsen, N. S., and Neutzel, J. A. Resistance to small doses of insulin in various clinical conditions. *J. Clin. Investigation*, 29:862, 1950.

21. Pfister, H. O. Disturbances of the autonomic nervous system in schizophrenia and their relations to the insulin, cardiazol and sleep treatments. *Am. J. Psychiat.*, 94: (Suppl.) 109, 1938.

22. Freeman, H., Rodnick, E. H., Shakow, D., and Lebeaux, T. The carbohydrate tolerance of mentally disturbed soldiers. *Psychosom. Med.*, 6:311, 1944.

23. Hinkle, L. E., Jr., and Wolf, S. The effects of stressful life situations on the concentration of blood glucose in diabetic and nondiabetic humans. *Diabetes*, 1:383, 1952.

24. Harris, M. M. Insulin sensitivity of patients with mental disease. *A.M.A. Arch. Neurol. & Psychiat.*, 48:761, 1942.

25. Nadeau, G., and Rouleau, Y. Insulin tolerance in

schizophrenia. *J. Clin. & Exper. Psychopathol.*, 14:69, 1953.

26. Hauz, E. A. Present status of insulin resistance. Report of a case with autopsy. *A.M.A. Arch. Int. Med.*, 83:515, 1949.

27. Root, H. F. Insulin resistance. Editorial. *Pennsylvania M. J.*, 57:1098, 1954.

28. von Braunmühl, A. *Die Insulinschockbehandlung der Schizophrenie.* Berlin: Verlag von Julius Springer, 1938.

29. Mansour, T. E., and Hewitt, W. F., Jr. Sensitivity to insulin during adrenocortical response to cold stress in rats. *Endocrinology*, 54:20, 1954.

30. Bond, E. D., and Shurley, J. T. Insulin therapy and its future. *Am. J. Psychiat.*, 103:338, 1946.

31. Gellhorn, E., Feldman, J., and Allen, A. Effect of emotional excitement on the insulin content of the blood. *A.M.A. Arch. Neurol. & Psychiat.*, 47:234, 1942.

32. Scheflen, A. E., and Reiner, E. R. Sensitivity in insulin coma therapy. *J. Clin. & Exper. Psychopathol.*, 13:225, 1952.

33. Patterson, E. S. Psychophysiologic resistance in insulin coma therapy. *J. Nerv. & Ment. Dis.*, 125:547, 1957.

34. Meduna, L. J., Gerty, F. J., and Urse, V. G. Biochemical disturbances in mental disorders. I. Anti-insulin effect of blood in cases of schizophrenia. *A.M.A. Arch. Neurol. & Psychiat.*, 47:38, 1942.

35. Meduna, L. J., and Vaichulis, J. A. A hyperglycemic factor in the urine of so-called schizophrenics. *Dis. Nerv. System*, 9:248, 1948.

36. Goldner, M. G., and Ricketts, H. T. Significance of insulin inhibition by blood of schizophrenic patients. *A.M.A. Arch. Neurol. & Psychiat.*, 48:552, 1942.

37. Morgan, M. S., and Pilgrim, F. J. Concentration of a hyperglycemic factor from urine of schizophrenics. *Proc. Soc. Exper. Biol. & Med.*, 79:106, 1952.

38. Marsh, J. B., and Haugaard, N. The effect of serum from insulin-resistant cases on the combination of insulin with the rat diaphragm. *J. Clin. Investigation,* 31:107, 1952.

39. Moya, F. Mode of action of the hyperglycemic-glycogenolytic factor from urine. *Endocrinology,* 56:312, 1955.

40. Lerman, J. Insulin resistance. The role of immunity in its production. *Am. J. M. Sc.,* 207:354, 1944.

41. Corwin, W. C. Decreased resistance to hypoglycemia on successive days of administration of insulin. *Am. J. Physiol.,* 125:227, 1939.

42. Naatanen, E. K. The paradoxical effect of giant intravenous insulin doses on rabbits. *Ann. med. exper. et biol. fennial.,* 32:186, 1954.

43. Berson, S. A., and Yalow, R. S. Insulin antagonism, insulin antibodies and insulin resistance. *Am. J. Med.* 25:155, 1958.

44. Berson, S. A., Yalow, R. S., Bauman, A., Rothschild, M. A., and Newerly, K. Insulin-I[131] metabolism in human subjects: demonstration of insulin binding globulin in the circulation of insulin treated subjects. *J. Clin. Investigation,* 35:170, 1956.

45. Horvath, S. M., and Friedman, E. The effects of large doses of intravenous insulin in psychotic nondiabetic patients. *J. Clin. Endocrinol.,* 1:960, 1941.

46. Arquilla, E. R., and Stavitsky, A. B. The production and identification of antibodies to insulin and their use in assaying insulin. *J. Clin. Investigation,* 35:458, 1956.

47. De Bodo, R. C., and Altszuler, N. Insulin hypersensitivity and physiological insulin antagonists. *Physiol. Rev.,* 38:389, 1958.

48. Hökfelt, B. Selective depletion of the adrenaline content of the suprarenal gland by the injection of insulin in the cat. *Endocrinology,* 53:536, 1953.

49. Tietz, E. B., Dornheggen, H., and Goldman, D. Blood adrenalin levels during insulin shock treatments for schizophrenia. *Endocrinology,* 26:641, 1940.

50. Weil-Malherbe, H., and Bone, A. D. The effect of insulin on the levels of adrenaline and noradrenaline in human blood. *J. Endocrinol.,* 11:285, 1954.

51. Holzbauer, M., and Vogt, M. The concentration of adrenalin in the peripheral blood during insulin hypoglycemia. *Brit. J. Pharmacol. & Chemotherapy,* 9:249, 1954.

52. Millar, R. A. The fluorimetric estimation of epinephrine in peripheral venous plasma during insulin hypoglycemia. *J. Pharmacol. & Exper. Therap.,* 118:435, 1956.

53. Von Euler, U. S., and Luft, R. Effect of insulin on urinary excretion of adrenalin and noradrenalin. *Metabolism,* 1:528, 1952.

54. Gray, W. D., and Munson, P. L. The rapidity of the adrenocorticotropic response of the pituitary to the intravenous administration of histamine. *Endocrinology,* 48:471, 1951.

55. Bliss, E. L. Migeon, C. J., Eik-Nes, K., Sandberg, A. A., and Samuels, L. T. The effects of insulin, histamine, bacterial pyrogen, and the Antabuse-alcohol reaction upon the levels of 17-hydroxycorticosteroids in the peripheral blood of man. *Metabolism,* 3:493, 1954.

56. Billig, O., and Hesser, F. H. Histamine content of the blood during insulin shock therapy. *A.M.A. Arch. Neurol. & Psychiat.,* 52:65, 1944.

56a. Papacostas, C. A., Mozden, P., and Loew, E. R. Effect of histamine and histamine liberator, Compound 48/80, on blood glucose. *Proc. Soc. Exper. Biol. & Med.,* 97:297, 1958.

57. Bowman, K. M., Miller, E. R., Dailey, M. E., Simon, A., Frankel, B., and Lowe, G. W. Thyroid function in mental disease measured with radioactive iodine, I^{131}. *Am. J. Psychiat.,* 106:561, 1950.

58. Bowman, K. M., Miller, E. R., Dailey, M. E., Simon,

A., and Mayer, B. F. Thyroid function in mental disease. *J. Nerv. & Ment. Dis.*, 112:404, 1950.

59. Batt, J. C., Kay, W. W., Reiss, M., and Sands, D. E. The endocrine concomitants of schizophrenia. *J. Ment. Sc.*, 103:240, 1957.

60. Kay, W. W. The endocrinology of deep insulin coma therapy. In Reiss, M. (ed.), *Psychoendocrinology.* New York: Grune & Stratton, 1958, Ch. 12.

61. Best, W. R., Kark, R. M., Muehrcke, R. C., and Samter, M. Clinical value of eosinophil counts and eosinophil response tests. *J.A.M.A.*, 151:702, 1953.

62. Tsai, S. Y., Bennett, A., May, L. G., and Gregory, R. L. Effect of insulin hypoglycemia on eosinophiles and lymphocytes of psychotics. *Proc. Soc. Exper. Biol. & Med.*, 74:782, 1950.

63. Mann, A., and Lehmann, H. The eosinophil level in psychiatric conditions. *Canad. M.A.J.*, 66:52, 1952.

64. Alexander, S. P., and Neander, J. F. Adrenocortical responsivity to electric shock therapy and insulin therapy. *A.M.A. Arch. Neurol & Psychiat.*, 69:368, 1953.

65. Freeman, R. V., Jones, T. E., and Palmer, J. J. Three-year follow-up of patients developing eosinophilia during insulin coma therapy. *A.M.A. Arch. Neurol. & Psychiat.*, 71:501, 1954.

66. Dohan, F. C., Winick, W., Purcell, M., Bennett, I. F., and Hecker, A. O. Response of blood eosinophiles and plasma 17-hydroxycorticoids to insulin shock therapy. *A.M.A. Arch. Neurol. & Psychiat.*, 73:47, 1955.

67. Tietz, E. B., and Birnbaum, S. M. Level of adrenocortical substance in the blood during hypoglycemic treatments for schizophrenia. *Am. J. Psychiat.*, 99:75, 1942.

68. Bliss, E. L., Migeon, C. J., Nelson, D. H., Samuels, L. T., and Branch, C. H. H. Influence of E. C. T. and insulin coma on level of adrenocortical steroids in peripheral circulation. *A.M.A. Arch. Neurol. & Psychiat.*, 72:352, 1954.

69. Marks, L. J., Weiss, D. M., Leftin, J. H., and Ross-

meisl, E. C. The adrenocortical response to insulin coma. I. Effects of an entire course of insulin coma therapy on the urinary excretion of 17-hydroxycorticosteroids and 17-ketosteroids and on circulating eosinophils. *J. Clin. Endocrinol. & Metab.*, 18:235, 1958.

70. Bennett, I. F., Letonoff, T. V., Winick, W., and Dohan, F. C. Relationship of blood glucose to changes in "insulin sensitivity" during insulin shock therapy. *A.M.A. Arch. Neurol. & Psychiat.*, 78:221, 1957.

Chapter 4

BIOCHEMICAL CHANGES IN THE BRAIN OCCURRING DURING INSULIN HYPOGLYCEMIA

WILLIAMINA A. HIMWICH, PH.D.

The early and undeniably beneficial effects of insulin therapy as reported by Manfred Sakel immediately caught the attention of neurochemists and neurophysiologists all over the world. Many studies were undertaken to explain the success of the therapy. Although we have learned much about the effects of insulin hypoglycemia on brain metabolism from these studies, we still do not have a definitive answer as to why the treatment works. The changes which have been described may just be concomitant or may be the ones essential to the success of the treatment. The crucial experiments are still to be designed. One problem hampering the elucidation of the changes in brain chemistry accompanying hypoglycemia in man is the impossibility of obtaining human brain samples for analyses. Since the development of true psychoses in animals is doubtful, the evaluation of any therapy in animals is impossible. Hence we can only deduce what happens in human brain on the basis of what we know occurs in animal brain. We can not as yet do more than suggest what may be the crucial chemical changes in the brain which determine the success of the therapy.

Even before the advent of the Sakel treatment scientists were interested in the effects of hypoglycemia on the brain. The discovery in 1929 by Himwich and Nahum[1] that the R.Q. of the brain is approximately one, and the conclusion that the glucose is the principal substrate used by that organ, started a series of animal researches. Today we may wish to modify the statement that glucose is the chief substrate of the brain to one that glucose is the chief metabolic support of the brain. This change is necessitated by the accumulation of data suggesting that the brain continuously metabolizes other substances than glucose, such as amino acids.[2] These substances, however, can be maintained at their normal levels only if sufficient glucose is also used.[2] This elucidation of the role of glucose in no way minimizes its importance to the brain.

Studies on the cerebral metabolic rate (CMR) in patients undergoing insulin therapy have in general been lower than normal irrespective of the manner in which blood flow was measured.[3, 4, 5] Cerebral blood flow apparently is little altered by insulin hypoglycemia and the reduction in CMR depends largely upon the decrease in oxygen utilization by the brain.[5] Brain metabolism may be reduced by this method to less than one-quarter of normal. Himwich[6] suggests, however, that such low values continued for any prolonged period of time are not commensurate with life. During this time the electroencephalogram shows a pronounced shift with a decrease of alpha rhythm and an increase of the delta waves (Fig. 1). These changes correlate with the fall in blood sugar and the EEG is restored to normal by the administration of glucose.[7]

Kerr and Ghantus[8] demonstrated that glycogen and lactate fell in the brain in both dogs and rabbits after the administration of insulin and showed that this fall was due to the hypoglycemia, not to epinephrine production stimulated by the low blood sugar. In view of the possibility that hypoglycemia may release catechol amines in the brain and that these neurohormones may work directly on the brain, this finding may need to be re-evaluated.

The early work of Kerr and his colleagues has been confirmed by Stone[9] for lactic acid and by Olsen and Klein,[10] for lactic acid and glycogen. The latter workers extended these observations to show that in the adult cat not only do glucose, glycogen and lactate fall during hypoglycemia, but also pyruvate and the energy-rich phosphates. These results might be expected since the maintenance of a normal level of these substances depends largely upon a normal metabolic rate.

Chesler and Himwich[11] followed the loss of glycogen in various parts of the brain of adult dogs subjected to varying degrees of hypoglycemia. Glycogen fell first in the parts of the central nervous system which had the highest metabolic rate, i.e., caudate nucleus.[12] The decrease in glycogen of the corpora quadrigemina, cerebral cortical gray, thalamus, cerebellum, and medulla occurred in that order (Table 1). Thus it appeared that even though the cerebral gray matter had originally the highest glycogen content the depletion depended principally upon the metabolic rate in the part rather than upon its initial content of glycogen. In the human patient undergoing insulin therapy the march of symptoms can be ascribed to a metabolic depression, first of the cerebral cortex, followed by glycogen loss and metabolic depression in the other part of the brain extending in a caudad direction.[6] These findings in man and dog are not as contradictory as they appear. Although it has never been conclusively demonstrated, it is probable that in man the cerebral cortical gray matter has the highest respiration of any part of the brain, while in the adult dog the caudate nucleus is the most active (Fig. 2). Ferris and Himwich[13] also found that the effects of hypoglycemia upon the glycogen distribution in the brain were related to age as well as to the degree of hypoglycemia. In the newborn dog, in whom the caudad areas of the brain show the highest metabolic rate[12] (Fig. 2) the glycogen depletion occurred first in the spinal cord, cerebellum and medulla. These data confirm the earlier suggestion that during insulin hypoglycemia the primary factor determining the order of glycogen loss in areas of the brain is the relative metabolic rates of the parts. However, in young animals the glycogen content of the caudad areas such as medulla is greater than that in the cephalad ones,[14] e.g., cerebral cortex (Fig. 3).

The Russian worker Goncharova[15] followed the changes in total and bound glycogen in the brains of rabbits subjected to insulin convulsions and in those given 0.3 to 0.5 units of insulin per kg. of body weight daily for four to six weeks. In those animals that convulsed glycogen dropped to 35% of the normal level. The bound glycogen fell to 37% of the total as compared to 55% in the normal animal. No significant changes could be demonstrated in the enzymes which synthesize or break down glycogen. As might be expected no change occurred in the brains of those animals receiving relatively small doses of insulin for several weeks.

On the basis of these investigations there remains no doubt that during insulin hypoglycemia the brain is deprived of its normal sources of energy. Before we look at the metabolites used by this organ in the absence of glucose, we will turn a moment to the changes in mineral metabolism. Yannet[16] studied mild and severe hypoglycemia in cats by determining extracellular water, potassium, sodium, non-lipid nitrogen, and phosphorus. Recent findings with the electron microscope suggest that the brain has no extracellular space. If this is true, then Yannet's data on the shifts in water and electrolytes between the cells and extracellular space need to be re-evaluated. However, his general conclusions on electrolyte shift probably still stand. A loss of intracellular potassium occurred in those animals that survived a large dose of insulin without demonstrable neurological or histological change (Table II). The cats that survived but showed marked neurological involvement had an even greater loss of cellular potassium. W. A. Himwich and Sullivan[17] produced deep hypoglycemia in rabbits by a standardized technique which avoided the complications of anoxia or those due to the muscular components of convulsions. The animals were maintained in deep insulin hypoglycemia until the heart showed signs of failure as evidenced by dysrhythmia and marked slowing. These rabbits were sacrificed 3-6 hours after the beginning of the experiments and at least two hours after the cortical electroencephalogram showed a disappearance of brain waves and became flat. The procedure used to sample brain has been described in detail in that paper. Under these circumstances there was a significant fall in potassium and an equally significant rise in sodium in the brain. They concluded on the basis of Yannet's experience[16] that these animals if they had not been sacrificed would have shown permanent neurological damage.

Using a microincineration technique, Liebert and Heilbrunn[18] studied the change in total ash and in water in brains of guinea pigs subjected to more than fifteen insulin convulsions. There was no actual loss of mineral substance but merely a shift from the ganglion cells "probably to the glial apparatus." These authors found, as did Yannet,[16] no change in the total water content of the brain between the control animals and the hypoglycemic ones.

More recent investigations have followed the changes in amino acid content of the brain during hypoglycemia. Dawson[19] found that rats subjected to various degrees of hypoglycemia had a marked reduction in free glutamic acid of the brain but no change in glutamine. The hypoglycemia he produced was neither very deep nor prolonged; only two animals showed convulsions. On the basis of free amino acid nitrogen and of free glutamic acid, he concluded that the loss of the free acid accounted for the fall in amino acid nitrogen. Cravioto and his colleagues,[20] using paper chromatography, demonstrated that while glutamic, glutamine and γ aminobutyric acid decreased, free aspartic acid increased under insulin treatment. They suggested that aspartic acid rose due to transamination between glutamic and oxalo-acetic acid. ∝-Ketoglutaric, one of the products of this reaction, could then enter the tricarboxylic cycle to yield energy. This increase in aspartic acid may explain Dawson's failure to find a greater change in free amino-acid nitrogen.

W. A. Himwich and Petersen[21] using rabbits prepared in essentially the same way as those described by Himwich and Sullivan,[17] were able to show that both free glutamic acid and glutamine fall to half their normal values during prolonged hypoglycemia. The administration of glucose or glutamate by intravenous drip restored the brain levels of glutamic acid and glutamine toward normal; the glutamic acid recovering its normal level before glutamine (Table III). Since in the normal rabbit the injection of much larger quantities of glutamic acid does not influence brain glutamate, these data suggest that the so-called blood-brain barrier to glutamic acid has been destroyed either by the destruction of cells or by the reduction of glutamic acid in the cells. If the controlling factor which prevents the free entrance of the amino acid into the brain is nothing more than a given cellular level of this substance, during insulin hypoglycemia the reduction of free glutamate would permit free entrance of the amino acid from the blood. The possibility of an actual change in the permeability of cells cannot, however, be overlooked in animals such as these who are subjected to long, deep insulin hypoglycemia. The shifts in potassium and sodium in the rabbits described by Himwich and Sullivan[17] suggest that they too, like the cats reported by Yannet,[16] suffered severe neurological and histological changes. Samson and his colleagues[22] using cats prepared in the same fashion as Himwich and her co-workers[17] found with paper chromatography that glutamic, glutamine, valine γ-amino butyric, serine, and alanine all fell progressively with the duration of hypoglycemia. Conversely free aspartic rose markedly, glycine perhaps a little. Cravioto's published chromatograms[20] could also be interpreted to show that he also found a decrease in serine, alanine and valine in his rats. Samson's data[22] suggest that aspartic acid finally falls if hypoglycemia is sufficiently prolonged. Essentially negative results have been reported by these authors[22] as to changes in total desoxyribonucleic acid, total pentose nucleic acid, "protein-side-group-ionization," total nitrogen and acid-soluble nitrogen during prolonged insulin treatment.

Not much is known of the effects of hypoglycemia on the lipids of the brain. Randall[23] showed that repeated convulsions induced by insulin caused a small but significant decrease in phospholipids and in neutral fat but had no effect on cholesterol in the brain. McGhee and her colleagues[24] confirmed Randall's data on phospholipids and showed that even if enough glucose was given to maintain blood glucose at normal levels after insulin, brain phospholipids still fell (Table IV). The administration of lecithin likewise had no effect.

No consideration of the effects of hypoglycemia would be complete without appraising the important data collected by Geiger and his associates[2] on the perfused cat brain. By perfusing the brain with a glucose-free medium he obtained information on how the brain attempts to maintain its energy needs without glucose. His results suggest that amino acids, phospholipids and nucleotides are used to furnish energy and that in the continued absence of glucose these materials cannot be rebuilt. The shifts in potassium and sodium in such an aglycemic preparation are similar to those reported above for animals in deep insulin hypoglycemia.[25]

There seems little doubt that the brain deprived of glucose is forced to use its own structural materials for maintenance. Figures published by W. A. Himwich and Sullivan,[17] although obtained microbiologically, suggest that bound glutamate may be destroyed to help maintain free

glutamate during hypoglycemia. It is interesting to speculate that if memories and patterns of behavior are stored in
the brain as chemical templates, such chemical models may
be destroyed as the brain frantically attempts to fulfill its
energy needs without glucose. Such changes would be too
minute to be detected by histological technics and as yet by
chemical ones. It is also possible that the more newly
formed templates may be more labile or may lie spatially in
a better position for metabolism. Thus hypoglycemia might
remove recent schizophrenic behavior patterns and allow
older and more normal patterns to reappear or permit the
building of new normal patterns. These are interesting
speculations but we will require more knowledge not only
of neurochemistry but also of neurophysiology and of the
behavioral sciences than we now have to answer them.

Costa and Himwich,[26] using animals prepared as described by Van Meter et al.[27] and essentially the same as
those used by Himwich and her co-workers,[17] have followed
the changes in serotonin content of the limbic and sensory
cortex, as well as the amygdala, hippocampus and other
brain areas as insulin hypoglycemia progressed. After a
short period of hippocampal convulsions a significant increase in serotonin occurred in the hippocampus, dience-
phalon and telencephalon. The medulla-pons area showed
no difference from the normal. If convulsions in the hippocampal area were allowed to continue for a longer period
of time the values for serotonin tended to return to normal.
It is difficult to explain the early increase in serotonin in
some parts of the brain. The authors argue that it can not be
due to blood-carrier changes since all areas then would be
expected to increase. The most likely possibility, they suggest, is a change in enzyme activity due indirectly to a decrease in energy-rich phosphate compounds. An impair-
ment of energy in this way would result in a failure of the
brain to form pyridoxal phosphate which is necessary for
the activity of the enzyme which destroys serotonin. It
would be expected that all enzymatic reactions which re-

quire energy such as is usually supplied by adenosine triphosphate would be inhibited during insulin hypoglycemia. Another example of the far reaching effects of a depletion of energy stored in the phosphate compounds is the report by Elliott, Crossland and Pappins[28] that acetylcholine is decreased in hypoglycemia. In this case the enzyme which synthesizes acetylcholine is dependent for energy upon adenosine triphosphate. A decrease in this latter substance then would lead to an inability of the brain to maintain normal levels of acetylcholine. Such derangement of the normal enzymatic patterns and metabolic balance have widespread effects. Some of these shifts in metabolism may have great therapeutic importance and may relate only indirectly to lack of glucose. Further research is needed to clarify these points.

Data on the effects of insulin hypoglycemia on the neurohormones were published by Paasonen and Vogt[29] for substance P and for serotonin. They found no significant changes. However, their data are fragmentary and the insulin dosage was small—2-3 units per kg. of body weight. Vogt[30] found that even a lower dose of insulin (1.5-1.8 units per kg. of body weight) caused a significant fall to 66% of the normal level of noradrenaline in the hypothalamus of dogs.

A not infrequent accompaniment of insulin hypoglycemia in human beings is the occurrence of moderate epileptiform convulsions. It is important, therefore, to clarify in our thinking what changes in neurochemistry may be due to the convulsions *per se* and thus may be expected to follow the use of convulsant agents such as electroshock and metrazol. Himwich and Fazekas[31] have concluded that all shock therapies have an element of cerebral metabolic depression. It may be argued that in the convulsive therapies such as electroshock, localized areas, which are convulsing violently, have a sharp increase in metabolism. If in these areas not enough glucose is available to support the metabolism, regional hypoglycemia would occur. In this way, insulin therapy and convulsant therapies could be expected to produce similar changes. Stone[32] found that in mice picrotoxin and metrazol caused an increase in brain lactic acid. The same group of investigators showed that dogs given convulsant agents when under curare and artificial respiration showed a decrease in cerebral phosphocreatine, an energy-rich phosphate compound. In cats[33] similarly treated, glycogen in the brain as well as energy-rich phosphates fell while lactic acid increased in that organ. Thus apparently while insulin hypoglycemia causes a fall of brain lactic acid due to the lack of available substrate for its formation, convulsions cause an increase in this substance as a result of the sharp acceleration of metabolism which they evoke and of a failure of the blood to supply sufficient oxygen to support the increased metabolism of overactive parts of the brain. In these areas anaerobic metabolism might increase even though arterial oxygen remained at normal levels.

Colfer[34] showed that convulsions produce a redistribution of sodium and potassium between neurons and extracellular fluid but found no change in total brain sodium or potassium with convulsions due to sound or metrazol.[35] With picrotoxin convulsion lasting for thirty minutes, Himwich and Sullivan[17] reported a significant increase in sodium in the brain. This increase in sodium ($P = <0.05$) was not as large as those induced by deep insulin hypoglycemia ($P = <0.01$). The change suggests a shift in cellular permeability if not an actual destruction of cells.

It can be seen, therefore, that convulsions *per se* differ from insulin hypoglycemia in neurochemical effects mainly in the change in lactic acid. In both cases there is a deprivation of energy to the brain and a resultant cerebral depression. As has been suggested by Himwich and Fazekas,[31] this factor is the common denominator in all successful shock therapies for mental diseases. The generally greater beneficial effect of insulin shock in schizophrenia and conversely the effectiveness of electroshock in depressions but not in schizophrenia suggest that something more specific than depression of cerebral metabolism is the crucial factor in determining the success of the therapy.

Summary

Insulin hypoglycemia deprives the brain of glucose which is needed for energy and for the rebuilding of other substances destroyed by metabolism thus enforcing a restriction in the exogenous energy supply. In an attempt to maintain itself the brain uses its stored energy—glycogen. This substance is withdrawn first from those parts of the brain which have the greatest activity. In the absence of glucose other substances such as amino acids and lipoids which are being constantly metabolized cannot be kept at normal levels. If the hypoglycemia continues, the brain then breaks down part of its cell structure. These changes are reflected in a loss of amino acids and a shift in salts, sodium, and potassium with the amount of sodium being increased and the level of potassium falling. With the lack of glucose the over-all metabolism of the brain decreases. The reduction of energy also upsets the balance between the various enzyme systems which depend upon the energy obtained from metabolism. This change undoubtedly has far-reaching consequences. One result found so far is a change in acetylcholine and serotonin both of which play important roles in the normal function of the brain. In hypoglycemia the former decreases due to lack of energy required to build it in the brain, the latter increases because the enzyme which destroys it also needs energy.

The effectiveness of insulin shock therapy depends upon the fact that the brain is temporarily lacking in glucose and hence in energy. This deficiency produces widespread alterations in the brain metabolism. We cannot as yet say which of these changes are essential for the beneficial effects. It seems probable, however, that the therapeutic results depend not upon the lack of glucose *per se* but upon the far reaching effects which the lack of energy has upon the hormones and enzymes of the brain. Research is just beginning to explore these possibilities.

Bibliography

1. Himwich, H. E., and Nahum, L. H. The respiratory quotient of the brain. *Amer. J. Physiol.,* 90:389-390, 1929. Ibid, 101:446-453, 1932.

2. Geiger, A. Chemical changes accompanying activity in the brain. In: Richter, Derek (ed.), *Metabolism of the Nervous System.* New York: Pergamon Press, 245-256, 1957.

3. Ferris, E. B., Jr., Rosenbaum, M., Aring, C. D., Ryder, H. W., Roseman, E., Hawkins, J. R. Intracranial blood flow in insulin coma. *Arch. Neurol. Psychiat.,* 46:509-512, 1941.

4. Himwich, H. E., Bowman, K. M., Daly, C., Fazekas, J. F., Wortis, J., Goldfarb, W. Cerebral blood flow and brain metabolism during insulin hypoglycemia. *Amer. J. Physiol.,* 132:640-647, 1941.

5. Kety, S. S., Woodford, R. B., Harmel, M. H., Freyhan, F. A., Appel, K. E., Schmidt, C. F. Cerebral blood flow and metabolism in schizophrenia. The effects of barbiturate semi-narcosis, insulin coma and electroshock. *Amer. J. Psychiat.,* 104:765-770, 1948.

6. Himwich, H. E. *Brain Metabolism and Cerebral Disorders.* Baltimore: Williams and Wilkins Co., 1951.

7. Himwich, H. E., Hadidian, Z., Fazekas, J. F., Hoagland, H. Cerebral metabolism and electrical activity during insulin hypoglycemia in man. *Amer. J. Physiol.,* 125:578-585, 1939.

8. Kerr, Stanley E., Hampel, C. W., and Ghantus, Musa. The Cardbohydrate Metabolism of Brain. IV. Brain glycogen, free sugar, and lactic acid as affected by insulin in normal and adrenal-inactivated cats, and by

epinephrine in normal rabbits. *J. Biol. Chem.*, 119: 405-421, 1937.

9. Stone, W. E. The effects of anaesthetics and of convulsants on the lactic acid content of the brain. *Biochem. J.*, 32:1908-1918, 1938.

10. Olsen, Norman S., and Klein, J. Raymond. Effect of insulin hypoglycemia on brain glucose, glycogen, lactate and phosphates. *Arch. Biochem.*, 13:343-347, 1947.

11. Chesler, A., and Himwich, H. E. Effect of insulin hypoglycemia on glycogen content of parts of the central nervous system of the dog. *Arch. Neurol. Psychiat.*, 52: 114-116, 1944.

12. Himwich, H. E., and Fazekas, J. F. Comparative studies of the brain of infant and adult dogs. *Amer. J. Physiol.*, 132:454-459, 1941.

13. Ferris, Shirley and Himwich, Harold E. The effect of hypoglycemia and age on the glycogen content of the various parts of the feline central nervous system. *Amer. J. Physiol.*, 146:389-393, 1946.

14. Chesler, Annette and Himwich, Harold E. The glycogen content of various parts of the central nervous system of dogs and cats at different ages. *Arch. Biochem.*, 2:175-181, 1943.

15. Goncharova, E. D. Effect of insulin and adrenalin on the polysaccharide metabolism in the brain. Reports of the Acad. Sci., Ukrainian USSR, 183-185, 1957. Translation Center, John Crerar Library, Chicago.

16. Yannet, Herman. Effect of prolonged insulin hypoglycemia on distribution of water and electrolytes in brain and muscle. *Arch. Neurol. and Psychiat.*, 42:237-247, 1939.

17. Himwich, Williamina A., Sullivan, W. T. Chemical constituents of brain as affected by insulin hypoglycemia, convulsions and fever. *J. Nerv. Ment. Dis.*, 124:21-26, 1956.

18. Leibert, Erich and Heilbrunn, Gert. Mineral content of

the brain. *Arch. Neurol. and Psychiat.*, 43:463-471, 1940.

19. Dawson, R. M. C. Studies on the glutamine and glutamic acid content of the rat brain during insulin hypoglycemia. *Biochem. J.*, 47:386-391, 1951.

20. Cravioto, R. O., Massieu, G., and Izquierdo, J. J. Free amino-acids in rat brain during insulin shock. *Proc. Soc. Exper. Biol. and Med.*, 78:856-858, 1951.

21. Himwich, Williamina A., Petersen, Jo Ann C. Recovery from insulin coma and hematoencephalic exchange. *Dis. Nerv. Sys.*, 19:104-107, 1958.

22. Samson, F. E., Jr., Dahl, D. R., Dahl, Nancy, and Himwich, H. E. Studies of the hypoglycemic brain. The amino acids, nucleic acids, total nitrogen and side-group-ionization of proteins in cat brain during insulin coma. *Arch. Neurol. and Psychiat.* Inpress.

23. Randall, L. O. Effect of repeated insulin hypoglycemia on the lipid composition of rabbit tissues. *J. Biol. Chem.*, 133:129-136, 1940.

24. McGhee, Eva C., Papageorge, Evangeline, Bloom, W. L., Lewis, G. T. Effect of hyperinsulinism on brain phospholipide. *J. Biol. Chem.*, 190:127-132, 1951.

25. Geiger, A., and Geiger, R. S., and Magnes, J. Survival of perfused cat's brain in the absence of glucose. *Nature*, 170:754-755, 1952.

26. Costa, E., Himwich, H. E. Brain serotonin metabolism in insulin hypoglycemia. Presented at the International Biochemical Congress, Vienna, Austria, 1958.

27. Van Meter, W. G., Owens, H. F., Himwich, H. E. Cortical and Rhinencephalic Electrical Potentials During Hypoglycemia. *Arch. Neurol. Psychiat.*, 80:314-320, 1958.

28. Crossland, J., Elliott, K. A. C., and Pappius. Acetylcholine content of brain during insulin hypoglycemia. *Amer. J. Physiol.*, 183:32-34, 1955.

29. Paasonen, M. K., and Vogt, Marthe. The effects of drugs on the amounts of substance P and 5-hydroxy-

tryptamine in mammalian brain. *J. Physiol.*, 131:617-626, 1956.

30. Vogt, Marthe. The concentration of sympathin in different parts of the central nervous system under normal conditions and after the administration of drugs. *J. Physiol.*, 123:451-481, 1954.

31. Himwich, H. E., and Fazekas, J. F. Factor of hypoxia in the shock therapies of schizophrenia. *Arch. Neurol. Psychiat.*, 47:800-807, 1942.

32. Stone, W. E., Webster, J. E., and Gurdjian, E. S. Chemical changes in the cerebral cortex associated with convulsive activity. *J. Neurophysiol.*, 8:233-240, 1945.

33. Klein, J. R., and Olsen, N. S. Effect of convulsive activity upon the concentration of brain glucose, glycogen, lactate and phosphates. *J. Biol. Chem.*, 167:747-756, 1947.

34. Colfer, H. F. Studies of the relationship between electrolyte of the cerebral cortex and the mechanism of convulsions. In Epilepsy, Res. Pub. ARNMD, 26:98-117, 1947.

35. Colfer, H. F., and Essex, H. E. The distribution of total electrolyte, potassium, and sodium in the cerebral cortex in relation to experimental convulsions. *Amer. J. Physiol.*, 150:27-36, 1947.

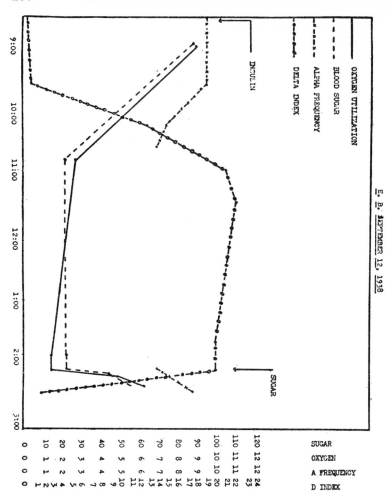

Figure 1. The cerebral arterio-venous oxygen difference, blood sugar, and brain waves during insulin hypoglycemic treatment for schizophrenia. After insulin effect
takes hold, the alpha frequency decreases, the same as cerebral arterio-venous oxygen difference and blood sugar. At
the time when the alpha frequency has disappeared, the
cerebral arterio-venous difference and blood sugar have
fallen to a low level, and the patient is no longer in contact
with environment. During the subsequent period of hypo-

glycemia coma, the arterio-venous oxygen difference falls somewhat, and blood sugar remains low. When the treatment was terminated by the oral administration of sugar, the alpha waves reappeared, cerebral arterio-venous oxygen difference and blood sugar rose, and the patient aroused. Taken from reference 7.

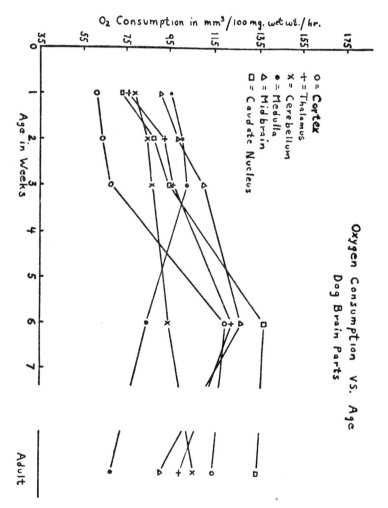

Figure 2. The changes in oxygen consumption of the various parts of the dog brain at 1, 2, 3, and 6 weeks and in

adulthood. In general, the cerebral metabolism increases during the first six weeks and then reverses slightly. Taken from reference 12.

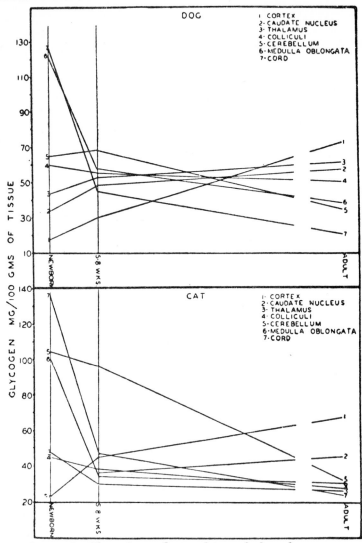

Figure 3. Changing relationships of the glycogen content in the various parts of the neuraxis during growth. Taken from reference 14.

TABLE 1

Glycogen content (mg. %) of parts of the central nervous system of hypoglycemic dogs.*

No. of Exper.	Caudate	Corpora quadri-gemmina	Cerebral grey	Thalamus	Cere-bellum	Medulla	Cord
			Hypoglycemia				
1.	8	26	56	45	40	35	46
2.	12	28	33	40	32	26	14
3.	8	32	21	27	33	24	14
4.	1	8	16	8	30	49	122
5.	20	0	11	18	18	36	45
6.	12	13	19	20	8	19	16
7.	6	15	10	8	1	31	43
8.	0	0	2	0	1	31	32
9.	0	2	6	0	6	13	26
			Normal				
Aver.	58	50	73	62	35	37	29
Range	44-71	37-60	45-108	41-68	23-46	21-47	15-31

* Taken from Chesler and Himwich.[11] The observations of nine experiments are presented in the table. A heavy line has been drawn to separate the glycogen contents of the animals into two divisions. The values to the left of the heavy line are significantly lower than the lowest values for the normal range for that same part, while those to the right are not significantly lower than the normal. In general the upper parts of the brain lose their glycogen deposits before the lower areas are depleted.

TABLE 2

Average Content of Water, Chloride, Sodium, Potassium Per Kilogram of Fat-Free Brain of Control and of Experimental Animals Given Insulin.*

(1) No. of Animals	(2) Water, Gm.	(3) Chloride, mM	(4) Sodium, mM	(5) Potassium, mM
Group 1. Control Animals				
20	862 ± 1.1	48.0 ± 0.70	61.2 ± 0.66	101 ± 0.73
Group 2. Animals During Hypoglycemic State				
15	857 ± 2.2	44.7 ± 0.53	57.9 ± 0.87	102 ± 0.88
Group 3. Animals Which Survived with No Demonstrable Evidence of Involvement of Central Nervous System				
12	857 ± 2.4	45.1 ± 1.6	63.4 ± 1.3	99.3 ± 1.8
Group 4. Animals Which Survived with Evidence of Involvement of Central Nervous System				
10	868 ± 2.8	54.7 ± 2.1	77.9 ± 3.2	83.0 ± 2.4

* Taken from Yannet.[16]

TABLE 3

Free Glutamic Acid and Glutamine in Brain Parts*

	Glutamic Acid Hemisphere Samples		Glutamine Hemisphere Samples	
	Right mg %	Left mg %	Right mg %	Left mg %
CONTROL:				
(7)**	97.3	(7) 100.0	(7)* 46.7	(7) 44.3
HYPOGLYCEMIC:				
(10)	59.5	(10) 54.9	(9) 19.4	(9) 17.4
HYPOGLYCEMIC & GLUCOSE:				
SubQ (6)	100.3	(6) 101.8	(5) 28.8	(5) 27.4
Drip (5)	84.8	(5) 89.4	(4) 22.2	(4) 20.2
HYPOGLYCEMIC & GLUTAMATE				
Drip (5)	93.2	(5) 84.6	(5) 23.8	(5) 27.4

* Adapted from Himwich and Petersen.[21]
** No. animals used.

TABLE 4

Changes in Brain Lipide P with Hypoglycemia*

Experiment	No. of Animals	Lipide P per 100 gm. fresh tissue		t value**	p**
		Mean	Standard deviation		
		mg.	mg.		
Normal control	12	263	17.3		
Insulin	12	241	20.2	2.797	0.02
Insulin-lecithin	6	233	10.8	3.677	0.02
Insulin-glucose	6	237	12.8	3.152	0.02

* Fisher.

* Taken from McGhee et al.24

Chapter 5

ELECTROENCEPHALOGRAPHIC CHANGES IN THE BRAIN DURING INSULIN HYPOGLYCEMIA*

CHARLES H. SAWYER**

In the late 1920's, when Sakel[1] was first testing insulin hypoglycemia in the treatment of schizophrenia, Berger[2] was making his initial recordings of brain waves known as the electroencephalogram (EEG). It was natural that the effects of hypoglycemia should be studied by the new recording technique, and this was soon done in patients by such pioneer electroencephalographers as Hoagland, Rubin and Cameron[3] in this country and Berger himself[4] in Germany. These investigators described a widespread slowing of the brain waves, the disappearance of the alpha (10/sec.) rhythm and the prevalence of the very slow delta waves, as assessed by a "delta index," during the depths of hypoglycemia.[3] During the past twenty years, these findings have been amply confirmed in countless publications, many of which were reviewed by Engel, et al.[5] in 1954. However, in spite of the number of studies on hypoglycemia and

* The new research reported in this review was supported by a grant from the National Institutes of Health, B-1162.
** Fellow of the Commonwealth Fund, 1958-59.

mechanisms of insulin action by EEG and other techniques, Sakel, in his 1954 reappraisal,[1] admitted that the rationale for the proved effectiveness of insulin shock therapy was still unclear.

Basic studies on the effects of hypoglycemia in experimental animals followed the early clinical EEG reports. Moruzzi[6] correlated blood sugar levels with EEG waves in the rabbit and found that the high-amplitude slow waves gave way to low-amplitude activity prior to motor convulsions. Goodwin, et al.[7] compared insulin and metrazol seizures in the rabbit and suggested that the former might be caused by a purely subcortical disturbance. In 1939, Hoagland, Himwich, et al.[8] introduced an important innovation in technique when they recorded simultaneously from the cerebral cortex and the hypothalamus in the dog. They reported that during hypoglycemia, the cortical potentials disappeared before the hypothalamic waves were affected and that extremely high-amplitude EEG activity, accompanied by convulsions, cardiac or respiratory changes, might occur in the hypothalamus after cortical failure (Fig. 1). From these and related data, Himwich[9] developed a concept of successive horizontal levels or layers within the brain which were affected sequentially by internal environmental conditions, such as by hypoglycemia, anoxemia or drug action.

According to the useful doctrine of phyletic layers, the idea for which Himwich[9] credits Hughlings Jackson, the cerebral cortex is depressed before the subcorticodiencephalon. In turn, the mesencephalon, the rostral medulla and then the caudal medulla are released from the restrictive influences of the superior layers. Symptoms of the related stages of hypoglycemia include drowsiness and loss of contact with environment as the cortex becomes depressed; motor restlessness, exaggerated reflexes, sympathetic symptoms and even convulsions as the second level is released; paroxysmal tonic and torsion spasms accompanied by increases in blood pressure and heart rate as the midbrain is

BLOOD SUGAR mgm.%	TIME
95	10:05
45	11:00
33	12:40
26	2:30
	5:00
22	7:15
	9:06
179	9:20
179	9:25

POSTERIOR HYPOTHALAMUS

ANTERIOR HYPOTHALAMUS

CORTEX

1 second

Calibration 50 microvolts

Fig. 1. Records from cortex, posterior hypothalamus, and anterior hypothalamus in the dog during insulin hypoglycemia and recovery. (From Hoagland, *et al. J. Neurophysiol.*, 2:276-288, 1939.)

released; and decerebrate rigidity and parasympathetic phenomena as the medullary layers take over and are in turn depressed. The concept of successive functional layers has been helpful clinically in analyzing the relative depth of hypoglycemia.

However, developments in neurophysiology within the past ten years have given strong support for a vertical stratification of the brain, a concept developed by Livingston, *et al.*[10] According to this scheme, three vertical columns extend the length of the neuraxis. On one side is an afferent column made up of the direct ascending paths to sensory areas of the cortex. On the other side, an efferent column includes the cortical motor areas and descending motor pathways. Between the two is a vertical column composed of indirect or relayed connections, the center of which consists of multiple, short neuronal collections of neuropil which comprise the interneuronal systems and association regions of the cerebral cortex, the nonspecific and diffusely projecting nuclei of the thalamus, the reticular formation of the brainstem and the interneuronal gray matter of the spinal cord. It is in this central column, which includes the reticular activating system of Magoun, Moruzzi and Bremer,[11] that depression or facilitation by pharmacological agents is especially to be sought.

The reticular activating system was introduced by Moruzzi and Magoun in 1949,[12] and since that time it has come to be associated not only with sleep and wakefulness but also with integration of changes in blood pressure, respiration and pulse; secretion of pituitary hormones; initiation or inhibition of movement; and alteration in signals conducted by the primary sensory system.[11] Through its close connections with the rhinencephalon and hypothalamus, to be discussed further below, it undoubtedly influences emotional expression.[13, 14] The reticular system is especially sensitive to anesthetics,[15] and its destruction results in complete, permanent coma.

In their study on brain stem arousal mechanisms in the cat, Arduini and Arduini[16] found that hypoglycemia, like hypoxia and anesthesia, blocked auditory evoked potentials (click stimuli) in the reticular formation, while they proceeded to the auditory cortex via the classical auditory pathway with undiminished amplitude. More recently, Fernandez and Brenman[17] reported that such auditory evoked potentials reached the cortex even though the blood sugar level was depressed to 5 mg. per cent. In the pentobarbital-treated cat, Grenell[18] has reported that intravenous insulin in high dosages facilitates cortical responses evoked by direct electrical stimulation of the cortex but only if the ascending reticular activating system is intact. Insulin applied locally to the cortex is ineffective. Quite recently, Van Meter, Owens and Himwich[19] have reported that the cortical and subcortical alerting response to painful stimuli disappears in the hypoglycemic rabbit. These authors found that responses to light flashes were lost in the visual cortex as early as or earlier than in the midbrain following insulin treatment. In unpublished work in collaboration with Berkowitz and Sundsten,[20] we have measured the threshold of arousal by direct electrical stimulation of the reticular formation of unanesthetized rabbits with chronically implanted electrodes (Fig. 2). It is evident that when the blood sugar is markedly depressed the threshold of arousal is elevated and that it returns to normal rapidly after treatment with glucose. The bulk of the evidence, then, supports the hypothesis that the midbrain reticular system of the middle column in the vertical scheme of neuronal organization is profoundly affected by hypoglycemia as early as stages one and two of the horizontal phyletic layer concept.

Another neuronal system which has received considerable attention recently is the rhinencephalon or limbic lobe.[21]

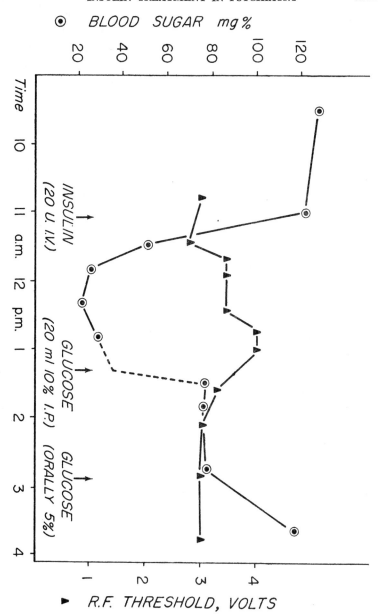

Fig. 2. Relation between insulin hypoglycemia and EEG-arousal threshold following direct electrical stimulation of

the midbrain reticular formation in the rabbit. A motor convulsion occurred just prior to injection of glucose. From Berkowitz, *et al.* (Unpublished data, 1958.)

Subcortical and allocortical in its organization, it belongs largely to the middle column of the vertical schema.[10] Included in the rhinencephalon are the olfactory bulb and tubercle, the septum, the hippocampus, the amygdala and their connections. Twenty years ago, Papez[22] proposed a circuit of rhinencephalic structures which, he suggested, might serve as the anatomical substrate for emotion. According to his scheme, impulses passed from entorhinal area to the hippocampus and then successively via the fornix to the mammillary body, the anterior thalamus and the cingulate cortex, finally returning to the entorhinal area through the cingulum and longitudinal striae. Adey[13] has presented new anatomical and electro-physiological evidence that the Papez circuit can also project in the reverse direction, with impulses going via fornix to hippocampus to entorhinal area and thence to the midbrain reticular formation. Green and Arduini[23] and Nauta[14] have published physiological and morphological evidence, respectively, of transmission pathways from midbrain reticular formation to septum, from which the precommissural fornix can relay data to the hippocampus. Hippocampal arousal, like neocortical arousal, is controlled by the reticular system, but it is characterized by a synchronous theta (4-7/sec.) rhythm as compared with neocortical asynchrony.[23] It is clear that the rhinencephalon is functionally closely related to the reticular activating system.

The neuropathological literature contains numerous references to damage incurred in rhinencephalic areas, especially the hippocampus, as a result of prolonged insulin hypoglycemia.[24-7] Several authors have considered seizures necessary for the production of these pathological changes.[25]

To determine the occurrence, severity and localization of cortical and subcortical seizures during hypoglycemia,

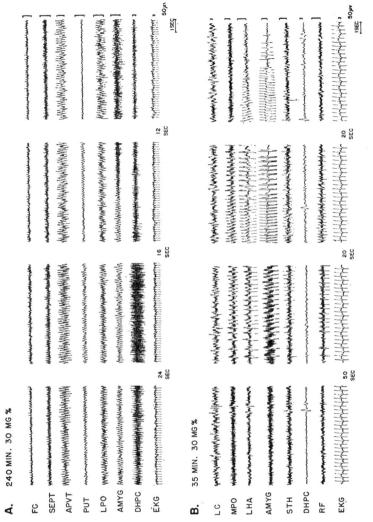

Fig. 3. A. Hypoglycemic seizure involving dorsal hippocampus and amygdala. B. Characteristics and sites of pro-
jection of an amygdaloid seizure in the dorsal hippocampus.
From *AMA Arch. Neurol. & Psychiat.* Tokizane and Sawyer,
March 1957.

Abbreviations employed in this and in subsequent Figures are as follows: AMYG, amygdala; APVT, anterior para-

ventricular thalamic nucleus; DHPC, dorsal hippocampus; DMT, dorsomedial thalamic nucleus; EKG, electrocardiogram; FC, frontal cortex, GP, globus pallidum; LC, limbic cortex; LGV, ventral part of lateral geniculate body; LHA, lateral hypothalamic area; LPO, lateral preoptic area; MPO, medial preoptic area; OB, olfactory bulb; PUT, putamen; RF, reticular formation; SEPT, septum; SN, substantia nigra; STH, subthalamic nucleus; VPM, ventroposteromedical thalamic nucleus.

Tokizane and Sawyer[28] studied the effects of high insulin dosages on the EEG of acute rabbit preparations with electrodes stereotaxically placed in a wide variety of subcortical centers as well as the frontal and limbic cortical areas. In 10 of 24 rabbits, the blood sugar was lowered below 50 mg. per cent, and eight of these suffered EEG seizures starting invariably in rhinencephalic structures and seldom progressing to the cortex. Fig. 3 illustrates the characteristics of typical hypoglycemic seizures in two of their rabbits. The animal in Fig. 3A revealed seizure activity only in the hippocampus and amygdala. The rabbit in Fig. 3B had sustained a hippocampal seizure just prior to the record illustrated. During post-seizure depression in the hippocampus, an amygdaloid seizure was seen projecting to the preoptic regions, the subthalamus and the reticular formation, but not to the cortex.

In similar acute rabbit preparations, Van Meter, Owens and Himwich[19] have also observed subcortical EEG seizures in the hippocampus and amygdala, not associated with movement, which might progress to the cortex or remain isolated subcortically. Motor seizures appeared to originate simultaneously in cortical and subcortical leads, but the motor artifact obscured any localization of the origin of such seizures.

Recently, in collaboration with Berkowitz and Sundsten,[20] we have reinvestigated the effects of hypoglycemia, using unanesthetized "chronic" rabbits with electrodes permanently implanted in multiple regions of the brain instead of acute preparations. Such animals are free to move about, and their behavioral activities can be correlated with EEG alterations and blood sugar levels. Since they are not under surgical trauma at the time of recording, hypoglycemia can be induced by low insulin dosages. It is possible to compare the effects of high vs. low insulin dosage in a given animal. EEG correlates of the effects of irreversible brain damage may also be sought in such chronic rabbits. As mentioned above, arousal thresholds were recorded following direct stimulation of the midbrain reticular formation (Fig. 2).

Ten chronic rabbit preparations have thus far been studied in this way, and rhinencephalic EEG seizure activity has been observed in seven of them. The other three succumbed, probably to the combined effect of hypoglycemia and the stress of experimental treatment, before exhaustive studies had been made. Typical examples of the EEG characteristics and related behavior in two of the seven "seizure" rabbits will be presented below (Figs. 4-6).

In Fig. 4 are seen some of the EEG changes in a fasted rabbit that received a total of 480 units of insulin over a three-hour period. Blood sugar data are not available for this animal. At no time did this rabbit exhibit motor convulsions, but it lay quietly in a comatose state throughout most of the first post-insulin day. It could not be induced to eat but was maintained by parenteral injections of glucose for three days. During this time it remained reasonably alert and responsive to stimuli until several hours before death when it lapsed into an extremely lethargic condition. Within 30 minutes of the injection of the first 160 U. insulin (A), the olfactory bulb (OB) showed marked depression, and by 45 minutes (B) it had started spiking. In less than 2 hours (C), EEG seizures starting in OB but progressing to the lateral hypothalamic area (LHA) were observed, with occasional spiking in the amygdala (AMYG). Isolated EEG seizures were common in OB (D), and by

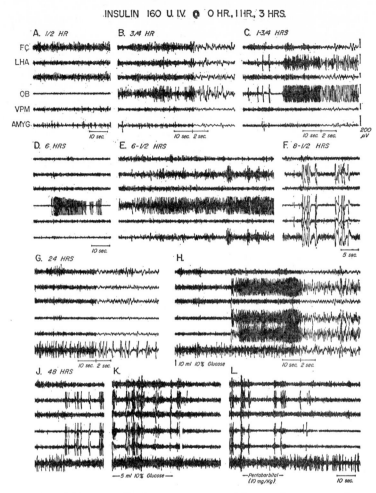

Fig. 4. Sites and characteristics of hypoglycemic subcortical EEG seizures in the rabbit. Note the irreversible change in amygdala (AMYG) after 24 hours. The electrode site for channel 3 was lost in the process of histological confirmation. For further explanation, see text. From Berkowitz, *et al.*[20]

6½ hours they often progressed through LHA and AMYG (E). By 8½ hours (F) the thalamic nucleus VPM was also involved, and amygdaloid EEG activity had become quite conspicuous. By the end of the first day the seizure activity in AMYG had become most prominent, and at the start of the second day (G), it became apparent that irreversible

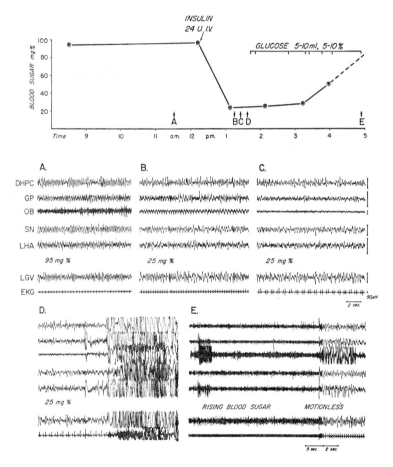

Fig. 5. Changes in the blood sugar level and associated alterations in subcortical EEG tracings following low insulin dosage in the rabbit. The motor convulsion in D is mostly movement artifact as revealed in the EKG channel. Further explanation in text. From Berkowitz, *et al.* (Unpublished data, 1958.)

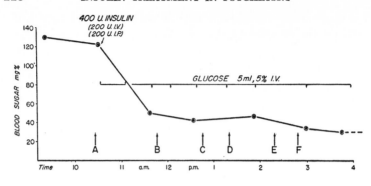

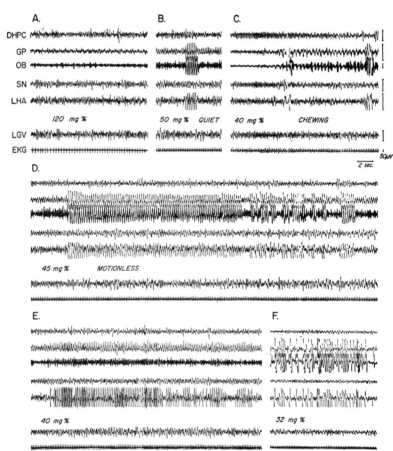

Fig. 6. Subcortical EEG changes at various times, indicated on the blood sugar curve, following high insulin and weak glucose treatment. The seizures appear to be triggered in the olfactory bulb and to involve principally the globus pallidum and the lateral hypothalamic area. From Berkowitz, *et al.* (Unpublished data, 1958.)

changes had occurred in AMYG. Injections of glucose did not eliminate the abnormal spiking in AMYG, but, as seen in H, they occasionally triggered seizure activity in the other sensitive areas, LHA, OB and VPM. Apparently, the blood sugar level was critical in these regions showing reversible seizure activity, for on the third day (K) injection of glucose quieted their seizures without affecting AMYG. Pentobarbital (L) also reduced the seizures in the active channels, but spiking continued in the amygdala. On the fourth day of recording (not shown), prior to death, seizures were absent from channels 1-5, but AMYG continued spiking to the end. At no time did the cortex (FC) show independent seizure activity, and not until 48 hours after insulin was there any suggestion that the rhinencephalic seizures might involve it (K, L).

Figs. 5 and 6 illustrate the effects of low and high insulin dosage in one fasted rabbit on consecutive days. Fig. 5 shows the slowing of the EEG, alteration of the EKG and depression, especially in OB, before the motor convulsion in D. Most of the convulsion record is movement artifact as indicated in the EKG channel, but spikes in channels 2, 3 and 5 preceded the motor seizure. Interestingly, these channels (E) revealed subcortical EEG seizure activity, unrelated to movement artifact, during the rising phase of the blood sugar after glucose administration. These regions, GP, OB and LHA, were the areas to show prolonged EEG seizure activity on the following day with high insulin dosage (Fig. 6) and periodic weak glucose injections. Various patterns of EEG seizure activity were observed (B-F) with very little movement and practically no motor artifact. At one stage

(E), the hypothalamus (LHA) appears almost to "solo" in its seizure activity. Glucose injections were terminated and the rabbit died that night.

Motor convulsions of the type illustrated in Fig. 5D were common within 90 minutes after weak (20-25 U) insulin injections, and they would be classified as in stage 2 of the phyletic hypoglycemic levels.[9] Such motor seizures are considered teleologically an attempt on the part of the animal to raise its own blood sugar, and they are accompanied by signs of sympathetic discharge.

The subcortical seizures represent a greater degree of hypoglycemic involvement, even though they may appear on the rising phase of the blood sugar curve. If there are motor concomitants, they are of the tonic-clonic or torsion type with the animal exhibiting a slow writhing activity, but usually they are absent. Possibly with the high insulin dosage the stage of motor convulsions is bypassed rapidly and without incident; however, further effects of the high insulin dosage, e.g., dehydration,[29] may contribute to the subcortical seizure activation.

Tokizane and Sawyer[28] have reviewed the unique features of the amygdala and hippocampus, the natural high-amplitude of their activity and their low threshold to seizures in response to electrical, drug or chemical stimuli. These authors suggested that subcortical seizures involving these areas but undetected in the absence of subcortical electrodes might constitute a key reaction on which the beneficial results of shock therapy depend. Van Meter, Owens and Himwich[19] have reaffirmed this suggestion, proposing "that the mechanism of the therapeutic action of insulin hypoglycemia includes a change in rhinencephalic function."

There is increasing evidence that at least some of the tranquilizing drugs exert similar influences on the rhinencephalon. MacLean, et al.[30] reported that in the cat insulin seizures and reserpine treatment had similar effects on behavior and on protein synthesis in the hippocampus. The

Killams[31] and Sigg and Schneider[32] have shown that reserpine lowers the threshold of rhinencephalic seizures. Preston[33] and Stewart[34] have presented similar evidence for chlorpromazine. A comprehensive review of the action of psychopharmacologic drugs has been contributed by Himwich.[35]

A unified theory of the action of therapies involving shock, coma, tranquilizers or lobotomy has been proposed by Fink.[36] He relates the efficacy of therapy with the ability to induce a persistent change in cerebral function, two indices of which are a delta shift in the EEG spectrum and an increase in incidence of seizures. The present insulin data are consistent with this theory, and they suggest that the delta shift reflects underlying involvement of the reticular formation, while the seizure incidence reflects a change in rhinencephalic function. Further study of the interrelations between the reticular formation and the rhinencephalon with respect to subcortical seizures is indicated.

Summary

Insulin hypoglycemia induces a marked slowing of the cortical EEG, an effect which has been described as a "delta shift" since the resultant waves are of the slow delta variety. In experimental animals it is apparent that accompanying this shift and perhaps responsible for it is a severe depression of the reticular activating system; the change is characterized by a rise in the arousal threshold and a failure of the reticular system to transmit evoked afferent potentials. The state of deep insulin hypoglycemia is often attended by EEG seizure activity, usually originating in subcortical centers of the rhinencephalon and often not progressing to the neocortex. A single course of insulin treatment may cause permanent localized damage in subcortical nuclei, characterized by continuously spiking EEG activity. A tendency towards seizure activity in these centers is also promoted by certain tranquilizing drugs, and it is suggested that these changes in rhinencephalic function may represent one common mechanism of action of the latter therapies and insulin shock treatment.

Literature Cited

1. Sakel, M. The classical Sakel shock treatment. A reappraisal. *J. Clin. Ex. Psychopath.*, 15:255-316, 1954.
2. Berger, H. Uber das Electrenkephalogramm des Menschen. *Arch. Psychiat., Berlin* 87:527-570, 1929.
3. Hoagland, H., Rubin, M. A., and Cameron, D. E. The electroencephalogram of schizophrenics during insulin hypoglycemia and recovery. *Am. J. Physiol.*, 120:559-570, 1937.
4. Berger, H. Uber das Electrenkephalogramm des Menschen. *Arch. Physchiat., Berlin* 106:165-187, 1937.
5. Engel, R., Halberg, F., Tichy, F. Y., and Dow, R. Electrocerebral activity and epileptic attacks at various blood sugar levels. *Arch. Neuroveget.*, 9:147-167, 1954.
6. Moruzzi, G. Action de l'hypoglycémie insulinique sur l'activité électrique spontanée et provoquée de l'écorce cerebrale. *Compt. rend. Soc. Biol.*, 128:1181-1184, 1938.
7. Goodwin, J. E., Kerr, W. K., and Lawson, F. L. Bioelectric responses in metrazol and insulin shock. *Am. J. Psychiat.*, 96:1389-1405, 1940.
8. Hoagland, H., Himwich, H. E., Campbell, F., Fazekas, J. F., and Hadidian, Z. Effects of hypoglycemia and pentobarbital sodium on electrical activity of cerebral cortex and hypothalamus (dogs). *J. Neurophysiol.*, 2:276-288, 1939.
9. Himwich, H. E. *Brain metabolism and cerebral disorders.* Baltimore: Williams and Wilkins, 1951.
10. Livingston, W. K., Haugen, F. P., and Brookhart, J. M. Functional organization of the central nervous system. *Neurology*, 4:485-496, 1954.
11. Henry Ford Hospital, International Symposium. *Retic-*

ular Formation of the Brain. Boston: Little, Brown and Co., 1958.

12. Moruzzi, G., and Magoun, H. W. Brain stem reticular formation and activation of the EEG. *EEG Clin. Neurophysiol.*, 1:455-473, 1949.

13. Adey, W. R. Organization of the rhinencephalon. In Henry Ford Hospital International Symposium, *Reticular Formation of the Brain.* Boston: Little, Brown and Co., 1958, Chapter 31.

14. Nauta, W. J. H., Kuypers, H. G. J. M. Some ascending pathways in the brain stem reticular formation. In Henry Ford Hospital International Symposium, *Reticular Formation of the Brain.* Boston: Little, Brown and Co., 1958, Chapter 1.

15. French, J. D., Verzeano, M., and Magoun, H. W. A neural basis of the anesthetic state. *AMA Arch. Neurol. & Psychiat.*, 69:519-529, 1953.

16. Arduini, A., and Arduini, M. G. Effect of drugs and metabolic alterations on brain stem arousal mechanisms. *J. Pharmacol. & Exper. Therap.*, 110:76-85, 1954.

17. Fernandez, C., and Brenman, A. Effect of hypoglycemia on auditory cortex and cochlear receptor in the cat. *Am. J. Physiol.*, 188:249-254, 1957.

18. Grenell, R. G. Mechanisms of action of psychotherapeutic and related drugs. *Ann. N. Y. Acad. Sci.*, 66:826-835, 1957.

19. Van Meter, W. G., Owens, H. F., and Himwich, H. E. Cortical and rhinencephalic electrical potentials during hypoglycemia. *AMA Arch. Neurol. & Psychiat.*, 80:314-320, 1958.

20. Berkowitz, E., Sundsten, J. W., and Sawyer, C. H. Unpublished data, 1958.

21. Kluver, H. Brain mechanisms and behavior with special reference to the rhinencephalon. *Journal-Lancet.*, 72:567-576, 1952.

22. Papez, J. W. A proposed mechanism of emotion. *AMA Arch. Neurol. & Psychiat.*, 38:725-743, 1937.

23. Green, J. D., and Arduini, A. A. Hippocampal electrical activity in arousal. *J. Neurophysiol.*, 17:533-557, 1954.

24. Stief, A., and Tokay, L. Beiträge zur Histopathologie der experimentellen Insulinvergiftung. *Zeitsch Neurol.*, 139:434-461, 1932.

25. Lawrence, R. D., Meyer, A., and Nevin, S. The neuropathology of hypoglycemia. *Quart. J. Med.*, 35:181-202, 1942.

26. Hicks, S. P. Brain metabolism in vivo. *Arch. Path.*, 50:545-561, 1950.

27. Zeitlhofer, J., Tschabitscher, H., and Wanko, T. Zur Pathologie des protrakierten Insulin schocks. *Wiener Zeitsch Nervenheilkunde*, 9:445-458, 1954.

28. Tokizane, T., and Sawyer, C. H. Sites of origin of hypoglycemic seizures in the rabbit. *AMA Arch. Neurol. & Psychiat.*, 77:259-266, 1957.

29. Billet, J., Lafon, R., and Billet, B. Modifications biologiques apportées par une injection de haute doses d'insuline chez des sujets non diabétiques. Hypothése sur la pathogénie du coma insulinique. *Ann. méd-psychol.*, 1:175-196, 1953.

30. MacLean, P. D., Flanagan, S., Flynn, J. P., Kim, C., and Stevens, J. R. Hippocampal function: tentative correlations of conditioning. EEG, drug and radioautographic studies. *Yale J. Biol. & Med.*, 28:380-395, 1956.

31. Killam, E. K., and Killam, K. F. The influence of drugs on central afferent pathways. In *Brain Mechanisms and Drug Action*, W. S. Fields, Ed. Springfield: Thomas, 1957, pp. 71-98.

32. Sigg, E. B., and Schneider, J. A. Mechanisms involved in the interaction of various central stimulants and reserpine. *EEG Clin. Neurophysiol.*, 9:419-426, 1957.

33. Preston, J. B. Effects of chlorpromazine on the central nervous system of the cat. *J. Pharmacol. & Exper. Therap.*, 118:100-115, 1956.

34. Stewart, L. F. Chlorpromazine: use to activate electro-

encephalographic seizure patterns. *EEG Clin. Neurophysiol.*, 9:427-440, 1957.

35. Himwich, H. E. Psychopharmacologic drugs. *Science*, 127:59-72, 1958.

36. Fink, M. A unified theory of the action of physiodynamic therapies. *J. Hillside Hospital*, 6:197-206, 1957.

DISCUSSION

DR. RALPH W. GERARD: I've had a wonderful time hearing of the things that agitated us a quarter of a century ago. This is confessing to an emotional retrogression, just as Joe Wortis did in discussing the events of a quarter century back.

I had not planned to discuss this presentation, so these comments are completely off the cuff; but, as Dr. Williamina Himwich was offering interpretations of these newer findings, I was thinking that it is only the *findings* that make progress. The theories have changed very little; every one of the suggestions made now was offered quite fervently at the beginning of the insulin hypoglycemia era. I was guilty of the suggestion that the shock therapies resulted from a burning out of the clinkers in the metabolic furnace. There was, under the action of insulin—and possibly even under metrazol, which led to an anoxia for a while—an initial decrease in cell metabolism with a subsequent rebound to increased rates and so to a cleaning away of the bad material residues in the nervous system. Speidel, observing transparent salamander tails, claimed to see the breaking of microscopic connections under some shock treatments. Gellhorn, on the contrary, interpreted shock effects in terms of the autonomic nervous system and endocrines, and these views are again before us, with the renewed emphasis by Dr. Sawyer that particular brain regions require attention.

This may sound as if I'm saying that no progress has been made, which obviously is false. What I am trying to say is that, until a certain level of factual achievement is attained, one is compelled to guess as to the meaning of it all, and that the guesses are likely to cycle in the same general circuit. When the facts finally reach a critical point for theoretical explosion, or crystallization, there is no longer any possibility of toying with other guesses and, at least for a few decades, only the one interpretation seems tenable. I am inclined to think that, in the whole area of neurochemistry and neural metabolism, we are rapidly approaching a point where some present guesses will become reasonable certainties and many others will be excluded. In the meantime, it still remains unfortunately true that clinical experience is ahead of laboratory analysis. Some of the most important things found in this area have resulted from accidental· observations and empirical experiments of clinicians. It is not quite yet possible for the laboratory worker to build his facts into a coherent and elaborate scheme of how the nervous system really works.

DR. BERNARD B. BRODIE: Today's discussion has been especially interesting to me because it has raised in my mind the question of why insulin-shock treatment and reserpine should both benefit patients with mental illness.

What I have heard leaves me with the feeling that it is not yet possible, on the basis of available data, to formulate a useful working hypothesis that will explain the therapeutic effectiveness of insulin shock—at least on a biochemical-physiological level.

Despite the fact that insulin causes convulsions and reserpine elicits sedation, the two substances induce in animals a number of responses in common: 1) Depletion of catechol amines from the adrenal medulla through control sympathetic stimulation. 2) Lowering of catechol amines in brain. In addition, the acute administration of reserpine can, like insulin, result in the release of ACTH. Whether or not these effects are concerned in the therapeutic action of the substances in mental disease is not known.

It is provocative that insulin shock lowers glutamic acid in brain, as pointed out by Dr. Williamina Himwich, since glutamic acid is a precursor of γ-aminobutyric acid which may have a role in the brain as an inhibitory hormone.

One observation which suggests that changes in levels of brain neurohormones may be involved in experimental convulsions is the well-known observation that reserpine enhances experimental convulsions in animals. We have found that raising the brain levels of norepinephrine and serotonin by giving monoamine oxidase inhibitors, antagonizes electroshock and metrazol convulsions. The effect of monoamine oxidase inhibitors on insulin convulsions should be studied.

DR. FREEMAN: I do not have any theory but I would like to ask Dr. Brodie and Dr. Williamina Himwich about the role of adrenaline in mental disease. We have insulin coma therapy which improves psychotic conditions and produces an excessive amount of adrenaline in the blood and presumably in the brain. On the other hand, there is lysergic acid which also stimulates the sympathetic nervous system and produces a pseudopsychotic state in normals. I would like to ask either of you to explain this contradiction.

DR. B. BRODIE: As a result of the administration of large doses of reserpine, adrenaline is liberated from the adrenal gland. Nonadrenaline in the brain is also eliminated. Therefore, the effect is to liberate enormous amounts of free catechol amines. But after the catechol amine stores are depleted, the secondary effect is the lack of nonadrenaline in the brain and the catechol amines in the adrenal gland.

DR. HAROLD G. WOLFF: My associates, Dr. Henry Dunning and Dr. Heloise Hough, made studies several years ago (1937 and 1939) on the relative vascularity of the various parts of the cat's brain, and came to the conclusion that within the neuraxis, neural surface area, oxygen consumption and vascularity vary directly in magnitude. Their observations were supported by the analyses of oxidase activity of nerve tissue by Campbell (1939). His data on the relative oxidase content of the dorsal root ganglion and the sympathetic ganglion were especially pertinent.

In both instances the cell bodies were rich in oxidase, but the intercellular nerve tissue of the sympathetic ganglion was far richer in oxidase than was the intercellular tissue of the dorsal root ganglion. Since glia contain no oxidase and the sympathetic ganglion is rich in terminal arborizations as compared with the dorsal root ganglion, it follows that the oxygen consumption is greater where the neural surface area is greater. It was also apparent that the vascularity was usually greater when the oxidase content was richest.

On the basis of their studies on relative vascularity of various parts of the nervous system, both Dunning (1937) and Hough (1939) concluded "because of the presence of dendrites and terminal arborizations of axons (structures having a great neural surface area) that a tissue containing these structures received a maximal blood supply." Since the synapse is among the structures in the neuropil, it was suggested that the synapse shares in this rich blood supply.

Now today we have heard again a review of such a hierarchy in the utilization of glucose and the effects of hypoglycemia. Is this earlier postulate of the relation between vascularity, i.e. blood supply, and total cell surface being restated, or are we now being asked to reconsider this matter and to suppose that one part of the brain regardless of synapse number has a greater glucose need than another part?

It would be much simpler if we could simply reduce this use of glucose and oxygen in the blood to the maintenance of cell membranes and not have to go into peculiarities of cell structure.

My second comment has to do with the very provocative suggestion reaffirmed by Dr. Williamina Himwich's observations that the change in the cell permeability is associated with hypoglycemia. For some time now we have been working on a proteolytic enzyme in the spinal fluid of patients. We find that individuals with degenerative or inflammatory disease of the nervous system have an increase of some proteolytic enzymes, and to our surprise and considerable excitement we also find that patients with schizophrenia have an increase in proteolytic enzymes.

This enzyme system is capable of combining with human serum or globulin to produce polypeptides which have a number of interesting properties, many of which resemble those of the vasodilator polypeptides derived from plasma proteins by Keele, et al.; and of "bradykinin," the name given by Rocha e Silva, et al. to the substance or substances produced on incubation of certain snake venoms or trypsin with serum, plasma or plasma globulins. Electrophoretic studies of serum proteins incubated with cerebrospinal fluid have shown that the enzyme attacks the alpha and beta bands. We therefore need to open up a new kind of questioning about the nervous system in schizophrenics, not that this protease elevation that we are able to measure is specific for schizophrenia, but that it indicates again that the schizophrenic brain is functioning in an unusual biochemical way. Perhaps what we are picking up are some of the epiphenomena that are the "ashes" of the process involved. It is conceivable that insulin is augmenting the reconstructive process of this altered metabolic state.

DR. W. HIMWICH: I want to comment on the last part of Dr. Wolff's suggestion first.

I think certainly you were right and that is one thing we have thought about. Incidentally in animals and humans too, if a high fever is produced and maintained for a long period of time, we also get changes in the permeability of the brain.

To get to your first question about the hierarchy of the parts of the brain, I would not want to say that we understand what this means. Certainly we must consider the number of synapses and capillarity. However, there are studies from some laboratories suggesting that gray cells *in vitro* from different areas of the brain have intrinsically slightly different rates of metabolism. One thing that we would like to be able to do would be to remove the longitudinal system that Dr. Sawyer was talking about, and work with those as well as the horizontal one.

DR. CHARLES H. SAWYER: I would like to comment that the lesions in the vertical organization that we mentioned do have a very high oxygen requirement, and that the reticular formation for instance, is depressed very rapidly by anoxia just as it is by drugs and chemicals.

The cortex of course has a very high oxygen requirement and I think there we perhaps will have to differentiate between intrinsic activity and evoked activity coming up from the afferent columns. It may be that we can pick up evoked activity at a time when the intrinsic activity of the cortex is completely gone.

DR. JOHN DONNELLY: I would like to give an account of some of the experiences we have had both in our clinical work and in our laboratories under Dr. Malcolm Gordon.

I had wondered for some years whether the therapeutic effects of insulin coma were in fact due to the occurrence of coma at all. Insulin after all is a substance which has marked effects on protein metabolism concurrently with the changes in glucose metabolism. We evaluated the amino acid nitrogen in the blood and found that with increasing doses of insulin there was a progressive fall in the amino acid which did correlate with the drop in the blood glucose. In fact the pattern of the curve of the amino acid nitrogen was such that an analysis for amino acid nitrogen in a blood sample enabled the laboratory to tell whether the patient was in coma.

Following this we administered glucose intravenously in order to maintain the fasting blood glucose level. We establish first the coma dose so that the patient has one definite coma, then increase the dose of insulin to a level to insure the equivalent of coma dosage and have studied the amino acid nitrogen changes in the blood. We have found that with blood glucose maintained at the fasting level, the patient clinically remains oriented and in contact; he has none of the effects of hypoglycemia but the amino acid nitrogen drops over the 3 to 4 hour period in exactly the same manner and to the same level as when the patient is going into coma.

With regard to the blood-brain barrier I do not think there is a passive transfer through the barrier, in agreement with Dr. Williamina Himwich. We also found fluctuations in the amino acid nitrogen in the C.S.F. which were independent of changes in the blood. The amino acid nitrogen in the blood may drop to 50 per cent of the fasting level whereas in the spinal fluid there are variations in the amino acids, some increasing 150 per cent, others decreasing.

Thus we believe that any changes which occur in or through the blood-brain barrier are on a dynamic basis; that these changes are not due to simple diffusion or osmotic pressure. Such processes might be important in ordinary insulin coma since the energy required to maintain concentration gradients of amino acid is compromised by the absence of glucose. In our experiments, however, glucose was present so that the normal enzymatic mechanisms could function. There is a positive dynamic change within the enzyme systems, probably within the cell membrane.

DR. W. HIMWICH: I would certainly like to agree with Dr. Donnelly. The only trouble is that we don't really have any good evidence for it.

DR. DONNELLY: No, the only evidence there is suggests that the change is not a simple one. The evidence indicates that all the amino acids decrease in the blood, but in the cerebrospinal fluid some increase and others decrease. Therefore it is not a matter of osmotic pressure.

DR. CAMERON: I'd like to make a comment on something that Dr. Williamina Himwich said in regard to memory. She made the suggestion that the memory traces laid down in terms of the schizophrenic process tend to be lost due to biochemical changes.

There are two points that I should like to make. They are both derived from electroshock work, but I think they are applicable to the insulin coma field as well. The first is that any hypothesis must take care of the fact that memories tend to be re-established after having been lost. They can be re-established, but they may not all be re-established.

The second point is drawn from observations which we have carried out during the last year or so which seem to indicate that the amnesia which is produced by massive electroshock, is differential; that is, while there may be a complete amnesia for, shall we say, the whole period of the stay in hospital, for a period of varying duration prior to this complete amnesia there is a differential amnesia. By differential amnesia is meant that those events which have nothing to do with the schizophrenic experience tend to be reasonably well remembered, whereas those events which are with reference to schizophrenic experience tend to be forgotten.

An illustration might be something like this. Let us say that two months before coming into hospital the patient already had delusions of persecution by the Treasury Department, and at the same time he made a journey for some other purpose entirely to New York City. Now, he would probably remember the journey to New York City, but forget entirely the delusions about the Treasury Department which he had entertained at that time. We have wondered about this, and our speculation is that the differentiation is not on a biochemical basis at all but, rather, comes about as follows: memories tend to be recovered more easily when they are congruent with the ongoing conceptual framework of the individual. After he is well again, the memories of those schizophrenic experiences which he had when he was sick do not easily fit into his now normal, day-to-day conceptual framework and hence will tend to be excluded. In contrast, those experiences of a normal nature which he had during the period of his schizophrenic illness will be perfectly capable of fitting into his current conceptual framework and hence can be quite easily remembered.

In considering this idea it is, of course, necessary for us to bear in mind the rather simple observation which our rather shorthand method of categorizing events causes us to forget, namely, that the schizophrenic individual does actually have a great deal of perfectly normal thinking. There is a high degree of probability that he will wash his hands, shave himself, eat his morning bacon and eggs, and recognize his friends in terms of normal functioning rather than in terms of schizophrenic thinking.

CHAIRMAN HIMWICH: I remember that when we were both members of the faculty of Albany Medical College you pointed out that the patients in insulin hypoglycemia treatment, while out of environmental contact, could still be awakened for a moment or so and sometimes even respond rationally to a question before returning to deep coma.

DR. O. H. ARNOLD. We were able to terminate the coma using only glutamic acid, pyruvic acid or succinic acid administered intravenously. Termination of prolonged coma was also accomplished by this method when high doses of glucose or fructose were completely unsuccessful, and also when adrenaline and noradrenaline failed to exert a satisfactory effect. With the use of C 14 labelled succinic acid we were able to demonstrate that the blood-brain barrier was passed, and that the substance had penetrated into some ganglion cells. The C 14 activity was found in all components of the "Krebs" cycle in the brain substance of a mouse. In another instance, brain substance from a lobotomized patient was examined by means of the CO scintillator counter method. We again found radioactivity was present in the brain tissue. The function of the blood-brain barrier was tested with Fluorscin and the result indicated normal function in both instances.

DR. FINK: I wondered if I could ask Dr. Donnelly what changes in behavior were observed in his experiments.

DR. DONNELLY: We have been unfortunate in some ways in that for us to build up a good list of patients takes a long time, but with regard to the clinical outcome—

DR. FINK: Any change in behavior in the different kinds of treatment?

DR. DONNELLY: Well, we have had six patients who have completed a course on this particular regime. We started only about two years ago so we do not have very good follow-up figures—only on six patients so far. Two of the six patients returned to college this year; one went back to work and a fourth returned home. The two other patients are still in hospital—one is more or less stationary.

DR. FINK: And of the six patients were any of them followed by any other courses of treatment such as drugs, electro-shock?

DR. DONNELLY: No, none of the four patients who left the hospital was on any other treatment. The other two had different types of treatment including modified electro-shock and tranquilizing drugs. We are not claiming anything very great with these figures but at least they do raise the question in our minds whether the coma treatment would have produced a greater number of remissions.

Our question is: Is the effect of insulin in schizophrenia due to its protein effect rather than the glucose effect?

DR. BRODIE: I would like to remark about the effect of insulin on the blood-brain barrier. Can we define this barrier precisely enough to be able to state that insulin changes its permeability on the basis of the change in penetration rate of a single substrate. It is probable that the penetration of lipid insoluble substrates like glucose and certain electrolytes requires a number of specialized carrier mechanisms, and that one of these mechanisms may be affected. Perhaps it is better to simply state that after insulin shock, the penetration of such and such a substrate is increased or decreased.

CHAIRMAN HIMWICH: I am sure everyone will agree with your remarks on the blood-brain barrier. The term blood-brain barrier is not adequate without qualifying statements. We must know the particular substance which is involved in this exchange between blood and brain as well as the conditions under which the exchange takes place.

The concept of the five phyletic layers has pragmatic

value. In general, it facilitates one kind of analysis of behavior. More specifically in regard to our present topic, it helps physicians in estimating the depth of coma, and, therefore, aids treatment procedures.

The longitudinal concept has been emphasized by Dr. Sawyer. There is still another concept: based on the different susceptibilities of brain cells in various areas to noxious substances, a viewpoint which cuts across both the longitudinal and horizontal method of behavioral analyses. Each viewpoint is helpful and each adds part of the truth to the total picture.

DR. RALPH GERARD: Two or three factual points, stirred up by Dr. Donnelly's comments, and by Dr. Brodie's, might be worth getting into the record.

I think it is very likely true that even in the presence of glucose the primary fuel of the brain is not carbohydrate but some of the amino lipoidal substances on which the Geigers are working, partly while I was still directing the laboratory at U. of Illinois. By chemical analysis in brain perfusion experiments and by visual study of microsomes in tissue culture, even with adequate nutrition, the microsomal lipo-proteins decrease under electrical, chemical or physiological excitation and are restored rapidly afterwards. Glucose may well be the essential mediate fuel but not the immediate one under most conditions.

Another finding in this earlier work was that the entrance of glucose into the brain may well depend on the presence of one or two substances produced in the liver. This comes back to the other argument, about the blood-brain barrier. Of course this is not a simple thing. What is important is that there is something, beside the cell membranes of neurones and interposed between the plasma and the brain mass, which behaves like another cell membrane. Moreover, this extra penetration barrier seems to become more permeable under abnormal conditions. With disturbed metabolism, in hypoxia and the like, glutamate and glucose may penetrate more readily; and substances given therapeutically may sometimes reach their target when there is a specific lack. I am intrigued with Dr. Donnelly's finding of low plasma amino acid nitrogen in hypoglycemic coma, in connection with these points.

Chapter 6

SUMMARY

CHAIRMAN HIMWICH: I shall include my discussion of Dr. Gerard's remarks in my final summary. You realize that so much of importance has been said, that it is impossible for me to cover the entire field. I shall, however, pick out a point here and there, especially if it has clinical significance.

First, in regard to the phenomenon of prolonged coma. It may be said that by taking into consideration the warning signs of the approaching depression in the vital medullary centers as indicated by the longitudinal concept, it is usually possible to avoid the prolonged coma.

Next, Dr. Gerard has said that some of Dr. Geiger's work reveals that noncarbohydrate substances can be oxidized in the brain. This is in accordance with Dr. Geiger's observations that noncarbohydrate substances are oxidized by the brain and under normal circumstances are simultaneously resynthesized in that organ.

But, Dr. Geiger says the energy for resynthesis can come only from carbohydrate oxidation. In other words, glucose can supply energy for the function of the brain and for the maintenance of brain structure, and noncarbohydrate substances can supply energy only for the function of the brain and not for its maintenance.

I remember a pithy remark of Professor Sir Joseph Barcroft. He said that the lack of oxygen not only stops the machine, but wrecks the machinery. We can say the same for too prolonged hypoglycemia. It not only stops brain function, but also damages brain structure.

First to be affected, as my wife said, are the energy-dependent enzyme systems, and then other components of brain structure, all oxidized to yield energy.

In the earlier stages of hypoglycemia it is easy to restore the brain by the administration of glucose, but if the damage is severe, enzymatic systems are destroyed, glucose can not be utilized, and then irreversible coma supervenes.

Dr. Gerard remarked that our philosophical conceptions remain approximately the same until the acquisition of many new facts. This is borne out by my wife's idea of templates being destroyed. The templates are formed of the very substance of the brain including nucleoproteins. The idea goes back to one of Dr. Sakel's.[1] He concluded that the anatomic substrate of schizophrenic thinking was more vulnerable than the older more rugged normal behavioral mechanisms. This idea has an even longer history, for Hughlings Jackson pointed out that the more highly developed, the more recently acquired brain functions are more susceptible to adverse influences than are the older ones.

I shall next consider Dr. Bennett's discussion on the contra-insulin system. We can all agree with him that the changes seen during treatment, the variations in the dosage of insulin required, can be imputed in large part to alterations in the contra-insulin mechanism including the anterior pituitary, the adrenal cortex, the adrenal medulla. But there is another kind, that of insulin resistance observed in some schizophrenic patients who have not received insulin. Not every schizophrenic patient shows this resistance. Schizophrenia, however, is not a homogeneous disease entity but represents a group of disorders.

Comparatively recently an objective method to study insulin resistance was developed. The diaphragm of a rat is used for this test. The diaphragm is placed in a Warburg respiration chamber and the consumption of glucose is followed. When insulin is added to the fluid in which the diaphragm is suspended, glucose is utilized faster. The addition of the pituitary growth hormone, corticosteroids or adrenaline slows glucose uptake. If the serum of a healthy person is added to this test, glucose consumption is accelerated.

Now it is very striking that with the sera of some schizophrenic patients this increase of glucose consumption is interfered with. There is something in the blood of some schizophrenics that diminishes the use of glucose by the diaphragm. One lead for an explanation comes from a reference in Dr. Bennett's paper, the work of Berson and his group,[44] in which they showed that some diabetic patients who have been receiving insulin for three months or longer developed a substance in their blood capable of binding insulin. This substance proved to be a gamma globulin that binds insulin in a sort of loose complex. The insulin is, therefore, held in this complex and rendered unavailable for the use of the body, possibly because its size prevents rapid passage through the capillary wall. This is one cause of insulin resistance.

A group working in Norway, Haavaldsen, Lingjaerde and Walaas,[2] report further observations on the rat diaphragm. They found that a fraction of the sera, an α_1-globulin of 4 of 9 schizophrenic patients caused an inhibition of the glucose uptake by the diaphragm.

In view of the interest in protein fractions of the serum, and especially the work performed at New Orleans by Dr. Heath and his associate on the role of ceruloplasmin, the Norwegian investigators also studied the effects of that substance. Ceruloplasmin has a similar if weaker effect to diminish glucose utilization but ceruloplasmin is an α_2-globulin fraction. The thought arises that this contra-insulin substance which appears after long series of injections of insulin in a non-schizophrenic, also occurs but without insulin treatment in some schizophrenics. Such a suggestion is in accordance with the statement made by Dr. Sawyer that there may be chemical differences between schizophrenics and nonschizophrenic individuals.

Finally I should like to take a leaf out of Dr. Sawyer's book on a subject that was touched on several times, namely the similarities among certain successful therapies for schizophrenia and other psychotic conditions. It was mentioned by Dr. Sawyer in his discussion of the subcortical electro-encephalograph changes observed in the similar treatment. This suggestion was also offered by Dr. Brodie in regard to brain neurohormones.

In general, the successful treatments of schizophrenia affect rhinencephalic structures in many ways. The rhinencephalon as you know is probably the anatomic substrate of the emotions, and is involved in the physiology of emotion. The Papez' circle includes subcortical rhinencephalic brain structures and also has cortical representations. When a component of the rhinencephalon, the hippocampus, is stimulated it gives rise to impulses which pass through other rhinencephalic areas to attain the cingulate gyrus. This functional circle is completed in fibers leaving that structure and returning to the hippocampus. The amygdaloid nuclei and the septal region are also involved in the function of Papez' circle. Specifically, seizure patterns of brain waves are observed in the hippocampus and amygdaloid nuclei during hypoglycemic convulsion in animals as mentioned by Dr. Sawyer. Convulsive patterns in these areas must surely interfere with their normal functions. During hypoglycemia Papez' circle may, therefore, be stopped by the failure of these two rhinencephalic components. Whether or not the cessation in function of the Papez' circle is necessary for the correction of the abnormal symptoms[3] it is still pertinent to point out that the Killams found similar convulsive patterns in the amygdala and hippocampus of cats injected with reserpine.[4] Preston[5] has also demonstrated that chlorpromazine produces convulsive brain waves in rhinencephalic structures. There are other similarities among these successful treatments as mentioned by former speakers. It was the brilliant intuition of Dr. Sakel, however, that led him in this correct direction. It will require much more work of basic and clinical nature before we will be able to evaluate the full significance of his great contribution.

References

1. Sakel, Manfred. "Schizophrenia." Philosophical Library, New York, 1958.
2. Haavaldsen, R., Lingjaerde, O., and Walaas, O. Disturbances of carbohydrate metabolism in schizophrenics. Confin. Neurol., *18:* 270, 1958.
3. Himwich, H. E. Psychopharmacologic drugs. Science, 127:59, 1958.
4. Killam, E. K., and Killam, K. F. "Brain Mechanisms and Drug Actions." W. S. Fields, Ed. (Thomas, Springfield, Ill., 1957), 71-78.
5. Preston, J. B. Effects of chlorpromazine on the central nervous system of the cat: a possible neural basis for action. J. Pharmacol. Exper. Therap. 118:100, 1956.

Part Three

CLINICAL RESEARCH

AND FOLLOW-UP STUDIES

Chapter 7

INSULIN TREATMENT IN ENGLAND AND
ITS RELATION TO OTHER PHYSICAL THERAPIES

WILLIAM SARGANT

I know my fellow countrymen in Great Britain would wish me, first and foremost, to take this opportunity of paying a very sincere tribute on their behalf to the memory of the late Manfred Sakel. Whatever place his insulin-coma treatment of schizophrenia will finally occupy in our future treatment methods, there can be no doubt at all that his name will always rank very high amongst those who have completely revolutionized psychiatric thought and treatment in our present day and generation. Sakel's discovery, along with Meduna's introduction of convulsive therapy, Moniz's leucotomy, and, more recently, the advent of all the new tranquilizing drugs, has completely altered the whole outlook and practice of psychiatry in my country. And it was Sakel's work which provided the first real breakthrough in this whole recent striking advance of the physical therapies in our specialty.

Use in England

I have been asked today to talk specifically about the use of Sakel's insulin-coma treatment in England, and how we related it there to the use of all the other physical methods of treatment now at our disposal in psychiatry. To get matters in proper perspective I think it is important to go over, very briefly, the history of the introduction of Sakel's method into England. Naturally, his first claims were greeted with considerable scepticism, and it was only when several psychiatrists from Great Britain went to visit him in Vienna, and actually saw the results being achieved, that interest began to be aroused in this new and then rather alarming therapy. An early and stimulating report on Sakel's method, published by Dr. Isabel Wilson of the British Board of Control, soon gave it respectability in the eyes of the then sometimes conservative administrators of English mental hospitals. Very soon, pioneers such as Freudenberg from Vienna, were being specially brought over to England to help to get insulin treatment started at such places as Moorcroft House. Russell at Hanwell, Pullar-Strecker at Edinburgh, and others, also began to introduce Sakel's method in other parts of Great Britain. I myself took up the practice of insulin-coma treatment shortly afterwards, in 1938. It is now, in fact, twenty years since I first started to use this treatment at the Maudsley Hospital together with Dr. Russell Fraser, and I have subsequently used it ever since in all the psychiatric hospitals and clinics where I have worked. This has given me a long continuity of personal experience with this method.

Right from the start, one saw patients starting to get better at the Maudsley Hospital with insulin-coma treatment, who might have been treated psychotherapeutically for months before, and on whom every other method of treatment available at that time had been tried, without any success at all. Whenever I hear people casting doubts on the value and efficacy of insulin-coma treatment of schizophrenia, I generally expect to find somebody who has either strong and limiting psychotherapeutic prejudices, or who has spent far too little time working and observing for himself in an actual insulin-coma ward. For one had only to watch then some of the startling remissions that were being obtained so quickly by this treatment, compared to the older long and more drawn-out spontaneous recoveries—which could be so painful to the patient and doctor alike—to realise how valuable Sakel's method was to become as one of the means at our disposal of speeding up remission in recent and recoverable schizophrenic illnesses, and in perhaps stopping some of these unfortunate patients from slipping into prolonged and avoidable chronicity.

Insulin had started to become fairly widely used in England in 1939, when electroshock treatment was developed by Cerletti and Bini in Italy as a substitute for cardiazol—and World War II also broke out in Europe. Claims began to be made that insulin-coma could be replaced by the use of electroshock, and such claims were too often based on crude, short-term statistics, rather than on a shrewd clinical comparison of both treatments at the bedside by those actually using both of them. There was also a great shortage of medical and nursing staff in mental hospitals in England after the start of World War II; and this, together with the temporary vogue for electroshock, meant that insulin-coma treatment suffered a severe setback.

However, I am glad to say that during the whole of World War II some clinicians managed to keep insulin units fully functioning. I well remember some of my own patients, who were on insulin-coma therapy during the Battle of Britain, coming to me and saying they did not mind going on with insulin treatment, but they did object to being asked to go into coma on days when our hospital was being subjected to daylight bombing. This perfectly valid objection helped towards the development of a new modified form of insulin treatment by Dr. Craske and myself. Later on in the war this became very popular in the treatment of the acute battle neuroses, and still remains widely used in the neuroses in peacetime practice. The reason why I and others kept on with the insulin-coma treatment in schizophrenia in England, at a time when so many were giving it up, was because insulin treatment often seemed to produce much better clinical remissions than when electroshock was used alone, despite what short-termed statistics suggested. And one should always refuse to be impressed by psychiatric statistics that fail to make clinical sense. I am glad to say that in England the wave of enthusiasm for the routine use of electroshock alone in the treatment of schizophrenia was fairly quickly over. But it went on long enough to leave a wastage of patients who may have slipped into quite unnecessary chronicity, and some consequently needed leucotomy later on.

At the end of World War II, and with the return of mental hospitals to something approaching normality, insulin started to be used in every public, or what you would call State mental hospital, in my country. I have recently made a written enquiry of 67 psychiatric hospitals in the southern part of England, which I shall refer to again later on in my paper. It seems that every hospital except one private mental hospital and two neurosis centres in this area have been using Sakel's insulin-coma treatment of schizophrenia during the last ten years, and I have no doubt that this finding is generally applicable to the whole of the country. The use of insulin by the equivalent of practically every state hospital in England is, of course, in very marked contrast to the American scene since World War II. Here very many state hospitals have not been using it at all, and patients have, I think, often been sacrificed on the altar of the supposed efficacy of long courses of electroshock. I believe that much better results are obtained more humanely in many patients by a far wider routine use of insulin-coma, combined with much smaller amounts of electroshock when needed, and I think this viewpoint is now also held by the majority of my fellow countrymen working in this field.

Clinical Indications

What then in England have we found clinically, over the past twenty years, to be the main indications for the use of insulin-coma therapy in the treatment of schizophrenia? Well, there has been a body of opinion in Britain for many years now which believes that every possible recoverable schizophrenic deserves a trial of insulin therapy, combined with electroshock if needed. The disease has seemed to many clinicians to be much too serious a one to leave any single stone unturned which may help to produce as early a remission as possible, and to diminish the chances of avoidable deterioration and chronicity. Confirmation of this viewpoint has now been forthcoming in an unexpected way. Dr. Freudenberg and his colleagues at Netherne Hospital, while examining the hospital's chronic schizophrenic population, found recently that, of all the 1,345 patients who had been given insulin-coma treatment at the hospital from 1942 to 1956, only *one* patient having combined insulin-coma and electroshock treatment had drifted into and remained in the lowest hospital category (Grade 5) as regards the presence of chronic schizophrenic personality deterioration. Freudenberg reported that the patients who had had combined insulin and electroshock were, in fact, found to predominate in the highest levels of social functioning in the hospital (Grade 1), and were very scarce in the lower levels. In some way it seems that the combined use of insulin and electroshock at Netherne prevented the extreme degrees of schizophrenic deterioration often seen with all other physical treatments, and where physical treatments have not been used. And it was thought very unlikely that this particular finding could be solely due to chance.

But it is not always easy to provide insulin and electroshock for every schizophrenic who might possibly benefit from it, and I, like many others, have mostly confined the use of insulin-coma treatment to patients whose illness was of less than two years' duration. One also likes to see the patient's general personality fairly well preserved; for once affective splitting has occurred between thought and emotion, and the emotional tone has become markedly incongruous, and there are also hallucinations present, then the outlook for insulin-coma treatment generally becomes very much poorer; especially is this the case when this kind of symptomatology is accompanied by the presence of a poor asthenic bodily physique. On the other hand, a strong muscular physique has proved a favourable prognostic factor, and I agree with those who have found that a large gain in weight under treatment is often of good prognostic import. Personally, I have never seen a lot of good come from the treatment of even acute schizophrenic patients with insulin-coma who have not gained any weight during their illness, though this is not, of course, a completely hard and fast rule.

I think it can be argued that many of the early cases that get well with insulin would get well spontaneously anyhow if left a long enough time to do so. And, of course, many excellent insulin remissions do relapse again later on. There is hope, however, that, since the advent of maintenance chlorpromazine therapy, some of these insulin relapses may be avoided, and this so far does seem to be happening clinically. One of the greatest advantages of insulin-coma, or of insulin-coma combined with electroshock, has always seemed to be that not only is the speed of remission greatly increased, but so often the quality of the remission is so very much better. This was one of the very first things I noticed in my own patients when starting insulin therapy twenty years ago. Furthermore, Polonio in Portugal has shown that insulin is capable of helping patients who, without it, would have very little chance at all of ever achieving any sort of remission. In other words, although many fewer patients with bad prognostic features and poor body-build finally do well with insulin-coma, nevertheless some are helped who would never have had any chance of remitting spontaneously without it. This is in marked contrast to Polonio's other findings in patients with a better prognosis for spontaneous remission. Recovery generally occurs here anyhow; insulin serves only to accelerate the processes of normal recovery, and so saves weeks or months of suffering for the patients concerned.

I, too, like others in my country, have found insulin generally best used combined with electroshock treatment, which should be given in light coma or deep sopor. I am sure that if insulin is used alone without electroshock fewer good results are obtained, especially if depressive or stuporose features are present in the total picture. Many of us have also found the occasional case in which insulin-coma combined with cardiazol achieves success, where insulin-coma alone, or combined insulin-coma and electroshock, have failed. And, of course, we all know of patients who, having failed with ordinary comas, and with insulin and electroshock combined, do finally stage a dramatic remission when a temporarily irreversible coma occurs, and the patient can be resuscitated from this sometimes alarming complication.

The manner in which insulin-coma is given is also of the very greatest importance. Unfortunately, some hospitals in my country allow insulin-coma treatment to be mostly given and supervised by nurses. Light comas, only sometimes amounting to sopors, may then be used. It is quite impossible to compare the results of this sort of insulin-coma unit with other units run by trained doctors, especially when these have spent the time needed to learn how to take patients really deep into coma, and have become confident enough to run risks when necessary. Again, one of the other drawbacks in my country is that insulin-coma treatment is too often handed over to untrained doctors who are just starting their training in psychiatry; these are again afraid of giving deep comas because they are quite inexperienced in them. I am sure that some of the bad results obtained are due, in fact, to the treatment being badly done. The general impression, too, is that the giving of modified insulin treat-

ment alone is of very little value at all in the treatment of
early acute recoverable schizophrenia.

The number of comas to use in any patient is still subject
to debate, but I do not think one should give more than
forty good comas if no results are being obtained. There is
certainly evidence that at least some patients do better with
longer courses than with shorter ones. But this may in part
simply reflect the fact that, with longer courses much more
weight may be gained, and gain in weight during insulin-
coma treatment can be a most useful stabiliser of improvement.

Mode of Action

There is quite a lot of evidence available now, I think,
that it is not so much the giving of the insulin itself that is
of value in treatment as the bringing about of states of both
severe brain excitement and deep coma and collapse. Recently at the Maudsley Hospital it has been suggested by
Ackner and his colleagues that the production of deep coma
by means of barbiturates rather than insulin, and then the
sudden reawakening of the patient with very large and
highly stimulating doses of benzedrine (a method which
has also been recommended for some time past as a treatment of schizophrenia in Russia) produces somewhat similar
results as those obtained with insulin. Certainly I, too, have
found the production of a lot of non-specific or abreactive
excitement during insulin-coma treatment to be very helpful. Perhaps this helps to break through the abnormal
thought patterns present more easily than when only quiet
and inert comas and awakenings are achieved. Both the
arousal of abreactive excitement in sopor, and the brain
excitement produced by the giving of electroshock in early
coma, seem equally helpful in this respect.

I cannot help feeling that Sakel's insulin-coma treatment
has several different factors contributing to its success.
There is, first of all, the breaking up of recently acquired

patterns of schizophrenic behaviour by the acute excitatory and inhibitory effects of the insulin-coma treatment on brain function. This same break-up of recently acquired brain patterns can also be brought about by other types of coma combined with other sorts of states of induced excitement, and I have discussed this whole matter in greater detail in a recent book "Battle for the Mind."

Another aspect which I feel to be important, and which I have already mentioned in this paper, is the effect of bringing about large gains in weight. Weight gains, when they occur, seem to act as a valuable stabiliser of improvement. I think electroshock alone can be helpful in achieving the first "disruptive" phase of treatment, but it can be singularly ineffective in restoring lost weight, and in providing a physique more resistant to later bodily and psychological stresses. This may also help to explain why relapse seems to be commoner when electroshock is used alone than when insulin and electroshock are combined.

Insulin Coma and the Tranquilizing Drugs

The present relation of the new tranquilizing drugs to insulin-coma treatment in England is another point which has to be discussed. Undoubtedly many more enthusiastic claims have been made for the value of the tranquilizers in the treatment of all types of schizophrenia in America than in my own country so far. This may in part be due to the fact that we have used all the other possible treatments in schizophrenia in Great Britain more intensively than in the U.S.A. As an example, although we are only a small country compared to yours, we have already done nearly 15,000 full and modified leucotomies, the majority of them in chronic schizophrenic patients. It has been found that a third of these, considered hopeless of cure, leave hospital subsequently, and many return to work of a productive nature; another third are also improved as regards their anxiety, agitation, and acute mental distress. They can then be moved from closed wards and seclusion into open unlocked ones. Another reason, already mentioned, is the very widespread use of insulin-coma in England in the early recoverable case, and the much more conservative use of long courses of electroshock which I think, in the long run, only further disorganize the schizophrenic brain rather than help it.

This does not mean that we have not had some very impressive results indeed from the new tranquilizers, such as chlorpromazine and reserpine. But many less agitated and violent schizophrenic patients remain in our mental hospitals because other treatments are so intensively used, and it is in this group that many of the good results have been reported from American State hospitals.

Before attending this Congress, I made written inquiries of 67 mental hospitals and neurosis units in the southern half of England about their use of insulin and the tranquilizers in the early recoverable patient. This seemed to provide what should be a good representative sample of the rest of the country. Very interesting findings were obtained. I have already mentioned the fact that every large public mental hospital in the south of England has used Sakel's insulin-coma treatment during the last ten years. And since the advent of the tranquilizers, only nine of these 64 mental hospitals previously using insulin have given it up entirely. Twenty-one of the hospitals reported that there has been no reduction at all in the number of patients needing insulin-coma since the advent of the tranquilizers. But there was another very substantial group of 34 hospitals in disagreement with this. Though still using insulin therapy, they reported that there had been decreases, amounting to up to 80 per cent in some hospitals, in the amount of insulin-coma used since the advent of the tranquilizing drugs. It was surprising to find out how few hospitals had, in fact, given up insulin entirely, and among the replies were several emphasizing as strongly as possible that insulin still seemed the most valuable of the clinical treatments of the early recoverable schizophrenias. With these disagreements it is obvious that we shall need a much longer period of careful observation at the bedside before becoming too dogmatic on the relative long term values of these new tranquilizers vis-à-vis the older forms of therapy such as insulin-coma, electroshock, and leucotomy.

I have had some quite interesting personal findings on this matter. In the years 1951 to 1955, 42 selected patients were admitted with schizophrenia for special investigations or treatment to the psychiatric unit at St. Thomas's Hospital. Other patients of mine were also admitted to longer stay beds at Belmont Hospital. I found that insulin-coma was used on 27 of these 42 patients at St. Thomas's, and that 14 of the 42 had for various reasons to be transferred later to mental hospitals or observation wards. With the advent of the tranquilizers, however, the whole overall picture has shown an interesting change for the better so far. It has been possible not only to admit many more cases of schizophrenia, but also to get them better more speedily. Of another 44 patients with schizophrenia, all admitted since 1956, and mostly given chlorpromazine in doses of up to 1,000 mg. a day, only 5 patients, instead of 27, have needed insulin-coma treatment. The rest did much better than was expected with varying combinations of chlorpromazine, electroshock, and modified insulin used to restore lost weight. And only two of the last 44 patients, as opposed to 14 of the first 42, needed transfer to observation wards or mental hospitals later, despite the fact that so much less coma had been used. One or two patients, who in previous attacks were given insulin-coma, got better more quickly in subsequent attacks when tranquilizers, electroshock, and modified insulin were used in combination instead.

It does seem important, if one is going to try to substitute the use of chlorpromazine for insulin-coma, to give some additional electroshock at the same time, just as one often has had to combine insulin-coma with electroshock to get the best results. And the weight should always be got back to above normal if possible by the additional use of modified insulin treatment. We have encountered none of the dangers reported in the U.S.A. in thus combining chlorpromazine with electroshock, provided that the patient is kept lying down when treatment is given, and he rests afterwards; but preferably no chlorpromazine should be given for around four hours before electroshock treatment. One possible drawback to such combined treatment is the need to keep such patients on maintenance doses of chlorpromazine afterwards to avoid what seems to be almost inevitable relapse later. However, chlorpromazine may also prove useful in preventing relapse in patients who have had insulin-coma treatment. So I am not now so sure that the need to use maintenance chlorpromazine for a year or two amounts in itself to any valid objection to the substitution of tranquilizers for deep insulin-coma if thought desirable and helpful in any particular patient.

Despite the fact that the tranquilizers may be able to replace insulin-coma in some patients, we should still be very cautious about the giving up entirely of any treatment, such as insulin-coma, which we feel will still help even a small group of patients to achieve quicker and better types of remission. One or two hospitals, in answering the inquiry, said that one of the reasons why they had stopped using insulin-coma was that they did not feel it economic now to run an insulin-coma unit for only small numbers of patients. But I feel that once one tries to measure one's treatments too much against the yardstick of pounds, shillings, and pence, it is starting on a road which would lead eventually to suggestions that euthanasia would, after all, be a far cheaper way of running our mental health services. I think we must still be prepared to pay a heavy price, if necessary, to save even one schizophrenic from the thirty years or more suffering and chronicity seen in the back wards of mental hospitals. Fortunately it seems from the inquiry that insulin-coma is proving a long time adying in England among the many clinicians who have had long personal experience of its value. Furthermore, we have certainly not found in England, as has been reported from the U.S.A., that the tranquilizers have also abolished the need for leucotomy in the treatment of schizophrenia. Certainly they have reduced the need for this operation in some patients. But satisfactory results are still being obtained with leucotomy where the tranquilizers have failed dismally to do anything but keep patients a bit quieter in a mental hospital, rather than, as with leucotomy, getting them home and possibly back to work again. We have found, however, that modified leucotomies together with the use of tranquilizers have largely abolished the need for the old, full and mutilating operations.

Conclusion

In conclusion, I believe that the whole relative importance of insulin-coma, the new tranquilizers, electroshock, and leucotomy, is now in the clinical melting-pot at the present time as regards their skilled individual and combined use in the treatment of all types of schizophrenia. Much more work needs to be done before we can be certain just where we really are. And we must continue searching for much of our information at the bedside, rather than in the statistician's office, or from the high-powered advertising of the drug houses, if we are not to be led too far astray. We have several times seen treatments put forward as possible substitutes for insulin-coma. Most of them have quickly faded away after critical bedside examination and later follow-up. Will chlorpromazine and Serpasil prove to be just such another of these temporary 'booms' which can end in such tragic 'busts' for the chronic patients that can get left behind in mental hospitals by them? I hope not, and I believe that they will turn out clinically to be real, even if somewhat limited, advances.

I believe we must go on being prepared to use all the treatments now available to us, and combine these when necessary, if we are really going to help the many schizophrenic patients entrusted to our care. And until we find a much more specific remedy for the treatment of schizophrenia, we must never deceive ourselves that any one method of treatment, physical or psychotherapeutic, is going to be sufficient to help all of our patients. Sakel's insulin-coma treatment has been of immense value in the past, and should still have a possibly more limited, but still very valuable, role in the future. And certainly the impact of Sakel's great discovery on our specialty will be with us in psychiatry for years and years to come.

References

Ackner, B., Harris, A., and Oldham, A. J. (1957) Insulin Treatment of Schizophrenia. A controlled study. Lancet, 1, 607.

Freudenberg, R. K., et al. (1957) The Relative Importance of Physical and Community Methods in Schizophrenia. Paper read at the International Psychiatric Congress, Zurich.

Polonio, P., and Slater, E. (1954) A Prognostic Study of Insulin Treatment in Schizophrenia. J. Ment. Sci. 100, 442.

Sargant, W. (1957) "Battle for the Mind." Wm. Heinemann. London.

Sargant, W., and Craske, N. (1951) Modified Insulin Therapy in War Neuroses. Lancet, 2, 212.

Sargant, W., and Slater, E. (1954) "An Introduction to Physical Methods of Treatment in Psychiatry." 3rd edit. Williams Wilkins, Baltimore.

Chapter 8

THE SAKEL METHOD IN THE ARGENTINE

GREGORIO BERMANN

The Sakel method is a favorite one in the Argentine treatment of major psychosis and especially schizophrenia, and is also employed in toxicomanias and certain psychoneuroses. It is used in its classic form, as described by its creator in 1934 in "Neue Behandlungsmethode der Schizophrenie." Even though twenty-five years have passed since then, very slight modifications have been introduced; this gives evidence of the extraordinary clinical qualities of its author.

It must be said, though, that the treatments are not always conducted with the proper technique, related to the time in which the patients are left in hypoglycemic state, to the depth of the comas, as well as to the number of the comas to be given. It is well known that very often the success or failure of the treatments by hypoglycemic shocks lies to a great extent in the training and the ability of the physician who administers them. Many deficiencies are noticed, also, because the teaching of the method is not well done. In relation to the depth of the hypoglycemic shocks, it isn't enough, as it often happens, to leave the patient in coma during half an hour or forty minutes. No standard duration of coma has been established; it has to be adapted to each case. One of the most serious points in the method is the moment in which the coma must be discontinued. "The proper timing in terminating the hypoglycemia," insisted Sakel, "is the most important part of a successful treatment." Stopping the coma before the precise moment means an incomplete treatment, and prolonging it over the time required can produce disastrous results. The procedure demands great clinical subtlety, and an almost surgical precision. While in surgery and in other aspects of medical sciences a more perfect technique is required every day, in our specialty we haven't reached a similar degree of perfection and synchronization; this is a clear demonstration of the lack of maturity of psychiatry.

On the other hand, I have seen that the treatment was not always prolonged in cases in which it was necessary, that is to say, when the seriousness or the duration of schizophrenia required it. When I was working with Sakel, I saw patients treated not just for a few months, but for six months, a year or even more. Related to this aspect, Sakel had always in mind the anxious mother who forced him to continue the hypoglycemic shocks for much more time than he had planned, fighting his own will and pessimistic impression; success crowned the treatment, surprising Dr. Sakel himself.

Among my Argentine colleagues, I have insisted upon the necessity of having always in mind Sakel's teachings, who changed his method in three types of schizophrenic reaction: (1) in the *paranoid form* a classic treatment must be used with deep comas, to the end, during one, two or more months; (2) in the *catatonic excitation*, superficial comas, with a much longer duration of the treatment than in the former form; (3) in the *passive catatonic stupor*, the method must be adapted to each case; some times metrazol shocks must be added to insulin coma; in other cases, only hypoglycemic shocks are needed, terminating the coma in the activation acme.

I will summarize some of the experiences and contributions made in the Argentine to the Sakel method, which are not new to you.

1. Better results have been obtained when the patients are well prepared, physically and psychically.

2. With Dr. Hector Lestani, we presented a paper about intentionally prolonged coma in difficult schizophrenia cases to the First International Congress of Psychiatry (Paris, 1950). We had started from the verification of the benefits resulting in some cases of accidentally prolonged comas. Doctors Mario Machado and Juan Seggiaro, from Cordoba, systematized prolonged comas, and published their papers in different reviews, in *L'Encéphale* and *L'Evolution Psychiatrique,* of France (1952). They examined the physical condition, especially of the cardiovascular and neurovegetative system, which they watched constantly. They first produced a test hypoglycemic shock. After the third hour of hypoglycemia, they gave by tube hypertonic saline solutions, which they kept giving in intervals. "Par le moyen de l'administration répetée de solutions salines hypertoniques par sondage gastrique, ils disent, nous maintenons à tout moment la reversibilité de l'état du coma, et de cette façon il n'est pas necessaire de fournir des hydrates de carbone pour obtenir le reveil du patient." (Pathogénie et prévention du coma post hypeglicemique. *L'Evolution Psychiatrique,* 1952, p. 720.) Glycemia had to be maintained between 40-50 mgm o/o, not lower. Coma was prolonged during at least twelve hours. Not more than one prolonged coma a week should be given. This procedure has been almost abandoned on account of its doubtful results, and especially on account of the risks it carried.

3. As other authors, I have verified the successful results of Sakel's method in melancholic patients, especially in the involution period, in which electric convulsive therapy had failed.

4. I have employed with very good results, Sakel's method, in states of excitement in which it was dangerous to use other drugs or methods, performing two or even

three times a day hypoglycemic shocks up to sub-coma. Thus a sort of prolonged insulinic sleep was obtained.

5. Two colleagues have told me that they haven't obtained better results than those of the classic Sakel method, with the combination of prolonged sleep and insulin comas. This method, proposed by Pogorinski (*Korsakow Journal of Psychiatry and Neurology*, 1953), combines the inhibition of protection (cortical), with the mobilization of the vegetative mechanisms of defense that are supposed to contribute to destroy and neutralize the toxic substances which are supposed to produce schizophrenia.

6. Sometimes good results have been obtained from the combination of hypoglycemic shocks and pyrotherapeutic shocks interspaced twice a week, in schizophrenias refractory to the first method only.

7. Hypoglycemic shocks have been performed after lunch without any need of increasing the doses of insulin as used on a fasting stomach (Dr. Miguel Sorin).

8. Psychomotor excitation frequently observed in the precomatose period is controlled with the use of meprobamate given an hour and a half after the insulin injection.

9. The existence of fatal cases due to the simultaneous use of the Sakel method and reserpine makes it necessary to avoid the administration of reserpine under all circumstances while hypoglycemic shocks are being given.

10. The use of hypoglycemic sulphamidic derivates that reduce in about 50 per cent the necessary dose of insulin to provoke coma is being investigated. Before, and even now, barbiturates, ganglioplegics, Ampliactil, hyaluronidase (Nelson Borelli—Coma Insulinico y Hialuronidosa, "La Prensa Medica Argentina," 1957, page 1693), were used to diminish the number of insulin units used.

11. The Sakel method in schizophrenia must be complemented by other treatments (reserpine, convulsive therapy, occupational therapy, psychotherapy, etc.).

It is not exaggerated to assert that the Sakel method is

the greatest contribution to the progress of psychiatry in the twentieth century. Not only because of the mental recoveries achieved in thousands of patients, but because it has also contributed in a most outstanding way to fill the blank that existed—and that for many still exists—between medical sciences and psychiatry. The fundamental teaching that springs forth from his method—as Sakel himself put it in his most important paper to the International Congress of Psychiatry in Paris—is that schizophrenia, and in general, major psychoses, are mental symptoms of patho-physiological states. We can speak of somatic illness, of disease of a system or of an organ, but one cannot discuss the illness of something abstract like the "mind." A mental disease is the expression of the dysfunction of an organ of a diseased system. The study of the effects and the development of hypoglycemic shocks has contributed perhaps more than any other experience to underline the organic nature of mental disease, though the abundance of psychological symptoms has contributed to theoretical confusion.

How far we are from the point of view of Jaspers, of Binswanger or the analyst Harold Schultz-Henke, who in his vague book considers schizophrenia as a form of neurosis which can be cured through psychoanalysis! In the light of facts, how strange those pseudo-scientific fantasies sound. . . . As Foster Kennedy said long ago: "No matter what the verdict of the next ten years might be over the contribution of Sakel, we will no longer be satisfied handling sick minds with philosophy and words." (G. Bermann, El mayor progreso en Psiquiatria—*Rev. Latinoam. de Psiquiatria,* Buenos Aires, 1953).

Sakel wanted to write a patho-physiologic psychiatry, that would have crowned his scientific work. His work and his clear example, his effort and his ceaseless fight for a truly scientific psychiatry will last forever, and it will throw light on the work of the future generations.

DISCUSSION

DR. KALINOWSKY: I would like to say a few words on the papers of my old friends, Dr. Hoff and Dr. Sargant. You will hear more about the technique and its use in Vienna tomorrow morning by Dr. Arnold, because Vienna continues to be the center for insulin treatment.

Dr. Sargant and I of course had many discussions and fights about certain things which are details actually. However our basic philosophy is the same. We do need all treatments and that includes insulin, electric shock, tranquilizers and of course psychotherapy with it. This is particularly expressed in the Viennese Clinic. It was debatable if electric shock should be used alone with schizophrenics. Even though I feel that some schizophrenics can be treated with electric shock alone, there is no doubt in my mind that insulin is the most effective treatment combined with electroshock or other methods. There is also no doubt in my mind that insulin treatment gives the best quality of remissions, and I think the significance of this conference with the visitors from other countries is that I hope that insulin treatment will be stressed again more in our country here.

Thank you.

(Applause)

DR. BOND: Of course I come to this session with a very general and clinical question in my mind.

In 1936 after talking with Dr. Sakel, I set up an insulin unit and that's been functioning ever since. In that roughly 781 patients showed at first a recovery rate of 68 per cent full recovery plus 8 per cent fairly good recovery. If only acute patients had been taken in, that recovery rate might easily be 85 per cent.

Now the one question in my mind, the one question I have brought to this meeting is, how do you prevent relapses?

At first we were surprised at the recovery. It kept us perhaps from following up with other methods. This was so good, why try anything else.

Our methods were given a conditional approval by Dr. Sakel. I think he gave us a 90 per cent approval.

What bothers me is perhaps something you have heard before. What is schizophrenia? I have a very definite opinion that Bleuler's schizophrenia is not that schizophrenia that we are talking about.

I was glad to hear this morning that a chemical test is under way and it would be one of the great adventures of the future if we could make a chemical test and say this is schizophrenia and this is not. I should like to see that chemical test applied to some of the artists' paintings I have seen and some of the writers whose novels and poetry I've read. Almost all our electric shock and insulin shock have been given by psychoanalysts. If there's one thing I am sure about it's done the psychoanalysts a good deal of good.

(Laughter)

The question does remain, how do you prevent relapses in the insulin treatment of schizophrenia, and that's what I hope to go back home with a better idea of.

(Applause)

DR. RAYMOND WAGGONER: It has been a great pleasure to have had the opportunity to listen to such excellent papers as were presented this morning and this afternoon. I find myself in somewhat the same position as Dr. Bond and I'd like to echo his comments.

It appears to me as I have listened to the discussions that there is much semanticism involved in the diagnosis of the cases which have been described. In other words, it may be that many of these cases would be diagnosed as schizophrenia by some but as non-schizophrenic by others. This would help to explain the high rates of recovery which were reported.

It was my good fortune several years ago to refer a patient to Dr. Sakel for treatment and to treat the patient in association with him. I was very much impressed by his contagious enthusiasm for insulin therapy and his unique ability to treat patients with this method. It is my impression that the improvement which some of his patients experienced was the result of his boundless confidence as much as by the insulin he used. To me this implies that Dr. Sakel also used a very positive form of psychotherapy in addition to the insulin coma and this, it seems to me, should be always kept in mind. Patients should receive that therapy or combination of therapies which are most valuable to that patient as is determined from our experience with them.

Thank you.

DR. SIMON KWALWASSER: As I listened to Dr. Hoff and Dr. Sargant I couldn't help but be impressed with the enthusiasm that both these men have for the treatment they are giving. I followed Dr. Bond's results in his follow-up studies and I did a similar follow-up study in 1949 on 221 patients who were treated at Rockland State Hospital. I did this follow-up when I returned from the Army so that the last patient in this study had been treated at least five years previously and the earliest patients in this group had been treated as long as ten years before.

This study of 221 patients was made up of two groups. One group was treated by Dr. Holmes who started the unit at Rockland State Hospital after having taken the course with Dr. Sakel at Wingdale State Hospital. The group that Dr. Holmes treated was essentially a group of chronic schizophrenics. Since the treatment was so new at that time and the risks unknown, the only people who requested treatment were the relatives of the chronic patients. Dr.

Holmes' group consisted of about 60 patients. The insulin treatment was discontinued for about one and one-half years and in 1940 it was started again.

I treated 160 cases between 1940 and 1943 when I left for the Army and most of these cases were more acute than the first group.

And this brings us to what Dr. Bond has just said—that the more recent cases showed quite good results. Of our 160 cases, 87 per cent showed very remarkable improvement and left the hospital. In our study ten years later only 30 per cent of them were out of the hospital. If we are going to study the efficacy of any treatment for schizophrenics, we must study the long term results. I agree with Dr. Sargant when he says that maybe if these people could have had continuous treatment, this might have made a difference in the eventual result.

When I published the results of our metrazol treatment at Rockland State Hospital, I reviewed the literature and found that over the years many different treatments had been tried for schizophrenics and frequently the observers described remarkable results (and I think they really saw what they said they saw) which were soon followed by relapses.

When I interned at the Medical Center in Jersey City, they were still under the influence of Cotton and his theory of focal infection. Patients underwent extensive surgery in attempting to remove this focus of infection. Dr. Cotton at first reported a great many improvements but by now the theory of focal infection has been completely given up.

When I went to Hillside Hospital, where one would imagine that the results with insulin would have been much better because there was a great deal more time to work psychotherapeutically with patients as well, it turned out that it did not actually work that way. Since the emphasis was so much on psychiatry the organic approach was not accepted as readily by the therapists. So I think that the attitude of the institution towards the treatment, the enthusiasm and libidinal investment of the people who are giving it makes a considerable difference in the eventual result. I think we must take into account the psychological quality of what is happening as well as the organic quality of what is happening.

DR. SARGANT: One thing, Dr. Rinkel, that I would like to say is what a pleasure it has been seeing and hearing Dr. Earl Bond here today. Earl Bond's papers made all the difference to many of us at the start of our work on insulin. His findings encouraged us to keep going when some still doubted the efficacy of insulin. I would like to pay a tribute to Dr. Bond, not only for his pioneer work in this treatment, but also on behalf of the many patients and doctors in other countries who have also been helped by his work and example.

DR. HOFF: The 173 patients reported by Dr. Arnold had been under our observation and treatment for 5 years. A little over 80% of them are more or less normal; they have been discharged from the hospital and are now working again. Approximately 13% are living with their families, but are unable to work or to fulfill their social obligations. Only the remainder—a mere 7%—are still in hospitals, in chronic observation wards. All these patients were treated by insulin shock, sometimes combined with electroshock. All were also treated by group psychotherapy and occupational therapy. Sometimes group dancing and gymnastics were used. Furthermore, the relatives were taught in groups to be able to accept the patients' returning home and to understand the problems of the patients. In comparing Doctor Sakel's original group with ours we found that in the former only 42% were cured, while the rest underwent relapses. These figures, to be sure, are not completely accurate, as this group was terribly hit by the war. Many of the patients have simply disappeared. It is interesting to note that the number of remissions and relapses in this group is the same as given in Doctor Bond's report. We therefore believe that only by a combination of biological treatment, such as insulin and electroshock, supplemented by the use of tranquilizers, by psychotherapy (which we take very seriously), by occupational therapy, by psychological training of the relatives and by teaching better social adjustment on the part of all concerned (which is the task of our social workers) are we able to prevent relapses on the part of our patients.

I repeat: we believe in a many-sided cause of schizophrenia, because we believe both in organic and functional origins. We use biological treatment such as insulin and electroshock. We believe in psychological factors and therefore we use psychotherapy on the patients. We believe, also, that the disease is activated by catastrophic reactions and domestic exigencies. We therefore also treat the relatives of the patient in group psychotherapy. Another factor relates to the social background, and we try thus to attune our social workers accordingly. Sometimes our patients come in critical situations. At times during these 5 years they needed adjustment for a few days or weeks in our hospital. But there is obviously a great difference as to whether a patient is required to stay for 5 years continuously in the hospital, or whether he need stay merely for a few days or weeks. We must accept the fact that such patients may have relapses. It naturally makes a great difference, however, if we can shorten the duration of the relapse to a few days or a few weeks and thus prevent such patients from becoming inmates in our chronic wards. We have been accused of being too enthusiastic about the biological treatment of schizophrenia. If this were not so, it would mean that we should have been deprived of welcome criticism. I worked together with Doctor Sakel when we treated his first cases. At that time we were most enthusiastic, and such enthusiasm was very necessary. To be sure, we had many disappointments. But we see now clearly what the insulin treatment of schizophrenia can give us, and what we have to add to this modality. We believe that a combination of insulin treatment with organic and psychological measures represents the most effective weapon against schizophrenia. We will continue to adapt the treatment to the different forms of schizophrenia and to the need of the patient as an individual. We have also been accused of representing forms which are certain to undergo spontaneous remissions as being true schizophrenia. I am proud to call leading psychiatrists of your country my friends, and I am conversant with their diagnostic criteria. I am sure that we in Vienna are most conservative in our diagnosis of schizophrenia. We have emerged from a time when schizophrenia was a sentence of death, and we are therefore most cautious in rendering such a diagnosis. We are definitely certain that our patients would be given an identical diagnosis in this country.

Now, one word to Dr. Sargant. In the case of some of our patients we realize fully that we cannot hope to cure them. So we attempt to adapt them. This adaptation is accomplished by chlorpromazine or by neuroleptica. In many such cases we are able to discharge the patient from the hospital. They are able to dance or to work, but if we speak with them we know they are not cured. One has the feeling of coldness, that which Rümke calls "the feeling of schizophrenia." We call this process an adaptation, but not a cure of schizophrenia.

May I conclude: Schizophrenia to us is a serious disease, and we thus feel justified in using any and every method of treatment which offers promise of improvement. We feel no particular obligation to use insulin, but up to the present time we have no truly adequate substitute. We have developed a combined treatment, and we are temporarily satisfied with it. But in this combination, the insulin treatment plays an important part. Studies in the future will indicate more accurately which cases require insulin combined with electroshock, and which require neuroleptica. Perhaps we will exchange insulin for neuroleptica in some cases. We will always be guided, however, by the individual requirement of the patient in his disease.

DR. EARL BOND: I think Dr. Hoff is giving me an answer, how do you prevent the relapse. One important thing we want to know, whether we want to send the patient back home and back to work.

Chapter 9

TRENDS IN INSULIN TREATMENT IN PSYCHIATRY

Karl M. Bowman

History of the early insulin treatment in the U.S.A.

Shortly after I became Director of Psychiatry at Bellevue Hospital in February 1936, the late Dr. Paul Schilder suggested that we start insulin treatment of some of our psychiatric patients. He pointed out that one of our psychiatric residents, Dr. Joseph Wortis, recently graduated from the University of Vienna, had gained a good working knowledge of insulin treatment from Dr. Manfred Sakel. I must admit my first reaction was one of resistance but when Dr. Schilder persisted, I went to see the late Dr. S. S. Goldwater, then Commissioner of Hospitals. Back in 1936 we were not supposed to treat psychiatric patients, and so a program of therapy had to have official approval. After considerable time and effort we finally secured this permission and began treatment on September 1, 1936.

A large room on one of the men's wards was assigned for this purpose, with Dr. Joseph Wortis in charge. Bellevue was one of the first institutions to set up a real program of insulin treatment and we had doctors visiting us not only from all over the United States but from Canada and abroad. The late Dr. Frederic Parsons, Commissioner of the N. Y. State Dept. of Mental Hygiene, arranged with me to have several doctors and nurses work with Dr. Wortis and learn this new treatment. After we had carried out this program of treatment for some time, Dr. Manfred Sakel arrived in New York. I was somewhat surprised to discover how young he was. I found him very affable and pleasant and we became very good friends. Both Dr. Wortis and I wished to have Dr. Sakel work with us at Bellevue, but I could not secure an appointment for him. Nevertheless, he would visit our ward and give us friendly help and advice. Dr. Parsons quickly seized the opportunity and persuaded Dr. Sakel to take charge of a course of training in insulin therapy at one of the New York State hospitals. I did arrange for Dr. Sakel to talk at the 1937 annual meeting of the American Psychiatric Association, at which Dr. Wortis reported on the treatment of our patients at Bellevue.

Dr. Wortis translated Dr. Sakel's book, *The Pharmacologic Shock Treatment of Schizophrenia,* whose illustrative pictures of patients receiving insulin treatment were all taken from our Bellevue series. In the introduction, Dr. Sakel expressed his thanks to Dr. Wortis for translating the book and to me for my "support of the early introduction to America of this new approach to the treatment of the psychoses." There have been many variations and many theories of insulin therapy, and it is perhaps worthwhile to trace certain trends in its use. The original use of insulin seems to be linked up closely with convulsive treatment; indeed, convulsions were considered to be desirable and such measures as forced fluids and alkalinization of patients were used to produce convulsions. Later, when convulsions were thought to be harmful, patients were dehydrated, put into an acidotic condition and even given barbiturates to prevent convulsions.

Originally Dr. Sakel felt that psychotherapy played no role and he advised discharging a patient from the hospital as soon as coma treatment was finished. In our first demonstration of cases, which we held at Bellevue shortly after his arrival in New York, Dr. Sakel seemed upset that we should show these patients to an audience and spoke of the definite harmful effects. This intrigued me since if schizophrenia was considered an organic disease and treated by physiological methods without psychotherapy, a demonstration of the patient should not be expected to harm him. In my own experience, most psychiatric patients, if handled properly, can be demonstrated to medical groups not only with no harm to them but with actual benefit. However, there still remains much resistance to giving psychotherapy to insulin patients.

Soon we heard of the use of subcoma insulin with extreme claims as to what it accomplished. There still is considerable use of subcoma insulin in this country as well as in many other countries and we also find that small doses of insulin are used in internal medicine in order to stimulate the patient's appetite and to improve his nutrition and spirits.

After a time the view about convulsions again changed somewhat with the advent of electroshock therapy, and insulin coma was supplemented with electroconvulsions. These electroconvulsions were given at the start or at the end of coma or later in the day when the patient was no longer under the influence of insulin. Some groups routinely supplemented insulin coma with electroshock if the patient did not show definite improvement within about 15 comas. Time does not permit further discussion of the many other variations of insulin treatment.

Insulin Treatment in the Orient

I have made various trips to the Orient, starting in 1947. I have been interested to note that insulin was used a great deal in these countries. In 1947, when I was in China, I found, somewhat to my surprise, that insulin treatment was being used extensively. I then learned that the U. S. Armed Forces had left a large amount of medical supplies to the Chinese government and that considerable amounts of insulin were available for psychiatric treatment, although psychiatry was sadly lacking in equipment, personnel and buildings.

In Japan in 1950 insulin was used although electroshock, because of simplicity and cheapness, was employed extensively. In 1954-55, as Visiting Professor of Psychiatry at the University of the Philippines, I found that insulin coma treatment was accepted as the most valuable treatment for schizophrenia. In my few days' stopover there about six months ago, I found it was still being used. In my visit also to the University of Indonesia at Djakarta, Java, I saw the standard type of insulin coma treatment was being given and a recent check indicates it is still being used with the standard techniques. Some use of subcoma insulin occurs mainly on medical wards for its general tonic effect. In 1955 I also visited the two medical schools in Bangkok, Thailand and found the standard type of insulin treatment was being given. This past summer I spent some three months in Bangkok working at the two medical schools and visiting the government mental hospitals, where the standard type of insulin shock treatment is in use. There, too, I saw considerable use of insulin subcoma in both schizophrenic and non-schizophrenic patients.

Present Trends in Insulin Treatment

Many variations of insulin treatment have been introduced, often with claims of increased success, but usually these variations have not been generally accepted. Many believe that it is desirable to produce comas with as small a dose of insulin as possible. The so-called zigzag method has proved a valuable way of securing coma with lessened dosage. At one time there was considerable discussion of a type of prolonged coma in which the patient was nearly brought out of coma after the usual period and then put back into a second coma. The present time has seen a marked decrease in the use of insulin, with the claim that equally good or better results can be achieved with the new miracle drugs, and that they are less dangerous, require fewer trained personnel and are therefore less expensive. Undoubtedly, one disadvantage of insulin therapy has been the necessity of prolonged hospitalization, commonly a minimum of three months, and the setting up of an insulin ward with specially trained personnel. The dangers of insulin have also been argued. The reasons for discontinuing its use are somewhat contradictory. For example treatment is said to be purely empirical; without any understanding of the benefits, if any. Yet both medicine and surgery include many empirical treatments; and the use of psychotherapy involves much bitter controversy as to what is going on and what produces the improvement in the patient.

According to a second criticism, there are no adequate convincing statistics in insulin therapy. Without trying to go into all this, one can say that a few well-controlled statistical studies have indicated the value of insulin treatment and a few other well qualified ones have raised great questions as to its value. Indeed, similar argument can be raised as to psychotherapy; although most of us believe that psychotherapy has great value there are practically no adequate statistics as to its value. We also find many contradictory reports on the use of the so-called tranquilizing drugs and one can point to certain double-blind studies that show better effects from placebos than from drugs.

The present trend in the United States seems to be a very considerable replacement of insulin by the so-called tranquilizing drugs. The proponents of insulin treatment explain the reports of poor results in insulin treatment as being due to inexperience or not enough comas or long or deep enough comas. It is interesting that advocates of the neuroleptic drugs use exactly the same arguments. Dr. Lester Margolis, for example, maintains that those who favor older therapies such as electroshock and insulin treatment do so because they have not had adequate experience with newer drugs. He states, "The fact is, that with carefully administered, vigorous, neuroleptic therapy, with skillful coadministration of ancillary medications to control side effects, with dosage individualized to the patient's needs, tolerance and clinical response, the results in all but a few cases are decidedly superior to the traditional somatic therapies." He adds: "It must be recognized that the institution of a successful psychopharmacotherapeutic program requires much more effort on the part of the therapist, consumes more of his time and is far more complex than one employing the traditional therapies." If he assumes that those treating schizophrenics with insulin do nothing but administer insulin, that might be true. However, as far as I know, all the leading proponents of insulin therapy regard it as only a part of the patients' therapy program, which includes psychotherapy and the 24-hour management of the patient's life just as in a psychopharmacotherapeutic program.

Evaluation of New Therapies

In evaluating any new therapy, one has to discount the great enthusiasm of its proponents during the early days of treatment. We have seen a whole series of somatotherapies given with tremendous enthusiasm and elaborate claims which have not held up. Electronarcosis, carbon dioxide inhalation, ether inhalation and many others could be mentioned as examples. The present enthusiasm for the neuroleptic drugs should make us very cautious about passing any final judgment at this time.

The element of personal interest of the doctors and nurses and others concerned with the treatment, the special attention given to such patients and the therapists' enthusiasm and confidence will always be important factors in any evaluation. This criticism has been made many times about insulin treatment. It should be repeated in reference to the newer drug therapies.

Insulin and the New "Miracle" Drugs

The results of insulin treatment differ in many ways from the results claimed for the new miracle drugs. A proponent of the latter claims success if he is carrying a patient on a small dose of the drug after one, two, or three years of treatment and the patient can live outside in the community. If he is questioned more closely he is likely to admit that the minute he drops this dosage, the patient regresses. In other words, this is no curative treatment. It is primarily drugging a person to make him more comfortable and make him able to adjust outside of a hospital whereas he required hospitalization before such therapy. This is very different from the technique of giving insulin therapy, wherein after a certain period the patient is completely taken off the treatment and it is hoped that insulin per se will have had a certain curative value.

There appears to be less resistance to combining intensive psychotherapy with the newer drugs than there has been in combining intensive psychotherapy with insulin treatment. It is true that there have been a few articles protesting against psychotherapy with the patient "doped by drugs" but this is the exception. I have no objection to carrying a patient under drug therapy for one or five or ten years if one can get improvement in the patient by doing this. However, I do not believe that such a result should be equated with the patient who has had insulin treatment and is now out of the hospital with good social adjustment and essential cure.

Despite the great decrease in insulin treatment in schizophrenia, I believe it still has a definite place not taken by any other treatment. More effort should be made to combine insulin treatment with some of the newer drugs rather than merely to substitute the newer drugs for insulin treatment. Very little seems to have been done in this respect. I would further recommend that the various trials of combined treatment should include insulin in both coma and subcoma doses, the newer drugs and intensive psychotherapy and rehabilitation. It is too early to make any final comparisons between insulin therapy and neuroleptic drugs; it must be a matter of years before adequate controlled studies and statistics are available.

The Future of the Insulin Treatment

One may ask about the future of insulin treatment in schizophrenia. Historically we see many great discoveries in medicine which have been epoch-making but where this new method has later been supplanted by one superior to it. A classical example of this is the discovery of salvarsan (606) by Paul Ehrlich, which was a tremendous advance in the treatment of syphilis. But while salvarsan has been almost entirely supplanted by penicillin, this detracts nothing from the great value of Ehrlich's discovery. Similarly, if insulin were completely supplanted in the treatment of schizophrenia, it would not detract from the great value of Manfred Sakel's work. Already we hear of a pill being introduced which may be superior to insulin in the treatment of certain cases of diabetes. Even if insulin should be entirely supplanted by this new pill, it would not detract from the place in medical history occupied by Banting and Best. Probably it is only a question of time before some new chemical compound is discovered which will supplant all of the present treatments of schizophrenia. As one who regards schizophrenia as primarily a metabolic disorder, I think this seems quite possible. Some degree of psychotherapy will always be necessary, even if such a physiological treatment is discovered. However, I venture to predict that the long, drawn-out intensive individual psychotherapy will not be used except in a rare case.

I feel that we are on the verge of working out the physiological bases of schizophrenia and with a better understanding of them, newer and improved methods of treatment will quickly follow. I do, however, wish to end by paying tribute to Manfred Sakel for this great step forward in the treatment of schizophrenia which he developed.

Chapter 10

INSULIN THERAPY AS COMPARED TO
DRUG TREATMENT IN PSYCHIATRY

Paul H. Hoch

I do not wish to belabor the point as to what is better—drugs or insulin. Other speakers have expressed themselves on this point. I personally feel we will have to stop juggling this issue from one side to another. The question is not to determine if drugs are better than insulin or vice versa, but the seemingly naive issue comes up—what kind of patient responds to one treatment and what kind of patient responds to the other.

This discussion as to which treatment is better has been going on for many years, but without any research and without any—I would say—goal-directed information as to what kind of patient will respond to one and what kind will respond to the next treatment method.

It is not true that insulin is superior to the drugs in all patients. We have statistics, which will not be presented at this time, but which would indicate that some patients treated with insulin and did not succeed with it, were then treated with drugs and they are now out of the hospital and successfully adapting themselves in the community. We, of course, have many patients where the reverse is true. I personally have always insisted that insulin treatment should continue and should be given. Today perhaps the only difference in the application of insulin treatment is that we do not apply it as a primary treatment, but apply it in most instances with patients who failed with treatments which are easier to administer, less expensive, less dangerous, and less cumbersome.

Therefore, insulin treatment is retained as a part of the armamentarium and I have very similar reactions to it as described by Dr. Hoff. I would like to point out, however, there are certain similarities between insulin treatment and drug treatment which have not been mentioned but which I believe can give us clues for further research.

When Sakel introduced insulin treatment he quite correctly noted that the best candidates for this treatment are patients in an acute or sub-acute state of schizophrenia. He emphasized that some chronic patients benefit from this but he definitely mentioned a time limit, namely, that if this time limit was passed then probably the outcome of this insulin treatment would not be very successful. Our statistics compiled later on would bear him out on this.

Now we have a very similar situation in the use of the drugs. When the drugs were introduced it was emphasized that they were very helpful in practically every and any form of schizophrenia. Again, however, the issue is that acute schizophrenics and sub-acute schizophrenics respond well to the drugs and many of these patients respond as well to the drugs as they have responded to insulin.

When you encounter the chronic group of patients, however, some patients respond and many patients do not. Regardless of this we are probably all entitled today to be far more optimistic about acute and sub-acute schizophrenia. However, we are not entitled, neither based on insulin, nor on drugs, nor any other treatment at our disposal, to be very comfortable about the so-called chronic form of schizophrenia.

I may add that another issue is also unsettled. How many

patients who were treated successfully with insulin or drugs in an acute state will relapse? By relapse I do not mean returning to the hospital where they are retreated and emerge again more or less in a state of adaptability to the environment, but relapse in a true sense of the word, in that these patients remain in the psychosis.

This is a fundamental issue for which we do not have reliable statistics as yet, and actually I believe all our treatments in use today for schizophrenia will hinge on this issue. If we are able to treat a patient in an acute stage successfully and this patient does not become chronic, this is one thing. However, if we are able to treat him in an acute stage and later he becomes chronic, this is an entirely different story, and it is this that remains unanswered.

Another issue which I think would be of importance to mention and which is of great interest to me is the similarity of the responses of certain types of schizophrenics to insulin, drugs, and other forms of treatment. None of the speakers here today have broken down schizophrenia into its sub-groups. They have treated schizophrenia as a broad entity. This in itself of course is a problem, but I do not believe this is the main problem. The main problem is that the different clinical variations, the different clinical sub-groups are not followed sufficiently and as painstakingly as in the past.

Sakel has already pointed out quite correctly that insulin treatment was most effective in catatonic and paranoid schizophrenia, but far less effective in hebephrenics and even less effective in the simple form of schizophrenia. The drugs show exactly the same. I believe this is a clue which should probably be studied further. Are we dealing here with disorders that are different in quality or disorders that are different in quantity, and why is one individual influenced and the other not?

I believe it is time to break down our statistics and discussions on schizophrenia into different clinical entities within the framework of this disorder so that we will be able to do better comparisons clinically, statistically, and also prognostically than we are doing today.

I personally feel that the introduction of the drugs did not obviate the treatment with insulin. On the other hand, it contributed a great deal to psychiatry which insulin and the other treatment used before were not able to do. This is simply based on the fact that today you are able to treat a large number of patients simultaneously. I am completely unimpressed by treating a hundred, two hundred or three hundred schizophrenics, when we have 50,000 or 60,000 schizophrenic patients to be treated. Any manner which would permit us to reach at least a part of this large group of patients is welcome. Today I am not considering too much whether or not an individual case is helped better by insulin or the drugs. I personally feel there are patients who respond better to insulin than to drugs. But I am interested in applying treatment or some form of treatment to many unfortunate and helpless individuals who otherwise would receive nothing. Some of these individuals respond, some respond half-way, and some do not respond at all.

Dr. Hoff brought up an important issue, and this is probably the only point where I differ in this discussion. If I understood him correctly, he implied that insulin cures where the drugs are seemingly considered symptomatic treatments which suppress certain manifestations of the psychosis; these patients actually remain the same as they were before.

Now this, of course, may be true for some patients. I am sure I would be able to furnish him with the statistics and can show him that the patient under the drug properly treated made out as well as with insulin. Again the question arises what kind of patient, in what kind of constellation should this method be used. We have to be aware of the fact that we have at our hands today several empirical treatments. We do not know how they work, nor do we know how they influence a disease structure or a group of disease structures. Actually we are still groping in the dark, and as long as we are in such a situation I personally feel, as Dr. Hoff expressed himself, that all the treatments which are at our disposal should be used judiciously. I am especially concerned with the fact that if a patient is treated with one method and fails, the treatment should not be written off, but again and again other methods of treatment should be introduced. The yield in some such patients who did not respond to one treatment but who would respond to another form of treatment is rather impressive. For that reason we want and we will re-treat the chronic schizophrenics, and the many patients, with methods of treatment even though they fail with other methods.

I feel the contribution of Sakel was not so much the insulin treatment or its technique. In my opinion Sakel's great contribution was that against a prevailing trend, he perceived, based on the observations he made, the idea that we are capable of influencing schizophrenia. From that moment on schizophrenia or dementia praecox moved into the realm of the disorders which we were able to approach with treatment, and we visualized that treatments could be conceived and applied that are very similar to those applied to any other disease. This is a major contribution because most psychiatrists were without hope and quite helpless in relationship to the treatment of schizophrenia.

I believe the second contribution of Sakel which is of great importance, was that he pointed out that schizophrenia is probably not a reaction but an organic disease, and being an organic disease, it can be also approached in the same way as other organic diseases.

I am sure that continued research will probably modify many of our present concepts, and I am also sure that ten years from now, a conference like this probably will not discuss insulin and thorazine or anything that we have at our disposal today. Nevertheless, all these developments move toward a better understanding of a disorder which was considered more or less a puzzle, and we have the feeling that even though no solution has been offered as yet, our knowledge about schizophrenia is improving rapidly. With this knowledge we will be able to apply a basic etiological treatment that is lacking today.

DISCUSSION

DR. JACK R. EWALT: Like Dr. Hoff and Dr. Sargant, in Massachusetts we too regard schizophrenia as a very serious disorder. In our treatment of schizophrenia with "everything" however I believe our experiences reflect a little those of Dr. Sargant who stated he uses everything and then he gave us figures that would indicate that his present "everything" contains less insulin, more of the tranquilizing drugs, and in the short view with equally good and maybe a little bit better results. I don't think I could epitomize our experiences any better, although as you know, we have a very carefully constructed research program going on in insulin therapy in one of our institutions.

I would agree with Dr. Hoch that our research on these patients must be done on patients much more precisely defined than a diagnosis of schizophrenia. I think you are going to have to better classify patients so that when I talk about treating a schizophrenic or a hebephrenic schizophrenic, it is more nearly the same type of patient that you are talking about as hebephrenic schizophrenia. Some of the old-timers from Massachusetts can remember the famous fights that went on between Southard and May, I believe it was, about the diagnosis of manic depressive and schizophrenia, between the two hospitals. These are still famous in our archives.

I remember when I was a resident, the incidence of schizophrenia was much higher in Philadelphia than it was in Baltimore, during the time that Bond and Strecker were interested in schizophrenia in Philadelphia, and Dr. Meyer had a very conservative attitude toward schizophrenia over in Baltimore. For a westerner these places are pretty close together.

Now this means nothing except the word schizophrenia at least as used in the United States is a very imprecise term and a very dangerous thing on which to base research about which you are going to make projections.

I would like to take a moment to talk a little about the process of cure. Now as a matter of fact, no treatment ever cured any patient of anything, if you just stop a moment. Let's take something very simple like an open belly for an appendix. We don't cure the patient of the appendix, we take it out. We deprive him of it. It is still infected in the bottle or it is normal, depending on the indications for taking it out. But we didn't cure him of appendicitis. We took the appendix out. We stitched the belly together. If all goes well nature cures the patient.

We can only provide conditions that will enable the natural curative process of nature to cure the patient.

Now if we believe that schizophrenia is due to some combination of biological, psychological and sociological disturbances, which primary and which secondary, I leave to your own debate later, but I think you will all agree that fifteen minutes after it starts, all three of these things are all bound up, with each affecting the other in important ways. It is therefore to be expected that treatment directed towards the social factors, the psychological factors or the biological factors, will probably in proper cases, when properly administered, bring about beneficial results. One should not be confused by all these contrasting claims for treatment by these very things. Probably most of them are right in this short view.

And again I think in our structuring of these problems and in making up our protocols, we have to take a much shorter view in terms of time, and what's going to happen to the thinking processes, to the socialization process, the blood chemistry with the X factor in it; what happens to these over the short term as well as over the long term, in order to have any meaning come out of this chaos.

DR. MILTON GREENBLATT: Dr. Hoch's fine presentation, delivered with his usual tranquility and understanding, has prompted me to say something that has been on my mind all day. His judicious consideration of problems in this field make my remarks at this point relevant.

We must remember that when we talk of insulin treatment, Sakel treatment or insulin hypoglycemic treatment, we are considering a complex of factors. It is not simply the injection of a measured dose of insulin and then a prolonged period of unconsciousness, but many other factors; the patient may respond to any *one* or *all* of these factors. In the morning we omit breakfast, then we bring the patient down to a special therapy unit, there is specialized personnel ready to take care of him, administer "pharmacological" therapy, look after his physical needs, and over a period of weeks form an intensive and devoted relationship. There is a nurse, aide and doctor in attendance; the patient is put to bed, induced into unconsciousness; his vital signs carefully followed; he is fed; and there is the constant expectation of improvement as well as concern for his total psychophysiological state. That day, that night and the next morning he is more or less an object of special concern because of the possibility of delayed reaction. The staff is constantly alert for signs of improvement and expects and hopes for a favorable turn in his condition.

Now, Staff may be more or less enthusiastic and devoted and this will be a factor, as Dr. William Sargant has so well stated.

Further: insulin treatment is set in the hospital organization and it occupies a place in the hospital's hierarchy of treatments. In some hospitals, it may be the *principal modality*, the one in which superintendent and staff *believe*. In another hospital, insulin treatment may be valued much less, and patients receiving insulin treatment may even be considered as "déclassé" by other patients or staff.

We have had opportunity to observe insulin treatment in one hospital when it was first valued very highly and then when it was superceded by psychotherapy, drugs and other modalities. In the first phase, a patient wrote in the hospital newspaper, expressing, I think, the atmosphere of the hospital:

> "This is the Psycho, the
>   home of the buzz and the prod,
> Where the electric shock patients
>   speak only to the insulins
> The insulins only to God."

At this time, insulin was highly valued, we had enthusiasm for it, and results seemed satisfying.

Later, however, when psychotherapy became *the* treatment of value, interest in insulin declined and so did the results.

More than this is the feeling in the community about a specific therapy and how this gets communicated to the patient. If it is a relatively *new* treatment, and the rumors suggest great promise, relatives and friends bring into the hospital an added atmosphere of hope that the patient may pick up to good advantage.

Thus, insulin coma results depend on a multiplicity of factors and it is most difficult to unravel the effect of the one from the other. Here is where more research is needed, and certainly an attitude of open-mindedness.

We must remember, too, that insulin hypoglycemia, in many respects may act non-specifically, in terms of its ability to evoke psychophysiological *stress* response. Only a part of the insulin effect, perhaps a very small part can be *specific* to hypoglycemia *per se!*

Now, with all this, let us hasten to state that even if the insulin effect were not specific, any such treatment that brings so much devoted, detailed attention to the patient, and galvanizes and inspires the psychiatric and medical public, stands as a monument to its inventor, and easily wins a place in our heart. But let this not blind us to the scientific and research questions still remaining—questions that Sakel, too, would have wanted answered!

DR. D. EWEN CAMERON: I think these discussions have been extremely interesting.

One thing that came to my mind when I listened to Dr. Hoff and Dr. Hoch is that when we achieve a major advance in medicine, we tend to couch our thinking in terms of the ongoing premises of our time. For instance, it has been a serious handicap to psychotherapy and psychoanalysis that many of their basic concepts were couched in the then prevailing conception of determinism.

When somebody makes a real break-through, he does not actually break through all across the line. He breaks through in a particular area and carries with him ideas, some of which are already worn out. Some of the worn out ideas most of us carry with us are concerned with repair and recovery. The most prevalent idea of recovery is that it is analogous to the repair of a machine. Actually, recovery from schizophrenia is far more complex.

When we think about recovery, one of the things which we must take into consideration is that the human organism is an emergent phenomenon and that changes which we produce—perhaps by drugs, perhaps by other means—tend to have a momentum to carry on after the pharmacological action of the drug has ceased. That is why I am inclined to agree with Dr. Hoch in his summary of the importance of the use of drugs.

DR. SARWER-FONER: I just want to make a few comments which are really speculative. Dr. Greenblatt has said much of what I wanted to say, and Dr. Cameron dealt with some of the other things, so that I will content myself with several remarks.

I think it was Harry Stack Sullivan who said that any

method of assaulting psychotic defenses can at times be successful. Now in insulin coma we have a method which, from the discussion, seemed to have, at least for some patients, a physical or physiological, and a psychological substratum, which coincide or could coincide for the selected patient. It seems to me that because of this no matter what further advances are made against mental disease, unless they become specific, there will probably always be a place for insulin coma in some patients. One thinks of the stress that Dr. Bennett and Dr. Himwich mentioned, which has to do with carbohydrate metabolism, and you think of the interpersonal relationship factors that Dr. Greenblatt just mentioned, and you can add to this the need for care and for human contact.

At some level in the rhinencephalon or visceral brain, associative pathways and, perhaps, "unconscious" pathways (or "unreporting" pathways, as far as our awareness is concerned), must exist for early oral, olfactory, and visceral associations. When one thinks of some of the theories of child-mother relationships in regard to oral gratification, and oral deprivation, and the difficulties that schizophrenic patients have in interpersonal relationships in seeking some aspects of oral gratification, the possible importance of the olfactory brain associative areas is suggested.

Insulin coma produces a profound physiologic stress. This stress is, in its physiologic nature, on the substratum of cerebral carbohydrate metabolism, and as such may emotionally be linked with the visceral brain associative pathways, therefore possibly with early oral associative pathways.

In recovery from the hypoglycemic phase, the patient is orally gratified by being given food. He is also usually given i.v. glucose, and all of this usually involves personal and intimate care and attention to him, while he lies there very much in a dependent, regressed state (as to the physiological parameter).

Thus, the insulin coma treatment causes, for at least

some patients, the above-mentioned coincidence in oral dependency—oral gratification situations; coincident with severe physiological stress, again of an oral (carbohydrate metabolic) character; with a death threat, or symbolic dying, and on termination with a reawakening, a rebirth, or reliving. This latter is produced by the very personal care and ministration to the same basic oral needs (both physiological and psychological), by the significant adults of the patient's entourage.

It therefore seems to me that this remarkable coincidence of the above-mentioned factors can be exploited in a therapeutically beneficial way for at least the selected patient. Success depends largely on a properly trained team administering this expensive, elaborate, and at times dangerous, treatment. For the selected patient it may, it seems to me, always have a place despite the implied social shortcomings of expense, elaborateness, and its possible dangers.

Dr. Hoff's description of the catatonic patient who emerged from her catatonia eating food was, I think, a good case in point of all I have been trying to say. Renewed outward flow of energy, cathexising external objects, can follow this oral gratification.

DR. MANN: In my position, I think I have some appreciation for both sides of the problem. Speaking for psychiatry at a large state hospital in Massachusetts, both as a psychoanalyst and as a clinical director I would like to say first how much I enjoyed this session, and the review of the concept of Sakel's contribution in terms of the breakthrough in this sense, that for the first time it was possible to interrupt a process rather drastically, more abruptly and that this led to the very sensitive and careful biochemical etiological studies. I think many of you will agree with me that these studies led to the conclusion that we are still up against a big thick wall.

I would say that psychologically as well as biochemically we are up against the same wall. We have made some advances. We have found that many many things can influence the schizophrenic, can change him somewhat for the better and sometimes rather much for the better. I think none of us can speak of a cure in any schizophrenic, acute or chronic. I certainly agree that there is a great need for a much clearer definition of what we mean when we speak of any kind of schizophrenics, that our statistics are always open to question because the one who makes the statistics himself must be studied and known. But we are dealing essentially with an example par excellence of a psychophysiological disease. We are confused because, in contrast to all other diseases which are called psychophysiological, we have to deal—and here I repeat, the important thing is we have to deal with the psychophysiological disorder as it involves the whole person, in every sense of that word. We can't take out his appendix. We can't take out any organ.

This psychophysiological disease being so all inclusive involves all of the biochemistry, all of the physiology and all of society, and as I think of it, it probably confuses us too that we have to deal with the problems existing amongst ourselves and our society as well as with the schizophrenic who is somewhat isolated by being placed in a particular setting generally called a hospital. I think we see trends in the direction that the treatment of schizophrenia or at least the investigation of schizophrenia is going far beyond the chemical, the neurophysiological, the psychological, into the wider field of society itself.

Now I don't propose at all that there are any answers to the schizophrenia of society, but I do suggest that this is the overall problem in schizophrenia, that the study of schizophrenia is a study of the condition of man.

What I enjoy about a meeting of this kind is the opportunity to hear points of view of people who are interested in one particular aspect of the total problem. How we can bring together all these aspects, I think, is a problem for a schizophrenic society. And if we do that maybe we can get back to the less fortunate amongst us and see this problem as a classical psychophysiological problem involving not only individuals but all of our society.

DR. ALEXANDER GRALNICK: I'm sure that like many others I'm going to carry a lot more from this meeting than I have to contribute as a discussant. But I have been a little encouraged and fortified to say a few words that have been on my mind all day too.

I think I'm rather encouraged by the turn of events in the discussion. I'm not among the older people who came to have experience with the insulin treatment in the 30's and 40's. At that time, working at Central Islip State Hospital, we were among the first of the few who emphasized highly "the total treatment situation" and the place of the doctor-patient relationship in insulin therapy. It seems to me, if I may take off on Dr. Cameron's remarks, that Dr. Sakel gave us a total treatment procedure from which one had the choice of selecting out certain things which he might emphasize.

In reading Dr. Sakel's monograph of 1937, I happened to select out certain aspects of his personality. He was a very sensitive therapist, one who was very aware of his patient as a total human being who was perhaps not entirely an organic case. Some of us fortunately have chosen to select the doctor-patient aspect of the total treatment situation, mindful of course of the physiological changes which we are producing in the patient.

I think I would be among the last to say that the physiological changes which are produced are unimportant, but they help us only to set a stage in which the doctor-patient relationship can be studied. I think that one of the unfortunate things in the history of insulin treatment is that we haven't given this aspect of the treatment situation truly an objective study. If we do this in succeeding years, then we may begin to learn what Dr. Hoch was suggesting that we must learn, how to select the right treatment from a variety of modalities which come to our ken. If we study what goes on between the two human beings, namely the doctor and the patient, we will have a better chance of learning something of the psychology and the character structure, if you will, of the patient, and know what he responds to best. Only then will we be in a position to apply a particular type of treatment more successfully.

DR. HANS HOFF: May I say just a few words concerning an experiment now being conducted at our hospital—the Neuro-Psychiatric Clinic of the University of Vienna.

We are, of course, in complete agreement with the classical differential diagnosis of schizophrenia, which consists of three groups: the paranoid, the catatonic and the hebephrenic. We all know that the prognosis in these three groups differs. To these, however, we have added what we have termed the "pseudoneurotic group" of schizophrenia. But we have not been really satisfied with this differentiation and all it entails in the matter of prognosis and treatment, and accordingly we now offer a revised schema suggested by Doctor Arnold, based upon an experience of several hundred schizophrenic patients.

In our experiments patients are divided into two groups. One group is treated by insulin shock, supported by electroshock; the second group is treated by neuroleptica only. To both of these groups, psychotherapy—either the single or group form—is added. As a supplement, occupational therapy is introduced, and the relatives are adjusted in groups. This means, for example, that one patient is treated by insulin shock and psychotherapy, while an alternate patient is treated by neuroleptica plus psychotherapy. It is possible that in the near future we will introduce a group in which we will combine both treatments—insulin shock and drug treatment. We might already state that insulin shock treatment plus psychotherapy has proved to be the most effective in paranoid schizophrenia, while for catatonic patients in an acute phase electroshock, sometimes followed by insulin treatment, has proved to be superior. In hebephrenic patients a 3 months' treatment by neuroleptica combined with psychotherapy leads to a better adjustment and seems to be the best treatment. I believe that in 5 years we will have found an answer, and that we will then be able to decide which treatment has proved to be the most effective in any particular category of the disease.

I am not greatly concerned over whether or not we will continue indefinitely to employ electroshock or insulin shock treatment. I will always utilize—as I have in the past—such treatment as I believe to be most effective in each particular phase of my patient's disease. We still respect the necessity for employing the insulin treatment, but we also feel most emphatically that any kind of biological treatment signifies nothing more than a breaking through of the wall surrounding the patient's mind. After that door has been opened, somebody has to go through. Patients with schizophrenia need understanding and what is commonly called "the human touch." Such patients have lost contact with life, and only adequate psychotherapy, in addition to other forms of treatment, can restore their previous normal adjustment. This is the reason we combine biological treatment with psychotherapy. Although I have not yet had sufficient experience to warrant final conclusions, I believe that drug treatment, in selected cases, will substitute effectively for insulin shock treatment. I am in complete agreement with Dr. Sargant. We have applied psychotherapeutic treatment in schizophrenia for a considerable period, and we have also applied numerous other forms of treatment. We have also given up many difficult forms of treatment. These successes and failures, however, have led us to feel that a combination of biological treatment and psychotherapy offers the greatest chance of success in schizophrenia. We in Vienna, therefore, do not believe that the insulin treatment of schizophrenia should be discarded at the present stage of medical progress.

CHAIRMAN RINKEL: Dr. Conran (Senior Physician at one of the great state hospitals in the state of Massachusetts).

DR. CONRAN: I'd like to just make a brief comment. Hippocrates, I understand, the father of us all, believed that hemorrhoids were not present during any other illnesses and therefore he came to the conclusion that hemorrhoids cured a lot of ailments. I think we have advanced a great deal in wisdom and knowledge since then, to the extent that we now believe that the answer to many of our troubles is the atomic pile.

I think that we are not going to be as naive as this. I do want to emphasize or underline a great deal of what has been said today, a recognition for the need for objectivity. The reason I speak is that I have spent about eleven years trying to be able to adequately administer insulin coma treatment. This to me is quite an investment. It is difficult to be objective even here, and I am so aware of how much more investment there is in this meeting.

Today I feel quite happy in my investment. It has been adequately protected, so I have an innate sense of balance which forces me to just mention a therapeutic milieu structured on dynamic principles quite specifically as an aid to insulin therapy. Perhaps psychotherapy also may advance in effectiveness with time and experience. So that although prior to insulin there was no break-through, we would be I believe one-sided if we didn't hope for a sufficient advance in psychotherapeutic knowledge and skills to advance in this field as well.

Chapter 11

RESULTS AND EFFICACY OF INSULIN SHOCK THERAPY*

O. H. ARNOLD

This subject matter cannot be discussed before defining the term Insulin Shock Therapy (IST). Only the systematic and precise application of Insulin to obtain a series of hypoglycemic comas of sufficient length and frequency, under conditions which will be discussed later, can be described as IST, as we understand the term. In judging the results of IST, it is of great importance that the following details are observed: a) The technique of the treatment; b) Knowledge of the spontaneous courses which the schizophrenic psychoses take and their prognosis; c) The definite indications of IST.

a) *The technique of the treatment at the Vienna Clinic.* We begin the standard method with 30 units of Insulin which the patient receives at 6 A.M. on an empty stomach; this is followed by daily increases of 30 units until the patient reaches a coma. We recognize a state of coma at the moment when the patient is unconscious and cannot be awakened by external stimulations. During the first week the length of the coma should not be longer than 30 minutes and from the 10th Insulin Shock no longer than one hour. The amount of Insulin units used to produce coma

* Translation from the German submitted by the author.

is quite unimportant. Dosage must be increased very quickly to prevent the patient reacting with his total personality during the time of the basic disturbances of schizophrenia. If one doesn't do this, the psychotic impressions will be more intensive and enlarged and defense mechanisms of the personality in different states will be stronger and more intensive.

Daily application is necessary but hospital organization and the shortage of nurses force us to omit treatment on Sunday. During IST the patient should, however, never have more than one Insulin-free day a week. Should he contract an intercurrent infection he must have treatment for it by the latest methods, such as antibiotics, etc. But the IST must not be interrupted. If his life should be in danger the insulin treatment of course will have to be interrupted, but it must be repeated in all cases except with patients who have had more than 35 Insulin Comas (IC). After an interruption of 8 days or more we prolong the treatment by 10 or 20 insulin comas.

Normally, 50 insulin comas should be enough to cure the patient but in some cases it is necessary to continue up to 100 insulin comas or even more. It is axiomatic that the patient should not show any more symptoms of the process of schizophrenia during the last 20 insulin comas. If he does still show symptoms of schizophrenic process during the first 50 insulin comas then the treatment must be continued.

With our last 250 patients we have succeeded in freeing the "Prozess-Symptome" so that the actual rate of remissions is now 100%. It is only on reaching this figure of 100% (and this percentage only) that further conclusions can be drawn, and that statistics may be produced on the later courses of schizophrenic patients treated with Insulin-Shock. If this rate of remissions is not reached, the reason may be either false indications or incorrect treatment.

Successful treatment as described above is possible only with the new modifications of IST. The method of bringing the patient into coma has been changed. The "overstretching" and the "Zick-Zack method" were given up in favour of the drug Depressin. This is Hexamethonium, which breaks the regulatory mechanism of the organism against the effects of Insulin. By using this method the patient can be brought into coma within 4 or 5 days. The Insulin coma doses can be reduced to an average of 80 units of old Insulin. The combined method is now used in more than 80% of cases. Each primary process starts, in principle, after the 15th insulin coma combined with Metrazol Shock. Metrazol shock must be administered on two consecutive days in the middle of the week. It has been proved clinically and from the records of Electroencephalograms that the combination of IST with Metrazol is more effective than the combination of Insulin and Electroshock therapy.

In principle, all cases which are not free of "Prozess-Symptome" during the first 20 insulin comas must be treated by these combined methods. In those very rare cases which do not show remission in spite of a long application of Insulin, we use the intentionally prolonged coma, when the patient stays in a coma for 4 hours without getting a sugar solution. This treatment can be repeated up to about 10 times.

We wish to emphasize that this treatment should take place only in a ward which is specially organized for it. The patients should join a special group, sleep and work together in an atmosphere of recovery. The IST itself must be done under the supervision of the person in charge of the ward. The technical application of IST should be carried out by a group of one specially trained doctor and three specially trained nurses for every group of twelve patients. A psychiatrist who is also trained as an anesthetist must always be within reach owing to the complications which might occur during the treatment, and for the same reason, complete and modern anesthesia equipment is necessary.

b) *Knowledge of the spontaneous courses which the schizophrenic psychoses take and their prognosis* (Table 1).

TABLE 1

Type of Course	Frequency %	Prognosis	
1. Phase	15,6	±1,0	
2. Phase with transition into attack	4,0	+0,21	±0,016
3. Phase with transition into process	0,4		
4. Phase with transition into process and exacerbation	3,4	+0,21	±0,013
5. Attack	9,6		
6. Attack with transition into process	3,6	−0,31	±0,007
7. Attack with transition into process and exacerbation	14,0	−0,15	±0,018
8. Process	7,2	−0,58	±0,002
9. Process with Exacerbation	36,0		
10. Mixed psychosis	5,5	+0,67	±0,011
11. Mixed psychosis with transition into process	1,4		

The reference system corresponds to the average terminal stage of 500 schizophrenic disease courses.

Correlation coefficients and median error according to Brevais-Pearson.

Phase: Course which returns to the normal in a relatively short time.

Attack: Course which, despite considerable improvement, does not return to the normal in a relatively short time, but produces a defect—that is, a drop in general functioning level.

Process: Continuous progression of the disease process to a defect.

Exacerbation: An acute sudden deterioration from a normal level, attack, phase, or process with relatively quick return to the former level.

Mixed psychosis: Schizophrenic symptom formation combined with manic-depressive disease.

Reproduced with permission from O. H. Arnold, Schizophrener Prozess und schizophrene Symptomgesetze, Maudrich, Wien, Bonn, 1955.

The relationship between correlation numbers and words in general use is shown in Table 2.

TABLE 2

Full remission	up to	+	0,60
Social remission: i.e. the patient can support himself but the rest of symptoms remain	up to	+	0,20
Home care		0	
Change between home care and continuous stay in hospital	up to	—	0,25
Continuous stay in hospital	more than	—	0,25

c) *The definite indications of IST:*

Knowledge of the spontaneous course is the basis for the modern indication of IST. During recent years this knowledge has developed into a highly differentiated special system, which is shown in the following survey (Table 3).

TABLE 3
Indications

Type of Courses	Symptoms,* speaking for	against	Remarks	figures of prognosis	EST	Indication for Lobo. I + EST, Cardiazol
1. Phase	29-31, 33, 35		withdrawal of 50, presence of 1-4 and 36-39	all full recovery	10-20	
2. Phase with transition into attack	significant marked from 29-31, 33, 34, 35, 40-48, 17, further 20-22	34, 35, 40-48, 52.	does not speak against	+0,21 ±0,016	4-10	50 I+12 C late
3. Phase with transition into process	47, 48 and 56.					
4. Phase with transition into process and exacerb.			withdrawal of 52			
5. Attack	15-22, 36-39, 41, rare 1-14, 23-25	34, 35, 40 -47	withdrawal of 55, missing in 50%	+0,21 ±0,013	10-20	
6. Attack with transition into process	1-22, mainly 10-15			−0,31 ±0,007		50 I+12 C late
7. Attack with transition into process and exacerb.				−0,34 ±0,08		

						50	(+12 C) early
						50 I+20 C	late
						10-20	
8. Process	23-25, 36-42 with outstanding symptoms 40 and 42, 52.	1-22	no acute state in beginning, presence of singular sympt. 1-22	−0,15 ±0,018			
9. Process with exacerbat.	36-42 significantly marked, start in early age, 27-33, 35.			−0,58 ±0,002			
10. Mixed psychosis	29-33, 46, 54, 55	14-22, 34 43-45, 51, 52, 47, 48	improvement of symptoms in the MDK, rare 50	+0,68 ±0,013	+0,67 ±0,011		
11. Mixed psychosis with transition into process			add symptoms 47, 48.				

* Listed in Table 4

The meanings of the numbers 1 to 57 in Table 3 will be clear from the following survey of symptoms (Table 4).

TABLE 4

1. Transitory habit of the experience
2. Thoughts slipping away, interruption of thoughts, thoughts being pushed forward, thoughts in a film-like form
3. Double meaning
4. Ambivalence of feelings, mysticism
5. Disturbance and dissolving of moral and esthetic feelings
6. Change in codes and standards of values
7. "Philosophema"
8. Religious experiences
9. Experience in cosmogony, experiences related to creation and the end of the world
10. Feeling of sadness unrelated to environment
11. Feeling of losing control of thoughts, thoughts of being snatched away, diffusion of thoughts, telepathy
12. Strange thoughts of having thinking influenced by outside sources
13. Thinking out loud, echo of thoughts
14. The feeling of a voluntary freedom of being imprisoned
15. The feeling of being hypnotized
16. Disturbance of tenacity of attention
17. Vacancy, disruption of experiential world
18. Experience of thoughts of losing track
19. Substituting
20. The feeling of blocking of thoughts
21. Catalepsy
22. Tension, stupor
23. Lack of clarity of thinking, having a fog over the thoughts

24. Not to be able to think, we get stuck with thoughts, disturbance of concentration
25. Disturbance of dynamic feelings
26. Disturbance of vital feelings
27. Disturbance in organic feelings, disturbance of the body scheme and body image
28. Physical hallucinations
29. Skipping of thoughts
30. False associations
31. Sliding of wakefulness or of attention
32. Hyperkinesis
33. Raptus, compulsive lack of inhibition
34. Defect in the affective sphere
35. Stupor with relaxation
36. Disturbance in the mechanics of thinking because of the following interference and mixing of the thoughts
37. Thoughts being fused and condensed
38. Unreasonable feeling of a new meaning in experiences not related to the self
39. Experiences in connection with persecution without a system
40. Systemized facts
41. Moods of delusion
42. Tendency to dissimulation
43. Special characteristic disturbance of thinking: "Faseln," neologism, scattering of word associations
44. Disturbance in estimation of real values
45. Disturbance of the abstract performance within the field of attention
46. Tendency to visualize, pseudohallucinations
47. "Parabulien," "Parakinesis," "to behave as a fool"
48. Stupor with a tendency to negativism
49. Auditory hallucinations
50. Noises, imagining being called by name, singular voices
51. Imperative voices, threatening voices, the patient act-

ing as if he is providing a theme of discussion by strangers

52. Sensations as if being addressed in the third person, dialogues
53. Visual hallucinations
54. Possibility of observing and describing his own sickness, relative insight
55. Disturbance of the sleep
56. Somatic symptoms of acute form of disturbances of the vegetative and humoral function
57. Somatic symptoms of chronic form of disturbances of the vegetative and humoral function

The General Treatment Plan

During the course of long studies of schizophrenia, it was necessary to use the indications of IST as a frame for a general treatment plan. This plan includes the modern modified IST, occupational therapy, psychotherapy and the reorganization of the social milieu. The last factors are of course not of equal value.

Correctly indicated and conducted Insulin Shock Therapy is the basic treatment of schizophrenia.

The right terminal and organizational cooperation with the 3 other factors of therapy must all be based on the principle that the organic factor of schizophrenia must be treated first. The earlier effects of this treatment stop the process which goes on in a certain number of nerve cells in the brain before the other factors of therapy can be effective. The organic treatment should begin with the plan of an organized milieu of a group. The plan of general treatment should be designed by the doctor in charge of the ward. He supervises the whole treatment and must also take responsibility for the patient and his family. He has to maintain a firm attitude. He appraises the presumable duration of the disease. Only he can give information to the patient and his family about official actions concerning matters of internment, confinement, etc. and about hospital regulations. He also censures misconduct. The physician performing the actual treatment at the Insulin ward must behave in a neutral way.

The prospective psychotherapist starts his treatment when the patient becomes lucid and there is enough contact. In most cases this is possible during the IST, where the psychotherapist should have an informative conversation with the patient. From this first moment the doctor takes the position of a good father who sticks up for the patient for a speedy discharge. For instance, he takes care of small personal wishes and takes the patient's part against the head of the ward. He helps the patient step by step to obtain better conditions of accommodation, privileges for visiting the garden, watching television and for rebuilding good contact with his relatives. The polaric positions of these two physicians are chosen intentionally and proved to be an exceptionally good method of creating an atmosphere for making contact and preparing to build up a good and long-lasting transference to the therapist. Only in some cases can one speak of a deliberate psychotherapy during IST. Only in exceptional cases is it possible to start a classical psychotherapy immediately after completion of the IST. Sometimes at the end of an effective Insulin treatment the patient's organic psychosyndrome seems to fade away. The Psychotherapist must then decide whether the patient is able to join a psychotherapeutic group or whether single therapy is needed—or even none at all.

In the course of the development of our method a ceremonial order for the different groups receiving IST developed. This ceremonial was ground in and put into a rigid form. It consists of such things as the time for getting up in the morning, going to the Insulin ward and leaving it, being helpful to each other, eating, carrying out the different programs during the day, such as occupational and group therapy, walks, gymnastic hours, television, movies and visits. The content of this ceremonial order is not as important as the fact that it comes about. After the second (the prophylactic) phase of the IST there is an intensive effect on the psychosis and organic reaction of the brain. The patient receives such a shock in every dimension of his total personality that there is an absolute need to build up a primitive visible order before a system of norms can be restored in a higher and more complex field. The gradual re-individualization then permits a compensation so that these ceremonies and rituals are no longer needed.

The effects of occupational therapy must be seen from the point of view of the ceremonial order. This represents the phenomenon which in animal psychology is called a training effect. Another effect of occupational therapy is the tendency to take away basic energy from the contents of a psychotic process. This energy is needed to cope with occupational therapy. A much less important part of this effect can be seen directly under the special perspective of deep psychology. Finally the problem of resocialization depends essentially on the structure and the order of the outside environment to which he returns. The attitudes of the family and the people in his surroundings are an essential influence in this environment whilst the question of the patient's job is not as important. For this reason the members of his family should join a group and the therapist who treated the patient (in individual or group therapy) should also treat his relatives.

The discussion of this single factor of a planned general treatment shows first that IST is extremely important (it is a conditio sine qua non) but also that one cannot exclude the validity of all the other factors.

The level of the "immediate remission rate" depends almost exclusively on the indication, the technique and the consequence of the Insulin treatment. The level of "five years of remission" which can be accepted as a measure of long-lasting success depends to a certain extent on the other factors within the plan of the total treatment. The right time to start an Insulin treatment is limited to within

TABLE 5

Genesis of Schizophrenia

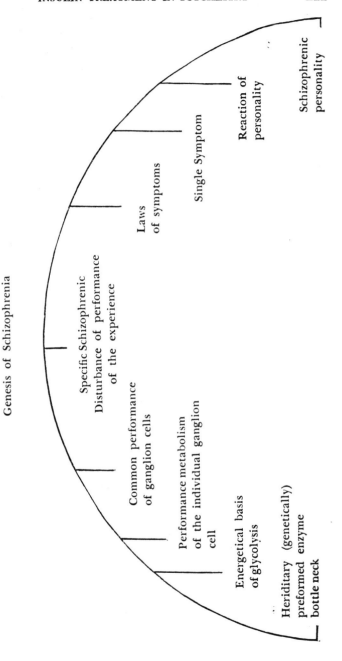

Schizophrenic personality

Reaction of personality

Single Symptom

Laws of symptoms

Specific Schizophrenic Disturbance of performance of the experience

Common performance of ganglion cells

Performance metabolism of the individual ganglion cell

Energetical basis of glycolysis

Heriditary (genetically) preformed enzyme bottle neck

a few months. This decision, which concerns the whole existence of the patient, has to be taken within this short period. It is understandable that compared with such a decision the actual length of the treatment (inpatient or outpatient) doesn't seem important even if it lasts 1 or 2 years or longer.

Theory of Insulin Shock Therapy

A theory of the efficacy of IST was developed at first on clinical material. With the time corresponding to the biochemical findings certain modifications of single factors changed without variation of the principal idea. This principal idea was pointed out by Professor Pötzl, the honorary president of this conference. He coined the word "Mauserung" (Moulting effect) to create a wide-ranging concept of thoughts concerning the effect of the IST. For the better understanding of this idea it is necessary to describe the basic concept of the process of the schizophrenic diseases.

The relevant point is the assumption of a dysfunction—reversible in its first stage—of single groups of ganglion cells and their performance which is responsible for the control of thalamo commissural function. The reason for this dysfunction lies in the development of a heredito-genetically preformed enzyme bottleneck. This bottleneck is either found in the anoxybiotic phases of the carbohydrate metabolism or in relation to the performance metabolism, which can be realized as the balance of the acceptors and donators of phosphates. This development leads to an excessive demand on the performance within this group of cells owing to a physiological or psychological overload (stress situation) of the patient.

In a later stage this disturbance of the performance metabolism in the singular ganglion cell leads to a process which successively decreases the differentiation stage of the common function. This forms the basis of a schizophrenic process or defective state.

Corresponding to the reserve of cells within the brain there is a possibility of repairing the performance of cell groups. Therefore the disturbed single cell in such a group must be destroyed.

To remove these disturbed members from the functional group is the problem of early causal treatment in schizophrenia. We must also do this because there is—according to up-to-date knowledge—no way to supply the missing control substances (enzymes) in such a disturbed cell.

Cori, Slein and coworkers pointed out that the effect of Insulin lies in a change of activity of the Hexokinase within the ganglion cells. Liebert thinks that Insulin works on the equilibrium which is at the connection point with pyruvic acid. The clinical observations prove that glucosis is not used by the ganglion cells after a certain period of Insulin effect. Glucose which is supplied via the vascular system in that stage is no longer absorbed. This is why those ganglion cells become necrotic and are destroyed. In this stage single intermediary products of the carbohydrate metabolism reorganize this metabolism. We could demonstrate that a coma can be stopped immediately with an intravenous injection of a 5% solution of succinic acid.

We can say that Insulin causes an acute disorganization of the carbohydrate metabolism within the ganglion cell. This disorganization leads first to a failure in the performance of the cell (see electro-encephalographic [EEG] studies), further on to a blockage of the respiration and finally to a destruction of the cell. Brain-anatomical and histological studies in animals and men who died after Insulin incidents showed that there was indeed a destruction of ganglion cells in large areas within the brain. Corresponding results are found after IST in the EEG records and in the psychological tests of the brain-performance. We could discuss the possibilities of the micromechanics of the Insulin attack but this would not be very relevant to the general aspect of its efficacy. In summary: Insulin is a drug which causes a tight stranglehold of an exactly determined strength on the life-function of a ganglion cell.

Considering that this stranglehold attacks all forms of ganglion cells, one may expect that those cells will successively be destroyed which have a heredito-genetical disturbance of the organization of their carbohydrate metabolism and which are in an actual state of injury, meaning that they are supporting the psychotic process. The ganglion cells without actual dysfunction, but having a potential trend to it, have more resistance to this destructive stranglehold. Healthy ganglion cells are affected, if at all, only in the final stages.

There are clinical reasons for the assumption that the efficacy of this stranglehold depends on the duration of the coma. After a coma, the ganglion cells recover in different time periods. The cells which are actually involved in the dysfunction recover last. The attack of insulin against the potentially disturbed ganglion cells seems to lead to further development of this disturbance before these cells are also destroyed.

Correspondingly we observed that under Insulin the psychotic syndrome temporarily flares up before a nonsymptomatic stage is reached. In that sense one can assume on the one hand that each flare-up of symptoms during IST is a sign of the existence of some of these potentially disturbed cells. On the other hand it is indicative of a prophylactic-effect of IST that the cell formations which are actually disturbed in their function are destroyed and all cells which could later on be actually disturbed (because of a potential dysregulation) are also destroyed by subsequent treatment. Therefore they cannot cause a new manifestation in case of a stress situation which might occur later on.

With the destruction of a certain number of ganglion cells in a common performance system, this performance will decrease to a lower level. Later on, cell formations from the big reserve within the brain join in the common function. So the "moulting effect" gives a chance to restore a disturbed general and common performance to a normal level.

With that theoretical discussion, it becomes clear why the Insulin treatment does not have any effect in such cases in which a spontaneous stabilization of the common function has reached a lower defective stage level. To be sure, there can be an effect in a prophylactic sense.

This point of view answers the question as to how long one should give Insulin treatment after the onset of a schizophrenic manifestation. According to this theory a general answer cannot be given. It depends on the level of the performance of the attacked cell groups and the stage of differentiation which manifests itself in the performance of the experience of the patient and the microsymptomatic mosaic.

Therefore it is necessary to analyze the mosaic structure of symptoms in their actual and longitudinal sense. The practical results of this analysis were shown in the schedule of indications.

To summarize the efficacy of IST, it is surprising that the substance itself is just one small link in a long chain.

The problem of IST is to find the right doses to produce the stranglehold effect of insulin on the individual cells. One must keep in mind that the objective of IST is the destruction of brain cells, in other words the production of a controlled brain lesion. If the treatment is not persistent enough, the effect will be insignificant and the rate of relapses will be high, not only because of failure to achieve an immediate effect but because prophylaxis has not been attained.

If one treats the patient without regard to any complication there is no case—assuming correct indication—in which the disease process cannot be removed and the danger of relapse cannot be prevented. But in many such cases we have to risk considerable organic brain damage (as we have seen it in intentional or unintentional cases of a prolonged coma).

All this experience points to the fact that there is a way between two extremes, which is not a well trodden road but a narrow path for the therapist during the whole period of IST. The right balance between these two possible effects of insulin (too little—too much) can be kept only with longlasting experience, correct indications and an excellent ward organization. There are reasons to believe that these concepts are recognized in only a very few IST wards in the world. That is why this method is not in favor in so many places. But in this sense we have to reorganize the program of the whole Insulin problem.

Results of Insulin Shock Therapy

All the concepts and facts must be kept in mind if the results of IST at the Viennese Psychiatric and Neurologic University Clinic over different treatment periods are to be presented. The result of each treatment in schizophrenia must be related to the course of the disease in nontreated cases. It is very important that the investigations of the spontaneous remissions and results of the treatment are made by the same person. This is the only way to guarantee the identity of all criteria of judgment.

The average spontaneous remission rate is given in the world literature as about 36%; a figure which in our own material is slightly higher because of the wide diagnostic frame in the definition of schizophrenia (Table 6).

TABLE 6

Results of the effect of Insulin shock therapy
(Viennese Psychiatric and Neurologic University Clinic)

Years	1933 - 1940	%	Course of 467 untreated cases 467	%	1952 - 1953	%
Number of cases	273		467		173	
Control time in years	18		9		5	
Full remission	117	42,4	67	14,3 } 40,6	81	46,8 } 80,3
Social remission	68	24,9	123	26,3	58	33,5
In observation of the family (temporary in hospitals)			143	30,6	22	12,7
Hospitalization	88	32,2	123	28,7	9	5,2
death, lost					3	1,7

The left side of Table 6 shows that with the beginning of Insulin treatment the spontaneous rate of remission (given in the world literature) is only slightly exceeded. Many authors thought that for the end results of a schizophrenic process the Insulin treatment had just a slight influence. The same authors thought the "five-years remission rate" would give a final result of the success of the treatment.

On the right side of Table 6 we find part of the results of the treatment during the years 1952-1953. These results are given because a reorganization took place in 1951. The 5 years' set term for a follow-up study should be observed. If one compares the amount of full remission and social remission—subsummarizing favourable ends—in spontaneous remission with the result of modified modern techniques of insulin treatment, both rates are in a proportion of 1:2.

This result is exceptionally good considering the sceptical attitude so often surrounding the treatment. It proves the efficacy of Insulin Shock Treatment.

Owing to the time taken in developing a good method the former results have been not so good.

With the onset of modern techniques in anaesthesia, including the use of Metrazol, it has become possible to increase the length and quantity of the coma to the optimal border of stress for the patient's organism. Only in that extreme form will the insulin treatment lead us to the success I have just mentioned. The number of incidents in the prolonged Insulin coma is in a special sense a measure for the energy which was used in the treatment. In our case material this number is 4%. The mortality is 2.4%. There is no more practical danger in prolonged coma using our technique of treatment with intubation and occasionally applied N_2O anaesthesia. We successfully used this method several times in exceptionally desperate cases.

Comparisons with the results of other authors are valueless so long as they do not apply the same treatment or use the indications under the same aspects and do not use a general plan for the insulin treatment.

Summary

I believe, and would like to point out, that IST by Sakel after it was developed according to the described technique has become, in our day, the standard treatment for all cases of schizophrenia. It developed exactly as Manfred Sakel indicated. I have had the honor of discussing this matter several times with him personally.

An exact knowledge of the microsymptomatics of the schizophrenic diseases, of the indications, of the theories of the efficacy, the techniques and procedures and a general plan for the treatment in connection with the theoretical background—all these factors have been the basis on which we have finally established the durable successes which this ingenious method deserves.

Literature

1. Arnold, O. H.: Zur Theorie des Insulinschock-Therapie der Schizophrenie. *Wien. Z. Nervenhk.* IV, 2-3 (1951)
2. Arnold, O. H.: Untersuchungen zur Frage des Zusammenhanges zwischen Erlebnisvollzug und Kohlehydratstoffwechsel. *Wien. Z. Nervenhk.* X, 1 (1954)
3. Arnold, O. H.: Zur Frage der multifaktoriellen Kausalität in der Psychiatrie. *Wien. Arch. Psych.* VI, 3-4 (1956)
4. Arnold, O. H. and H. Gastager: Insulinschockbehandlung trotz Diabetes. *Wien. Z. Nervenhk.* XIII, 3 (1957)
5. Arnold, O. H. and H. Hoff: Die Bedeutung der experimentellen Pharmakologie für die Neurologie und Psychiatrie. *J. M. Sinai Hosp.* XIX, 1 (1952)
6. Arnold, O. H. und H. Hoff: Die Therapie der Schizophrenie. *Wien. klin. Wschr.* 66, 20 (1954)
7. Arnold, O. H. and G. Hofmann: Untersuchungen über

Bernsteinsäure-effekte bei LSD-25 Vergiftungen und Schizophrenien. *Wien. Z. Nervenhk.* XI, 1 (1955)

8. Arnold, O. H., G. Hofmann and H. Leupold-Löwenthal: Untersuchungen zur Pathogenese der Schizophrenie III. Mitt.: Das Verhalten der C-14 radioaktiven Bernsteinsäure aus Kohlehydratstobwechsel der Gehirnnervenzellen. *Wien. Z. Nervenhk.* XIII, 4 (1957)

9. Arnold, O. H., G. Hofmann and H. Leupold-Löwenthal: Untersuchungen zum Schizophrenieproblem IV. Mitteilung: Die Verteilung des C-14 radioaktiven Lysergsäurediäthylamids im tierischen Organismus. *Wien. Z. Nervenhk.* XV, 14 (1958)

10. Arnold, O. H. und R. Schindler: Bifokale Gruppentherapie bei Schizophrenen. *Wien. Z. Nervenhk.* V, 2-3 (1952)

11. Bleuler, E.: Dementia praecox oder Gruppe der Schizophrenien, *Aschaffenburgs-Handbuch der Psychiatrie.* Leipzig and Vienna, 1911

12. Bleuler, M.: Das Wesen der Schizophrenieremission nach Schockbehandlung. *Z. Neur.* 173 (1941)

13. Bleuler, M.: Forschungen und Begriffswandlungen in der Schizophrenielehre 1941-50, *Fortschr. Neur.* 19, 9-10 (1951)

14. Von Braunmühl: *Insulinschock und Heilkrampf in der Psychiatrie.* Wissenschaftl. Verlagsgesellschaft, Stuttgart, 1947

15. Colowick, S. P., G. T. Cori and M. W. Slein: *J. Biol. Chem.* (Am) 168, 583 (1947)

16. Georgi, F., R. Fischer and R. Weber: Psychopathologische Korrelationen VIII. Modellversuche zum Schizophrenieproblem. Lysergsäurediäthylamid und Meskalin. *Schw. med. Wschr.* 81, 817-837 (1951)

17. Hoff, H.: Die organischen Grundlagen der Psychosen. *Wien. klin. Wschr.* 63, 1 (1951)

18. Leipert, Th.: Stoffwechsel und vegetative Regulation zur Frage der Insulinwirkung. *Acta neuroveg.* I, 1-2 (1950)

19. Mayer-Gross, W. W. McAdam and J. Walker: Lysergsäurediäthylamid und Kohlehydratstoffwechsel. *Nervenarzt* 23, 30 (1952)
20. Müller, M.: *Die körperlichen Behandlungsverfahren in der Psychiatrie I. Insulinbehandlung.* George Thieme, Stuttgart, 1952
21. Müller, V.: Katamnestische Erhebungen über den Spontanverlauf bei Schizophrenien. *Mschr. Psychiatr.* 122 (1951)
22. Pötzl, O.: Die Wirkungsweise der Schockbehandlung *Wien. Med. Wschr.* 97, 11-12 (1947)
23. Rinkel, M., Hyde, R. W. and Solomon, H. G.: Experimental Psychiatry III. A chemical concept of psychosis. *Dis. Nerv. syst.* 15 (1954)
24. Sakel, M.: *Neue Behandlungsmethoden der Schizophrenie.* Moritz Perles, Vienna-Leipzig, 1935.
25. Schindler, R.: Bifocal Group Therapy. *Progr. in Psychotherapie* vol. III (1957)
26. Schneider, C.: *Die schizophrenen Symptomverbände.* Berlin: Springer, 1942.
27. Slein, M. W., G. T. Cori and C. F. Cori: *J. Biol. Chem.* (Am) 186, 763 (1950)

DISCUSSION

DR. HOFF: I think what Dr. Arnold means when we think of the insulin shock treatment, has to be done by the destruction of cells; cells that are sick, and new cells which are potentially sick have to be destroyed. Otherwise relapses will come. That means that one of the most important things is to see that really every cell which is affected is really destroyed.

What Dr. Arnold tried to show you is that some clinical symptoms give us a hint if we want insulin shock treatment or even prolonged insulin shock treatment or a combination of insulin shock treatment and electric shock.

What he showed us is that after five years we were able to have more than 80 per cent people either completely recovered, meaning no more symptoms of schizophrenia whatsoever or adaptive ability which would allow them to live a full life. 81 per cent approximately are in that stage. Five years is a long time, and so if a patient has five years behind him and is still in a socially good condition or has no symptoms, we can assume that the number of relapses will be rather few.

What we really like to show is that if we try insulin treatment, we must go back to the original treatment of Sakel. That means it must be a treatment with the destruction of cells. Now that of course means that our indication of schizophrenia must be a very correct one.

As you have probably seen by the different symptoms which Dr. Arnold pointed out, all these cases are severe cases and would be known without doubt as schizophrenia.

Not a single case is only a schizophrenic reaction. I am definitely sure that every psychiatrist in any country in every circle would diagnose these cases as schizophrenia. We have seen spontaneous remissions in our cases, but we have double so many remissions, and that of course means that insulin shock treatment has had some success.

May I add only one word to what Dr. Arnold said. He mentioned that in all cases, psychotherapy and occupational therapy was given. There should be no doubt about that. I believe that insulin in combination with electroshock treatment, and of course with psychotherapy is the right means of treatment.

We have not divided the cases, as Dr. Sargant asked, into hebephrenic, catatonic and paranoid schizophrenic forms. I think it would be worth while, in a future time, if we would work on this kind of differential diagnosis.

DR. HERMAN C. B. DENBER: I would like to congratulate Dr. Arnold on the excellence of his presentation, the completeness and theoretical formulations. Certain points can be elaborated upon for discussion with the introduction of a cautious note. There are, firstly, the cultural factors with regard to a diagnosis of schizophrenia. It is believed in many quarters that schizophrenia is identical no matter where it is seen. There is, nevertheless, suggestive evidence that individual and cultural factors play a great role in the diagnosis of either a neurosis or a schizophrenic psychosis. These factors apply to the diagnosing psychiatrist as well. Unfortunately, Dr. Arnold has not provided us with the basis for his diagnostic criteria, particularly with regard to the various symptoms.

If I understood Dr. Arnold correctly, his concept is that schizophrenia is a hereditary disease in which one finds abnormal cells in the cerebral cortex. These are destroyed by anoxia as a result of the insulin coma treatment. It would appear that the deeper the coma, the greater the destruction of sick neurons.

This seems to lead to a rather nihilistic view: The brain

of a schizophrenic patient will eventually show wide acellular areas. If one should look at a biopsy of this brain, a picture would be seen resembling that of general paresis with its many acellular areas. In a study of brain biopsies on schizophrenic patients, using a silver staining technique, I have observed such extensive neuronal destruction with alterations at the synapse. The question arose at that time and now as well—were these primary changes; were these the result of the prolonged illness; or were these the result of the insulin coma, and/or electroconvulsive treatments? It was impossible at the time to entertain any of these hypotheses any further, and for this reason the work was never published.

One can ask, then, whether the anatomical changes Dr. Arnold speaks about are the result of anoxia due to insulin coma, or is this a non-specific action produced by any type of coma. There is a considerable amount of evidence to show that the presence of high voltage slow waves, of which Dr. Arnold spoke, can be produced not only by insulin coma but by many other types of treatment in psychiatry which give equally positive results. This holds for electroconvulsive treatment, and for some of the drugs which have anticholinergic properties.

I think that the theoretical concepts advanced by Dr. Arnold are fascinating. However, the implication that schizophrenic patients come out of insulin coma treatment with an organic defect should give us much to think about.

DR. KALINOWSKY: I only want to make some practical remarks.

I think it is very important for us to realize that we can get twice as many patients well with treatment as get well without treatment, and I want to point out that the figures which Dr. Arnold gave us are exactly the same as the figures of the larger statistics, including the ones with which Von Braunmühl came out during the war. We didn't get the literature from abroad then but had identical results and I hope that Dr. Arnold works up the statistics the same way as previous workers did.

One should point out that the statistical conclusions are often questionable, as we all realize. But it is a strange fact that in those hospitals where insulin is given properly (and this applies in this country to the Pennsylvania Hospital where Dr. Bond reported first and to the larger statistics and perhaps more suitable material in some typical mental institutions) results are identical. The confusion came from the fact that from many hospitals material was published which was not treated properly. The emphasis on the deep coma and the great number of comas cannot be repeated often enough.

I do think that we just have to have this goal in our treatment that whether we give more insulin or more electric shocks or more combined, we have to get twice as many patients well as we get from spontaneous remissions. And there are enough statistics on spontaneous remissions from the time before the somatic treatment in psychiatry.

I want to make one other remark. The agreement of those who were working in this field is significant. Those who have less experience in it feel that from a scientific standpoint they have to get statistical proof. They should realize that those who really know something about the treatment get the same results.

I want to make one more remark since I did get around in various countries. I want to support Dr. Hoff's statement that schizophrenia is the same in all countries and that cultural differences do not exist, as far as the cases of schizophrenia are concerned. In those various countries I saw patients undergoing insulin treatment, the more typical and more serious cases of schizophrenia were exactly the same. I never have any disagreements on the diagnosis of patients considered for insulin. The diagnosis of most schizophrenics is the same in all countries. It is some borderline group, some ten per cent of cases where you might call them pseudo-neurotic schizophrenics or severe neuroses or some special group. But the definite cases of schizophrenia like the ones presented by Dr. Arnold and the ones by Dr. Hoff and various others who have worked in this field are exactly the same in all countries.

CHAIRMAN RINKEL: Dr. Hoff always has pointed out that the deteriorated schizophrenic looks alike regardless of color, race, continent, country. There is no doubt about that.

DR. HOFF: I do not believe that organic changes in the brain cells are present in every case of schizophrenia. They are certainly not present in schizophrenic patients who die in an acute stage, but they are always present in old schizophrenics. They can be found in the 3rd to the 5th layer. Vogt thinks that certain pathological changes in brain cells are pathognomonic in schizophrenia. I am not certain of this. We believe that in the first stage there are only functional disturbances; that later on there is a true organic disruption of cell function, apparent not only clinically but visible in histological pictures as well. I do not believe that such changes are produced by insulin coma per se. I believe that such pathological changes appear first in a localized part of the brain as concomitants of the original schizophrenic process, and that at a later stage they spread throughout the cortex.

To repeat, I believe that specific cell groups are first involved in the development of schizophrenia. I would like to stress what my friend Kalinowsky has said. I have had the privilege of teaching psychiatry on 3 continents. I discovered that in the majority of cases we diagnose schizophrenia identically in Asia, America and Europe. We differ, apparently, only in so-called borderline cases. In the statistics of Doctor Arnold there is reported only a single case of doubtful nature. The other patients involved in Doctor Arnold's statistics would be diagnosed by everybody in this room, unquestionably, as schizophrenia.

DR. HAROLD HIMWICH: I have enjoyed Dr. Arnold's remarks. In fact, they agree very well with some of the data concerning the carbohydrate metabolism of the brain. The materials which constitute the cells, including phospholipids and amino acids, can be oxidized to yield energy. And that affords a basis for his conclusion that cells may be destroyed during hypoglycemia.

We would, however, welcome additional evidence for the suggestion that cells concerned with schizophrenic patterns are the ones most sensitive to hypoglycemia and, therefore, most likely to succumb to lack of energy.

Dr. Arnold used the term anoxia to include both lack of glucose and lack of oxygen. As a matter of fact, the hemoglobin of the arterial blood may be amply oxygenated during insulin hypoglycemia. But if respiratory difficulties occur, as may happen when the hypoglycemia becomes so profound that the medullary respiratory centers are involved, then anoxia can be superimposed on hypoglycemia. I wonder whether or not Dr. Arnold would consider the use of the expression *deprivation of energy* and thus render it possible to make a distinction between glucose lack and oxygen lack as causes of deprivation of energy. If the latter is added to the former, the total effect becomes more significant.

DR. NATHAN S. KLINE: I'll be very brief. I'd like to compliment Dr. Arnold too. I think the essence of progress is the ability to observe and describe and Dr. Arnold has done an excellent job.

There are one or two questions I would like to raise. Not all of them I think can be answered. In any treatment we tend to select patients. "Schizophrenia is schizophrenia is schizophrenia." We know that certain schizophrenics appear to have a better prognosis than others.

Now if there is only a certain amount of treatment available, the general tendency is to select those patients who have the better prognosis, so that we may not be able to fairly compare treated with untreated patients unless we select all patients who should be treated and then keep half as a control group.

The other questions refer specifically to Dr. Arnold's theory which to me is among the most interesting parts of the paper. I have no doubt that patients given insulin therapy respond better than those not given insulin therapy. Whether this means to what degree insulin affects the course of the disease, is difficult to tell. I ran an insulin ward at one time for two years and I have no question that insulin helped. But in respect to his theory about the cells, first of all I was not clear whether he had taken patients who had died during the course of insulin therapy and then had done cell counts on the brains of such patients as compared with others.

I would suggest, a more equitable way of doing it would be to take patients who had recovered following insulin therapy and then for one or another reason died and compare those with patients who had been given insulin and failed to recover. There should be theoretically a difference in the brains, in the cell count of these two different groups.

Also how within this framework can one explain spontaneous remissions. Do the defective brain cells somehow recover? If they do so I presume it must be through some physiological metabolic process, which means that there may be other factors which influence the recuperability of such cells.

The other brief observation refers to the Columbia Greystone Project with lobotomies. We did a cell count, a very tedious one, on the tissue of some of the schizophrenic patients and compared them with textbook norms of individuals who died in accidents and so on.

We came upon the interesting fact that the schizophrenics had many more cells per square centimeter than did the normal individuals. Our first conclusion was that schizophrenia was caused by too much brain power. But secondly on reviewing it, it appeared that there might have been differences in the sections of fixation and the count of the cells. But the thesis that Dr. Arnold presented is extremely interesting.

I am wondering if we couldn't compare other groups in order to establish it somewhat more firmly than it is at present. I do hope that perhaps Dr. Arnold would explain: 1) spontaneous remission; and 2) have there been comparisons of patients who recovered post insulin and those who failed. And also one final question: if it is a fact that brain cells are more sensitive, why would not repeated courses of insulin or more prolonged insulin comas manage to dispose of the still borderline cells, and thus bring about a recovery in this manner?

DR. DUSSIK: In order to save time, I want to point to a practical issue only. I assume that Dr. Hoff and Dr. Arnold do not mean that the patients reaching full remission show after the treatment evidence of an organic brain syndrome. I feel it is necessary to point out that their theory concerns the assumed mechanism of the curative insulin effect but that no symptoms of defect whatsoever result from this treatment after it has been successfully terminated.

CHAIRMAN RINKEL: Dr. Arnold, will you please close the discussion?

DR. ARNOLD: I thank very much all my discussants. The time is too short to answer all questions.

To Dr. Denber: I would prefer to discuss possibilities of our new diagnostic framework with him personally. There is no time to give more details for the diagnostic results on the basis of this study.

Next, the anatomical findings: Dr. Hoff has answered this question. We cannot say yet there are specific anatomical findings in the schizophrenic disease but we hope to develop a new microhistochemical method or microneurophysiological method. Just now we cannot say there are specific findings.

May I answer Dr. Himwich. It seems to me we use different words but the same meaning. First there is disorganization in the carbohydrate metabolism of the nervous cell. Next, the nervous cell starts a "Wot falls" function; and third, the cell will be disturbed. During this time, cells are also changed in the energy and in the performance metabolism. The details should also be discussed personally.

Dr. Dussik asked a very important question. Is in the fully remitted cases the defect a sign of a brain lesion, an organic brain lesion? I must say that this is not the case. In the time after the insulin shock treatment the patient shows Bleuler's syndrome during some months. In control examinations after five years we never can observe it. We never can realize any signs of a brain organic lesion.

To Dr. Kline, I thank him very much but it is also not time enough to discuss the details. Maybe we can do it personally.

I hope it was possible to bring a new approach with our ideas. I know I have difficulties to express myself in English. I beg your pardon, but I hope you will understand all things of importance.

Chapter 12

INDICATIONS OF INSULIN THERAPY

A. C. Pacheco e Silva

When the new drugs appeared, the so-called ganglio-plegic, neuroplegic or ataraxic, it was not long before numerous papers were published, in which the authors asserted that the use of shock therapies, including insulin therapy, was no longer justified since the new forms of treatment were superior.

However, as time goes by, observation and experience are showing that, notwithstanding the indubitably favorable results with the new drugs in the treatment of schizophrenia and other psychoses, their use does not, in our view, exclude the use of the shock methods, in particular insulin therapy. This conference organized for the purpose of evaluating the results obtained with insulin therapy, the merits of insulin treatment compared with other treatments, its indications, contraindications, and results obtained, is therefore justified.

When, in 1933, Manfred Sakel introduced insulin therapy, he called it shock treatment, because he did not fail to observe the intense physiological reactions which took place in the organism, during the period of hypoglycemia, causing an anabolic coma as well as a violent catabolic convulsion.

Almost immediately, two different types of shock were observed: the "dry shock," which ended in convulsion and the "wet shock," observed in the course of the coma. The technique originally recommended by Sakel consisted in the provocation of deep and prolonged hypoglycemic comas. Many authors, however, felt, after some experience, that this method was dangerous, requiring many precautions. As a result, it was not long before other modified techniques emerged using insulin in smaller doses, and not provoking more than a pre-coma, and even this of less duration than that recommended by the author of the method.

Lopes Ibor,[1] in approaching the question, comments: "The idea of intensifying the therapies is based on observation of great biological significance; it seems that those situations which place individuals before a maximum danger to life are capable of setting free compensatory 'curative' processes which would not otherwise come into action. Experience with prolonged comas, some observations on people who suffered strangulation or falls from great heights, support this opinion. The ideas of Selye on the 'adaptation syndrome' express the same fact. Is it therefore indispensable that the methods of treatment be necessarily brutal and even dangerous, in order to produce such an effect? Is there some relation between both the facts? It is possible that there is, but this does not exclude the possibility that human ingenuity can solve the problem by passing it. Cerletti[2] admits that the defensive substances, which have a beneficial action on the organism and explain the favorable results of the shock methods, are formed only during the comatose state, whence his designation of acroagonin (from the Greek *acros*, "supreme," and *agon*, "fight"), for a substance obtained from the brains of electroshocked pigs, which may have a beneficial action on various neuroses and psychoses. These reports unquestionably speak in favor of the original technique of Sakel, the prolonged and deep comas.

However, as P. Neveu[3] points out, various factors prevented, from the very beginning, the Sakel technique, as established by the author, to be rigorously applied.

Mayer-Gross, Sargant, Dax, Allan Walter, lamenting that

a wider application of Sakel's method had not been possible, suggested its centralization in "units" located in regional hospitals. The circumstances of the war and the scarcity of insulin caused difficulties which, unhappily, deprived many patients of this treatment.

The need of long experience of the psychiatrists as well as thorough training of the personnel collaborating in the use of this technique was pointed out in Holland and in Canada.

Delmas Mansalet,[4] deliberating on the same question, makes the following statement: "Without a doubt the majority of French psychiatrists dislike the use of insulin therapy in its phase called 'liminar' by Sakel in cases of simple neuroses, compulsions, slight excitations and toxicomanias. It is necessary, however, to point out that most of them are far from having applied the cure of Sakel over the long period of which the author of the method speaks."

Kalinowsky[5] comments, "Insulin coma treatment was unfortunately abolished by some hospitals due to the lack of personnel, and by others because inadequate treatment with not sufficiently deep comas or unduly short series of treatments, gave them unsatisfactory results."

The appearance of new therapeutic procedures, not requiring the same experience, care, and assistance, without the risks of insulin therapy in large doses, followed by deep comas, led many authors to progressively abandon the original technique of Sakel, substituting for it the gentler ones using subcomas of short duration. Few remained faithful to the classic formula of the creator of the method. The techniques in which reduced doses of insulin are used are generally employed according to an individual criterion, equally with respect to dosage, the duration of the hypoglycemic phase, the number of shocks and the combination with convulsive methods and the newer drugs.

In our opinion the modifications introduced into the original technique of Sakel, on the one hand had the advantage of not requiring such an exacting technique and not carrying so many risks, on the other hand brought the draw-backs of not causing such complete remission in schizo-phrenia cases, as had been observed previously when deep, prolonged, and numerous comas were provoked. Also the combination with other treatments as practiced almost every-where, creates a certain confusion in the statistics and pre-vents a definite conclusion as to the efficiency of the method.

Therefore it seems indispensable to us, in order to eval-uate exactly the effect of insulin therapy, that it be given especially to young patients, not previously treated by other methods, without combining it with other therapies, fol-lowing the technique of Sakel to the letter.

Principal Indications for Shock Therapies

The author presented[6] to the First International Congress of Psychiatry a table containing the principal indications for the shock therapies, pointing out the cases in which insulin therapy would be most precisely indicated as follows:

a) *Schizophrenia:* 1) Acute forms, less than one year old; 2) Paranoid forms; 3) Cases accompanied by psycho-motor excitement; 4) Forms which present a profound so-matic repercussion, with denutrition due to negativism and sitophobia.

The indications for (3) and (4) are based respectively upon the sedative effects of insulin and its effect on the general state of the patient. In certain cases when one wishes above all to improve the general conditions, sub-shock doses are sufficient and there is no need to proceed to coma.

b) *Manic depressive psychoses* (depressive and catato-nic forms).

c) *Psychoneuroses* (accompanied by intense anxiety).

In general, the results published by other authors and our own experience justify maintaining the same scheme, with slight modifications. Thus we feel that, in the **para-**

noid forms of schizophrenia, the therapy of impregnation with chlorpromazine is indicated.[7]

It appears to us that, in the other forms of schizophrenia, insulin therapy has its greatest and most decided indications. Mayer-Gross[8] stated: "Nevertheless the treatment by hypoglycemia introduced by Sakel at Vienna, in 1933, has found general recognition as the only effective method of treating early schizophrenia."

The same conclusions were reached by Delay, Jacobowsky, Sargant, Dax, Jones, Titeca, Pamboukis, Rouleau, Boschi, Bergmann, Diogo Furtado, and Pacheco e Silva, to mention only those who commented on the report of Sakel to the First International Congress of Psychiatry, in Paris. Few works have been published since then on insulin therapy, following rigorously Sakel's technique, in the treatment of schizophrenia.

The exception was made by F. H. West, E. D. Bond, J. T. Shurley and Meyers,[9] who published, in 1955, an interesting paper from which we quote: "The authors made a 14-year follow-up study of 781 persons who had received Insulin Coma Therapy. Aim of treatment was to produce as deep a coma for as long a period as is safe for the patient. Therapy was given 5 days a week; the average course required 3 months of hospitalization. The treatment considered ideal by the authors consists of 1½ to 2 hours of coma, of which an hour is in the second stage, a maximum of 1 hour in third stage, and a maximum of 25 minutes in fourth stage (extensor rigidity of arms and legs). The authors concluded that insulin coma therapy is effective in restoring patients to their prepsychotic level. It does not produce a permanent resistance to schizophrenia. Patients must be helped to maintain their adjustment through supportive psychotherapy, environmental manipulation, or further shock treatments. Intensive psychotherapeutic efforts must be made to correct the factors predisposing the patient to regress to psychosis. Insulin coma does not interfere with psychotherapy."

Insulin Coma Most Efficacious

From our personal experience we believe that insulin therapy (Sakel's technique) is the most efficacious treatment for the schizophrenic. The most complete and lasting remissions observed by us in schizophrenics were in cases submitted to insulin therapy with deep coma. Many of our cases treated over twenty years ago have not relapsed and others so far have such slight signs of the illness that only a meticulous examination, carried out by specialists, could disclose the schizophrenic residues.

In our first statistics published in September 1937,[10] in 104 patients treated, we obtained the following results:

Total remissions .... 33 patients—31.73%
Partial remissions .... 21 patients—20.19%
Improved .... 27 patients—25.96%
Unimproved .... 23 patients—22.12%

The results obtained since then agree in general with the first statistics, but the data can not be evaluated with certainty because unhappily we were forced, as were most of the psychiatrists of the world, to apply the technique of Sakel not in its true form which prevented us from judging its effects.

However, comparing the results obtained in the past with those of the present, it is our opinion that, in the treatment of schizophrenia with the insulin method of Sakel administered alone or combined with other shock methods and with various drugs, the best results were obtained with deep hypoglycemic coma.

Post-Insulin-Therapy Psychosis

We wish to mention certain changes observed in the typical picture of the schizophrenias, in some cases with changes in the personality of the patient, which led us to describe them, by analogy with the post-malarial-therapy psychoses, as post-insulin-therapy psychoses.[11]

Indications of Insulin Therapy

As to the indication of insulin therapy related to the different clinical forms of schizophrenia, we believe that this treatment is most to be recommended in its simple forms, in hebephrenia, in which there is intense psychomotor excitation. Insulin therapy has in these cases also a sedative action, calming the patients, facilitating the adaptation to hospital life, making possible the use of psychotherapy and occupational therapy.

In the depressive forms of the manic depressive psychosis, the method of Sakel is decidedly indicated because it helps to improve the general condition of the patients, besides acting in the psychic sphere. When uncontrollable ideas of suicide exist, which do not yield to insulin therapy, the combination with electroshock therapy is indicated, to remove with greater rapidity the ideas of self-destruction and avoid the patients carrying out this intention.

In the neuroses and the psychosomatic illnesses, in which there is a marked loss of weight, with nutritional disturbances, lack of appetite, repugnance to food, insulin therapy used in the form of sub-shocks is a very helpful therapy, improving the physical condition of the patient and also acting favorably on the mental picture.

Literature Cited

1. Ibor, Lopez. Thérapeutique biologique. In Comptes rendus des séances du Premier Congrès Mondial de Psychiatrie, Paris, 1950. Paris, Hermann et Cie., 1952. v.IV, p.28.

2. Cerletti, Ugo. Entrevue avec le Prof. U. Cerletti sur les "acroagonines." Attualita medica, no. 4, April, 1953.

3. Neveu, P. Thérapeutique biologique. In Comptes rendus des séances du Premier Congrès Mondial de Psychiatrie, Paris, 1950. Paris, Hermann et Cie., 1952. v.IV, p. 59.

4. Mansalet, Delmas. Thérapeutique biologique. In Comptes rendus des séances du Premier Congrès Mondial de Psychiatrie, Paris, 1950. Paris, Hermann et Cie., 1952. v.IV, p.101.

5. Kalinowsky, L. B. Thérapeutique biologique. In Comptes rendus des séances du Premier Congrès Mondial de Psychiatrie, Paris, 1950. Paris, Hermann et Cie., 1952. v.IV, p.104.

6. Pacheco e Silva, A. C. Thérapeutique biologique. In Comptes rendus des séances du Premier Congrès Mondial de Psychiatrie, Paris, 1950. Hermann et Cie., 1952. v.IV, p.79.

7. Pacheco e Silva, A. C., Carvalho, H. M., and Fortes, Roberto O. emprêgo da clorpromazina em doses macicas: síndromo de impregnação. Publicaçoes medicas, 198:49, §2, 1957.

8. Mayer-Gross, W., Slater, Eliot, and Roth, Martin. *Clinical psychiatry.* London, Cassell and Company, 1954. p.283.

9. West, Franklin H., Bond, E. D., Shurley, J. T., and Meyers, C. D. Insulin coma therapy schizophrenia. Am. J. Psychiat., 111:583-589, 1955.

10. Pacheco e Silva, A. C., and Ferraz, N. de T. O

método de Sakel nas esquizofrenias. Arquivos da Assistencia Geral a Psicopatas do E. de São Paulo, 2:499-516, 1937.

11. Pacheco e Silva, A. C. Psicoses post-insulinoterápicas. Arquivos da Assis. a Psicopatas do E.S.P., 2:265, 1937.

Chapter 13

NOTES ON THE APPLICATION OF THE SAKEL
METHOD IN MENTAL PATIENTS IN PERU

FEDERICO SAL Y ROSAS[*]

My observations relate to the application of the Sakel
method in the Victor Larco Herrera Hospital, the only one
for mental patients in Perú. As an introduction, I offer a
summary report on psychiatric care in Perú.

I. *Psychiatric Care in Perú*

Of the 181 public and private therapeutic institutions in
existence at the end of 1955, a mere six are for mental
patients; only one is a public institution, namely the Victor
Larco Herrera Hospital, maintained by the "Sociedad de
Beneficencia Pública de Lima" (Public Welfare Association
of Lima). Of the 18,701 public and private hospital beds in
existence at the end of 1955, a mere 1182, i.e., 6.3 per cent,
are for mental patients, whereas psychiatric beds represent
30 per cent of the total available in most European countries, and more than 50 per cent in the United States.

In 1954, there were altogether 1,934 physicians in all the
therapeutic institutes in Perú; the number in psychiatric
establishments did not, nor does now, exceed fifty. The Victor Larco Herrera Hospital has 102 nurses, male and female,
and only three social workers. Auxiliary personnel consists
of 301 persons, including student nurses and employees

[*] Translation from Spanish, approved by the author.

engaged in non-nursing duty. Preventive psychiatry has not yet been introduced. Nor is there any adequate legislation relating to the care and prevention of mental diseases.

II. *Frequency of Different Types of Mental Disease in Perú*

The data in this section are taken from my recent paper based on 9,117 new admissions to the Victor Larco Herrera in twelve years (1937-1949) and on the average population present in the hospital on December 31 for seven years (1938-44). (See Table 1.)

The endogenous mental diseases (manic-depressive psy-

TABLE I

Frequency of Mental Diseases in Perú
(Statistics of the Victor Larco Herrera Hospital)

	New Admissions		Average Population of the Hospital on December 31	
	Number	Per Cent	Number	Per Cent
1. Psychoses with syphilis of the central nervous system	608	6.66	581	5.65
2. With other infectious diseases	140	1.54	58	0.56
3. With circulatory disorders	65	0.70	13	0.12
4. Senile and involutional psychoses	550	6.03	264	2.56
5. Alcoholism	969	10.62	555	5.40
6. Various somatic changes	142	1.55	71	0.68
7. Total epilepsy	1132	12.48	1301	12.65
8. Neurosis	321	3.53	250	2.43
9. Manic-depressive psychosis	248	2.72	587	5.70
10. Schizophrenia	3339	36.63	4712	45.78
11. Paranoia and paranoid states	107	1.17	262	2.54
12. Psychopathic personality	287	3.15	446	4.34
13. Oligophrenia	587	6.34	954	9.27
14. Miscellaneous conditions not included in the above	626	6.86	239	2.32
A. Exogenous psychoses (1-6)	2473	27.12	1542	14.98
B. Endogenous psychoses (9, 10, 11)	3694	40.51	5561	54.02
C. Endogenous psychoses and psychopathies	3981	43.66	6007	58.36
D. Great endogenous circle (C-13)	4559	50.	6961	67.72
E. Infectious psychoses (1-2)	61	7.20	639	6.21
F. Cardiovascular plus advanced age	614	5.96	277	2.69
G. Exogenous psychoses plus epilepsy	3611	39.61	2843	27.71

chosis, schizophrenia, paranoia and paranoid states) account for more than 40 per cent of the first admissions and for 54 per cent of the average population of the hospital. This high proportion is due exclusively to the percentage of schizophrenia, which accounts for more than 36 per cent of the admissions and 46 per cent of the hospital population; whereas the frequency of manic-depressive psychosis is less than 3 per cent, and that of the paranoid psychoses less than 2 per cent of the first admissions. The exogenous psychoses account for 27 per cent of the first admissions and for 15 per cent of the total number of the patients hospitalized on December 31. Epilepsy, considered independently of the ailments mentioned above, accounts for 12 per cent of the admissions, of which 8 per cent are cases of epilepsy with psychoses. Generally, the inhabitants of Perú and those of the other countries of the torrid zone seem to be more prone to the endogenous and idiopathic forms of mental disease. The relatively higher frequency of the exogenous psychoses in the countries of the temperate zone is accounted for by the high mental morbidity springing from organic disturbances inherent in advanced age and linked with the increase in the average length of life (circulatory, involutional and senile psychoses), which occur on the largest scale in the United States.

III. *Data from My Experience with Insulin in Perú*

The Sakel method has been practiced in Peru since 1937. The data which I present are based on my general observations since that year, and specifically on my systematic observations in the Home for Women of the Victor Larco Herrera Hospital. In this hospital insulin is used in the Admissions Department, the Home for Women, the Home for Men, the Women's Ward, and the Men's Ward.

The insulin treatment is carried out independently in each building, under the supervision of a female or male nurse who is assisted by several nonskilled employees, male or female, or by students of the Co-educational School of Nursing. The personnel receive no special instruction in insulin therapy beyond that given in that nursing school. Moreover, due to a system of rotating the nursing staffs of the different departments, the insulin stations have no permanent staff. In order to obviate this drawback in some fashion, a short course for nurses in the Sakel method was given in my department by four physicians of the Home, in the last months of 1956; this must, however, be repeated from time to time, owing to the above-mentioned system of rotation, since nurses at one time trained in the department are no longer working with us.

Occupational therapy is carried out in each building in an as yet unsystematized form, for there are no specialized or permanent personnel available.

Mental diseases show similar characteristics among the population of Perú to those observed in Europe and in the United States. Our observations in this respect are still incomplete, and today all we can do is mention that the clinical pictures reveal a marked pathoplastic influence of the native mentality. A fact of interest in this respect is the very high frequency of the paranoid form of schizophrenia, which amounts to almost 60 per cent in the statistics of my Department. These cases are practically uniform, asthenic with deliriant ideas of persecution, whereas esthenic pictures with megalomaniac ideas are rare—which may also be related to the predominantly inhibited nature of the Peruvian native.

The insulin treatment technique followed by us is essentially Sakel's original one, to which we have adapted such later variations as we have regarded as helpful.

Following are a few specific facts of our own observing:

1. To this moment, the Sakel method is the essential and most efficacious measure in the treatment of schizophrenia, and is applicable to other syndromes as well, including manic-depressive psychosis. In the latter we do not resort to the use of insulin during states of manic excitation,

which are well controlled by electroshock and the tranquilizers, but we have done so in cases of depression which
resisted electroshock therapy.

2. The Sakel therapy really cures the patient. We do not
agree with certain authors (Heuyer is one of them) who
claim the contrary. We have kept track of schizophrenics
in whom complete remission was produced by insulin more
than fifteen years ago and no relapse has yet taken place.
This method seems to act not merely in shortening a phasic
schizophrenia, but by producing a structural change in the
patient.

3. The percentage of complete remission in the women
given the insulin treatment in my Department in recent
years is lower than that observed by us in previous periods.
Our present material shows a higher frequency of cases
which remain stationary on a level of a moderate or marked
improvement. Of seventy-three women patients treated with
insulin, thirty-four (almost one-half) have remained in a
state of slight improvement, and twelve in the state of social
remission. This picture is linked, in my opinion, with two
intimately interlaced facts: (1) my Department takes care
of paying patients, and (2) the Victor Larco Herrera Hospital closed its gates to nonpaying welfare patients in 1950,
pleading a lack of resources. Consequently, in our Home
there is a high percentage of very poor people whose families have made a veritable economic sacrifice to pay for
their care, but only when the patient has already become
gravely affected or dangerous—in other words, almost always belatedly. Of the seventy-three patients in this group,
only seventeen received insulin therapy sooner than one
year after the onset of the illness.

In the first group of seventy-three patients treated with
insulin in Perú by Honorio Delgado and his collaborators
(1938), complete remission was 87 per cent in the cases
where the illness had been present for less than six months,
63 per cent in the cases in existence for six to eighteen
months, and 9.5 per cent in the chronic cases. In the group

presented by us today, which happens by coincidence likewise to comprise seventy-three patients, complete remission
was achieved in merely nine cases (12 per cent of the total
number), in five of whom the illness had been present for
less than a year, in three for one to two years, and in one
for more than two years.

4. The combination of insulin with electroshock and
other therapeutic means, such as intravenous pyrotherapy,
according to Buscaino's method, and the various tranquilizers, has brought us generally good results. The addition of
electroshock seems to us to reinforce the action of the insulin, apart from its well-known effect on states of excitation.

5. Relapses were many after a complete remission produced by insulin, but always to a lesser degree than after
the use of electroshock. This is another of those matters the
investigation of which has been concluded. Table II reveals
that insulin was administered twice in nine cases, and three
times in three cases.

TABLE II

Distribution of the Material

	Cases
Age	
20 years or less	7
21-40 years	51
Over 40 years	15
Total	73
Race	
White	10
White plus Indian	35
Indian plus White	8
Indian	10
Other	10
Total	73

Region
Coast	44
Highland	24
Mountain	5
Total	73

Diagnosis
D. P. P. (Paranoid Schizophrenia)	43
D. P. H. (Hebephrenic Schizophrenia)	12
D. P. S. (Simple Schizophrenia)	4
D. P. C. (Catatonic Schizophrenia)	1
P. M. D. (Manic-Depressive Psychosis)	4
Others	9
Total	73

Duration of the Disease:
0 year	17
1-2 years	28
over 2 years	28
Total	73

Doses
15-50 units	13
60-100 units	28
110-200 units	28
over 200 units	4
Total	73

Therapeutic Results
Complete remission	9
Social remission	12
Slight improvement	34
No change	10
Turn to the worse	1
Interruption by death	4
Under treatment	3
Total	73

Number of series of Insulin

   No. One series 61

   No. Two series 9

   No. Three series 3

   Total   73

6. In connection with the view expressed by several authors concerning the need for a prolonged ("chronic") treatment as a guarantee of efficacy and dependability, we have applied a minimum of seventy comas, except in certain instances. If it was necessary, we continued to 100, 150 and up to 200 comas, the latter number being the maximum agreed upon in my Department. Thus we accomplished remissions which had not been brought about by the seventy comas. In forty-four cases, 100-199 comas were produced, and fifteen cases underwent 200 or more. Among the latter group (all chronic cases, except for one that had existed for less than a year), complete remission was observed in just one single case, in which the illness had been present for a year and a half, but an improvement occurred in more than half of the total number. Noteworthy is the fact that almost all the very painstakingly achieved remissions become lasting, and relapses are rare and very slight.

7. A deep or irreversible coma appeared in eight patients, in other words, in a little more than 10 per cent.

8. Three fatalities were observed: one owing to a mechanical accident (asphyxiation by sugar solution introduced with a catheter); the second fatality was caused by irreversible coma and terminal pneumonia, after nine days of a state of stupor; and finally, a third case of very grave coma led to a dextral hemiplegia, an agitated confusion, terminal bronchopneumonia and cardiac collapse. Another patient died from an intercurrent infection (typhoid fever) while she was under treatment. Naturally, this patient is not considered among the deaths connected with the insulin therapy. The proportion of these within the record of cases

presented (i.e., 4 per cent) is high in comparison with the figures given by Malzberg (1.29 per cent) and Müller (less than 0.5 per cent).

9. Other complications: We witnessed neither the activation of the psychosis nor the personality changes cited by other authors, but we did see three cases of passing disturbances of consciousness, apart from the two mentioned in paragraph 8. Local paralysis and paresthesia occurred in five cases, in three of which they were reversible. The cessation of movement was permanent in two; one of the latter was the case of the patient mentioned as last but none of the cases that terminated in death (see paragraph 8). In this patient a monoplegia of the right arm remained present until her death; the other one, forty-five years of age and afflicted for twenty-nine years, suffered a dextral hemiplegia in the fourth coma, which showed no improvement despite the interruption of the treatment, and still persists today. Skin-allergy was observed in two patients.

Convulsive attacks during the hypoglycemia were observed in eight cases, i.e., in more than 10 per cent. To Sakel and others such attacks are indicative of a favorable effect. Plattner, on the contrary, reports that in his observation such crises made their appearance in 1.6 per cent of the patients with complete remission, and in 4.3 per cent of the cases not favorably affected by insulin. In our material, the epileptiform attacks occurred in only one patient with complete remission and in five with slight remission; in the other two, no clinical change was produced by the insulin. In two other patients, convulsive attacks occurred during the afternoon hours. One of them had an epileptiform attack at 3 P.M., and later showed symptoms of hypoglycemia which made it necessary to give her an injection of sugar. She had no other attack. The other patient, however, had a prior record of clinical epilepsy; in our department, on the afternoon of the twenty-fourth day after the initiation of therapy, she showed symptoms of a coma and convulsive attacks which were not ended by the injection of dextrose, but did cease in response to the intravenous administration of two ampules (0.2 g) of somnifene (Diethylamine salts of diethyl and allylisopropyl barbituric acid).

We have observed psychomotor excitation in twenty-three patients, thirteen of whom were from the coastal region of the country, and nine from the highlands; these figures are not indicative of any influence of the native region, but Leonor Revoredo, who also works in the hospital, has found the patients from the coastal regions to be distinctly in the majority of those who show this symptom in response to insulin.

In two cases, we had to suspend the treatment because of an abrupt rise in the arterial pressure during the coma. In another patient, during the hypoglycemia, we observed an intense dyspnea, cyanosis and phases of apnea, which seemed to seriously imperil her life; fortunately, however, with an adequate adjustment of the dosage, the injection of antiepileptics and with antiallergic treatments, we were able to continue the therapy to the two-hundredth coma.

10. The minimum dose to produce a coma was 15 units in one case, and the maximum liminal dose was 240 units; the average minimum dose is 106 units. Most of the patients have a liminal dose that is higher than 100 units and less than 150. The highest dose applied in the course of the treatment was 500 units, given in a single case.

11. We have endeavored for the past five years to ascertain the influence of age, sex, region of origin (coastal or highland areas), race (white or Indian), etc., on such clinical data, as the liminal dose, degree of remission, sensitivity to insulin, convulsive attacks, etc. Our investigation is still in progress. Therefore we limit ourselves to pointing out provisionally a tendency in young persons to require high doses of insulin: of three patients whose liminal dose was more than 200 units, two were twenty-five years of age, and the third girl was twenty-one. A tendency to a high threshold is also observed in paranoid schizophrenia, and a tendency to low doses is noted in schizophrenia of the simple

form and in manic-depressive psychosis. It seems that recent cases require lower doses for coma than chronic ones; the lowest liminal dose recorded (15 units) was observed in a young hebephrenic whose affliction was less than a year old. The therapeutic result seems to be better in the paranoid and hebephrenic forms of schizophrenia and in the acute cases, which observation agrees with the already classic idea of the advantage of an early treatment.

DISCUSSION

DR. MILTON GREENBLATT: May I congratulate the speakers on the excellent papers and the stimulating problems raised.

I think it would be my function perhaps to point out difficulties in methodology. Many people have had intensive experience with insulin shock and claims regarding depths of coma vary as do the number of shocks. There are also many technical questions involved.

I think that what is needed is a simpler definition, within which you can define the optimal conditions, and then go on to a comparative study between insulin and other kinds of therapy.

I offer for your consideration one little study which attempted to assess the comparative value of deep and light insulin comas. This was done in our hospital a couple of years ago and was reported in 1957 to the American Psychiatric Association. Our comas were 35 in number in both groups. The coma's duration was 30 minutes and the study was done by three observers: a psychologist using the Rorschach test, a nurse and a doctor. It was interesting that we went into these studies believing that under those conditions deep coma was certainly expected. We found to our amazement that deep coma shows no marked advantages over light coma under these conditions.

The number of patients who improved and the number of patients who were discharged were essentially the same. A follow-up of these patients eighteen months later revealed that the deep coma had a very slight edge over the light coma but not significant.

I would like to submit this for your consideration and I would hope that the people with longer clinical experience would discuss it.

Chapter 14

INSULIN THERAPY OF SCHIZOPHRENIA IN PERU— OUR 20 YEARS OF EXPERIENCE

Honorio Delgado*

Introduction

In July, 1937, we initiated in Peru the treatment of schizophrenia with insulin in two groups, one in women and the other in men. At the beginning, we followed principally the method of Sakel[1, 2] and later the modifications introduced by Braunmühl.[3] Finally, we used the method of giving insulin in divided doses in insulin resistant cases. Thus we treated 76 patients till October of 1938. In the majority of these cases the illness was present for six months. The results of this work were published in December of 1938.[4] In 3 patients the treatment was discontinued because of intercurrent diseases. Of 73 cases of schizophrenia which received an average of 52 comas of one hour's duration, we obtained complete remission in 45 (61.6%), social remission in 9 (12.3%) and slight improvement or negative results in 19 (26.1%). Of the 73 schizophrenics, 31 were men and 42 women. Remissions occurred in 70.9% of the men (16 complete and 6 social) while in woman the rate was 76.3% (29 complete and 3 social).

In a previous study[5] we presented in detail the results in

* This paper was submitted but not read by the author—*Ed.*

a total of 100 schizophrenics: 91 cases received insulin alone and 9 insulin and metrazol. Remission was obtained in 70, complete in 56 and social in 14. No mention is made of this group of patients in the work that follows except in the first of the conclusions.

Materials and Methods

We are presenting 440 cases of schizophrenia of whom 335 were men and 105 women.* Of these cases, 317 (72.05%) were paranoid, 25 (5.68%) catatonic, 37 (8.41%) hebephrenic, 20 (4.55%) simple, and 41 (9.31%) atypical schizophrenics. With respect to age, the patients were divided in three groups: a. from 10 to 20 years, 69 cases (15.68%); b. from 21 to 30 years, 221 (50.23%); and c. from 31 years and up, 150 (34.09%). With respect to physical condition, the patients were classified according to Kretschmer's scheme: Asthenic 211 (47.95%), pyknic 74 (16.82%), athletic 33 (7.50%), dysplastic 4 (0.91%) and atypical 118 (26.82%).

Heredity: With regard to heredity we classified our patients in the following manner: a. patients among whose immediate relatives (parents and siblings) are mentally ill, especially schizophrenics, 80 (20%); b. patients whose distant relatives only demonstrated mental illnesses, 206 (46.82%); c. patients with no pathological heredity background, 146 (33.18%). With respect to premorbid personality, 177 (40.23%) were normal and 263 (59.77%) abnormal.

Duration of Illness: We date the duration of the illness from the time the first symptoms appeared until the first signs of cure with insulin, not taking into consideration the few previous cases that remitted with or without treatment but which we include in the analysis of the results of the therapy. Thus we have three groups: a. illness lasting

* Of these patients, 242 were of my service (male pensioners) of the Hospital "Victor Larco Herrera" and 198 of the private clinic "Santa Clara," which is directed by Professor J. O. Trelles and myself.

from 0 to 6 months: 151 (34.31%), b. from 6 to 12 months: 90 (20.46%), and c. from 12 months and up: 199 (45.23%).

Duration of Treatment: The duration of treatment was decided upon by the number of comas (of one hour's duration each), dividing the cases in three groups: a. First group up to 59 comas, 95 cases (21.60%); b. second group from 51 to 100 comas, 176 cases (40%), and c. third group more than 100 comas, 169 cases (38.40%). Simple crystalline insulin was used subcutaneously (in small doses) and intramuscularly. The coma was interrupted by the intravenous injection of a hypertonic dextrose solution and the oral administration of a dextrose syrup.

The *methods of treatment* we followed are four: a. Insulin alone, following the method of Sakel, the system of zig-zag of von Braunmühl and the procedure of divided doses that we introduced and described in our first paper[4] for the *insulin resistant cases:* 149 cases (33.86%); b. Mixed treatment, using insulin and electroshock or metrazol applied during the pre-coma period once or twice weekly (in some cases muscular relaxants and inhalation of oxygen in addition): 256 cases (58.18%); c. Insulin and chlorpromazine: 9 cases (2.05%), and d. Insulin, electroshock and chlorpromazine: 26 cases (5.91%).

The method of therapy was selected according to the clinical and physical state of the patient, duration of the illness, family and past personal history, previous treatments (if any) and the response to the latter. Thus, the paranoids were treated preferentially with insulin alone. The other types of schizophrenia were given more frequently mixed treatment. The combination with chlorpromazine in the therapy was used principally in chronic cases, of more than one year's duration, with strong hereditary tendencies or in cases that were not benefited by other types of treatment (insulin, electroshock, metrazol, chlorpromazine, reserpine, leucotomy, etc.). Patients with poor prognosis were given a combination of insulin with electroshock and chlorpromazine on the assumption that treatments became more effective by the simultaneous action of these therapeutic agents upon the cause of the disease.

The daily use of chlorpromazine ranged between 100 and 400 mg. having been administered orally in the majority of the cases and exceptionally intramuscularly. The average dose of insulin necessary to produce the first coma was 106 units. Two hundred and thirty-seven cases (53.86%) needed doses below this average value and 203 (46.14%) above. The minimum dose has been 15 units in a patient 28 years old, in whom 200 mg. of chlorpromazine was administered orally before and during insulin therapy. The maximum dose of insulin was 480 units, in a man 29 years old, castrated by self-mutilation during the illness. In patients treated with insulin alone the dose sufficient to produce coma varied up to 20 units more or less. In patients treated with chlorpromazine in addition, the effective dose of insulin always decreased progressively in the course of 1 to 4 weeks in quantities that varied between 20 and 80 units, arriving in some cases to half of the initial dose.

Results

We classified the effects produced by the four methods of insulin therapy as follows: a. *total remission* (TR), the mental state of the patient was identical or very similar to that before the illness, in any case, without symptoms; b. *social remission* (SR), if the patient's psychological condition allowed him to live with his family and carry out a type of work more or less similar to that before the illness; c. *improvement* (I) when such changes in attitude were obtained that were favorable to life within the hospital; and d. *without improvement* (WI), absence of favorable changes. To evaluate the results in relation to factors of the second order and to avoid excessive division in the total group we combined the four groups in two: *with remission* (R) to include cases with (TR) and (SR) and *no remission* (N) to include those with (I) and (WI).

It should be pointed out that in order to classify the patients according to their psychological condition at the time they leave the hospital or clinic, they are subjected to some tests during the last weeks of insulin therapy. After coming out of coma, the patients are given psychopathologic examinations with the object of finding out principally whether the mental derangements have disappeared and to see if the patient demonstrates acceptance of his illness.[6] In addition, we used, outside of the effects of insulin, narco-analysis with amytal, the tests by Rorschach, Wartegg or the test of pyramid by Pfister and the Thematic Appreception Test (TAT), besides the routine examinations. Patients with remission are discharged approximately one month after termination of therapy. Since the application of chlor-promazine, we recommended continuation of treatment with small doses of this drug for a prolonged period and under medical supervision.

TABLE I

Immediate Results and Diagnosis

Diagnosis	T R	S R	I	W I	Deaths	Total
Paranoid	116 (36.60%)	91 (28.71%)	45 (14.20%)	61 (19.22%)	4	317 (72.05%)
Catatonic	13 (52.00%)	4 (16.00%)	5 (20.00%)	3 (12.00%)	0	25 (5.68%)
Hebephrenic	7 (18.92%)	12 (32.43%)	11 (29.73%)	7 (18.92%)	0	37 (8.41%)
Simple	2 (10.00%)	7 (35.00%)	4 (20.00%)	7 (35.00%)	0	20 (4.55%)
Atypical	13 (31.71%)	14 (34.15%)	8 (19.51%)	6 (14.63%)	0	41 (9.31%)
Total	151 (34.32%)	128 (29.09%)	73 (16.59%)	84 (19.09%)	4 (0.91%)	440 (100%)

Legend: TR = total remission; SR = social remission; I = improvement; WI = without improvement.

Table I shows a summary of the results of the treatment according to the forms of schizophrenia. With respect to the various methods, even though the introduction of chlorpromazine is relatively recent, it appears that one can affirm that its combination with insulin and electroshock gives best results. In 24 paranoids with less than six months of illness treated in this fashion the following results were obtained: (TR) in 62.5% and (SR) in 25% (R= 87.5%).

With respect to age, a group of 150 patients of more than 30 years of age presented the larger proportion of remissions: 110 (73.33%). This is followed by the group of 10 to 20 years of age: 69 patients (15.68%), with 47 remissions (68.12%). Patients of 21 to 30 years of age presented less remissions: of 221 patients (50.23%) 122 had remissions (55.21%).

Patients in whose families mental or nervous illnesses were absent presented the larger proportion of remission: 67.81%; while in the group with strong hereditary familial background the remission rate was 59.09%. With respect to premorbid personality, between patients of normal and abnormal personality the difference in the proportion of remission was practically nil. The same was observed in cases that previously had attacks of schizophrenia and cases that became ill for the first time.

TABLE II

Immediate Results and Duration of Illness

Duration of Illness	R	N R	Deaths	Total
Under 6 months	119 (78.80%)	30 (19.87%)	2	151 (34.31%)
6-12 months	56 (62.22%)	34 (37.78%)	0	90 (20.46%)
12+	104 (52.26%)	93 (46.73%)	2	199 (45.23%)
Total	279 (63.41%)	157 (35.68%)	4 (0.91%)	440 (100%)

The results which compare the duration of the illness (Table II) agree, as one can very well see, with the results obtained universally. With respect to the effects of the duration of the treatment itself, our experience, contrary to prevailing opinion, favors prolonged treatment as shown in Table III.

TABLE III
Immediate Results and Hours of Coma

Hours of Coma	R	N R	Deaths	Total
Under 51	54 (56.84%)	39 (41.06%)	2	95 (21.6%)
51-100	129 (73.29%)	47 (26.71%)	0	176 (40.0%)
100+	96 (56.80%)	71 (42.01%)	2	169 (38.4%)
Total	279 (63.41%)	157 (35.68%)	4 (0.91%)	440 (100%)

Comparing the results according to sex, we considered only those patients that were treated in our private clinic under identical conditions. Of the 198 patients, 93 male and 105 female, the remission occurred in 64 (68.71%) males and 63 (60%) females.

Relapses

Relapse is considered when a patient becomes ill again during the first year after treatment. We verified 11 relapses (2.5%), the majority of them workers under social security who returned to the same hospital service for their condition. Of the 11 cases, 7 were paranoid, 3 atypical and 1 hebephrenic. Of those, 8 received mixed treatment (insulin and electroshock), 2 insulin alone and 1 mixed treatment plus chlorpromazine. The small percentage of proved failures is explained by the difficulty in following up patients who leave the hospital and the clinic. It wasn't possible for us to do a systematic follow up of our cases.

Complications

The following complications have been observed:

a. *Death.* During insulin treatment 4 patients died (0.90%), all paranoids: 1 of subarachnoid hemorrhage, 1 of pulmonary edema and 2 of cardiac failure.

b. *Prolonged Coma.* This unpleasant complication occurred in 15 patients (3.40%). The treatment we used consisted of injecting analeptics, Vitamin B_1, nicotinic acid, pyridoxin, small doses of insulin in hypertonic dextrose solution and above all, lumbar puncture repeated two to three times and removing from 50 to 80 cc of fluid. We also gave physiologic saline by nasal catheter and methamphetamine hydrochloride subcutaneously or intravenously 0.5 cc (10 mg) every thirty minutes. With these treatments, the patients responded slowly and the change in the conscious state lasted several days. In two cases we have tried a new treatment with surprising success. In view of the ineffectiveness of the therapeutic measures mentioned above, we administered co-carboxylase (Verolase) 50 mg in 2 cc of water intravenously. In one of the cases recovery from coma was immediate. Another patient, who was in a state of great psychomotor agitation, became tranquil, sat up in his bed after two hours but remained in a confused mental state that disappeared after three days following injection of 100 and 200 mg. of azacyclonal hydrochloride (Frenquel) intravenously every six hours. Both patients received mixed treatment and had prolonged coma with fever of 38.5° and 39°C, respectively.

c. *Coma with Agitation.* Here we refer to the psychomotor excitation that presents itself in the pre-coma as well as in the waking-up period of the insulin coma. It manifested itself in 123 patients (27.95%). The preventive treatment that proved to be most effective was the administration of chlorpromazine. The dose varied according to the cases.

d. *Epilepiiform Attacks.* They presented themselves during the actual effect of insulin in 77 cases (17.50%). The treatment was anti-convulsive. If administered in the morning, before insulin is given it is generally not effective. Therefore, it was necessary to administer it in addition both in the afternoon and at night in the majority of the cases.

Discussion

In comparing our results (Table IV) with those of other investigators such as those of von Braunmühl,[7] West, *et al.*,[8] Patterson,[9] Kolle,[10] and Feuerlein,[11] one sees that the incidence of the remissions, improvements and negative results of our findings approximates very much the mean of the above investigators.

TABLE IV
A Comparison of Immediate Results

Results	Braun-mühl	West *et al.*	Patter-son	Kolle	Feuer-lein	Delgado
Re-mission	73.3%	67.6%	64.3%	46.1%	79.3%	63.4%
Im-proved	15.0%	7.8%	....	37.2%	11.3%	16.6%
Not im-proved	11.7%	24.6%	....	16.7%	9.3%	20.0%

We want to comment especially on the results of the insulin therapy in relation to sex. Some authors, such as Gralnick,[12] Freudenberg[13] and West, *et al.*[8] obtained better results in women than in men. In addition, Freudenberg[13] gives importance to the role that the sex hormones play, citing that Houssay suggests that in the presence of insulin the estrogens have a sensitizing effect while the androgens have a de-sensitizing effect. According to our experience, using insulin alone, the major portion of remission occurred in women as was reported in our paper in 1938;[4] while in the patients treated at a later period, to a major part with insulin and electroshock, the proportion was inverse. We have proved indeed that the female is more sensitive to insulin to enter into coma. In effect, determining the dose capable in producing the first coma in the two groups of the private clinic, we found that the arithmetic mean for females is 115.9 units and for males 140.7 units. With respect to the argument offered by Freudenberg, we are inclined to doubt its value, taking into account the fact that of all our patients the one who required the largest dose of insulin was a castrated man.

Finally, we can generally affirm that according to the actual state of experience with respect to the treatment of schizophrenia the fundamental method is that of insulin therapy. In chronic cases and in those in whom insulin alone does not produce a progressive improvement the combination with electroshock and chlorpromazine gives the best results. This does not exclude the fact that once one of these treatments fails one can produce good results by the use of chlorpromazine combined with serpasil or serpasil alone in large doses. We have observed some remissions produced under the above conditions. Consequently, with the use of insulin and other new drugs, particularly chlorpromazine and serpasil, the therapeutic prognosis of schizophrenia is frankly pleasing, above all, with respect to immediate results.

Summary

1. We have treated 540 cases of schizophrenia: 100 from 1937 to 1939 with remission in 70% of the cases; 440 from 1939 to 1958 with remission in 63.4% of the cases. The following conclusions refer only to the above 440 schizophrenics.

2. With respect to the types of schizophrenia, the catatonic made up the major portion of total remissions (52%).

3. Among the four methods used, the one that gave the best results is the combination of insulin, electroshock and chlorpromazine.

4. In patients ill for less than six months, remission was produced in 78.80% of the cases; in those with six to twelve months in 62.22% and in those with more than twelve months in 52.26%.

5. Treatment associated with less than 50 comas pro-

duced remission in 56.84% of the cases; with 50 to 100 comas in 73.29% and with more than 100 comas in 56.80%.

6. With respect to sex, comparing two groups in equal conditions of care, remission was produced in 68.71% of the men and in 60% of the women.

7. Four of our cases died (0.91%). Other complications and the respective proved effective treatment are mentioned.

Acknowledgment

I would like to express my sincere appreciation to Doctors Miguel A. Chicata, Alfredo Saavedra and José L. Cunza for their valuable collaboration in the review of the case histories and the preparation of the material presented in this paper.

Bibliography

1. Sakel, M. *Neue Behandlungsmethode der Schizophrenie.* Vienna-Leipzig: Moritz Perles, 1935.
2. Sakel, M. Zur Methodik der Hypoglykämiebehandlung von Psychosen. *Wiener klinische Wochenschrift,* 2: 1278, 1936.
3. v. Braunmühl, A. *Die Insulinshockbehandlung der Schizophrenie.* Berlin: Julius Springer, 1938.
4. Delgado, H., Valega, J. F. and Gutiérrez-Noriega, C. Contribución al tratamiento de la esquizofrenia con insulina. *Revista de Neuro-Psiquiatría,* 1: 463, 1938.
5. Delgado, H. Tratamiento de la esquizofrenia con cardiazol e insulina. *Segunda Reunión de las Jornadas Neuro-Psiquiátricas Panamericanas.* Lima: Imprenta Torres Aguirre, 1939.
6. Saavedra, A. Algunas alteraciones psicopatológicas del despertar del coma insulínico. *Revista de Neuro-Psiquiatría,* 16: 1, 1953.
7. v. Braunmühl, A. *Insulinshock und Heilkrampf in der*

Psychiatrie (2nd ed.). Stuttgart: Wissenschaftliche Verlagsgesellschaft M.B.H., 1947, page 17.

8. West, F. H. *et al.* Insulin Coma Therapy in Schizophrenia. *Am. J. Psychiat.*, 111: 583, 1955.

9. Patterson, E. S. Effectiveness of Insulin Coma in the Treatment of Schizophrenia. *Arch. Neurol. & Psychiat.*, 79: 460, 1958.

10. Kolle, K. and Ruckdeschel, K.-Th. Erfolge der Insulinkur bei Schizophrenie. *Dtsch. med. Wschr.* 81: 89, 1956.

11. Feuerlein, W. Die Erfolgsaussichten bei der Insulinbehandlung der Schizophrenie. *Nervenarzt.* 29: 255, 1958.

12. Gralnick, A. A Seven Year Survey of Insulin Treatment in Schizophrenia. *Am. J. Psychiat.*, 101: 449, 1945.

13. Freudenberg, R. K. Observations on the Relation Between Insulin Coma Dosage and Prognosis in Schizophrenia. *J. Ment. Sci.*, 98: 441, 1952.

Chapter 15

MODIFICATION OF ANXIETY SUBSEQUENT TO INSULIN-INDUCED MILD HYPOGLYCEMIA

Andrew K. Bernath

Introduction

There is considerable evidence indicating that insulin induced hypoglycemia above the comatose level is effective in various psychopathologic conditions. It seems that the target syndrome is the anxiety which is always present in those disorders. No adequate explanation for the therapeutic results has been formulated. In this paper attempts will be made to answer the following questions:

1. What place has the mild hypoglycemia treatment in the psychiatric armamentarium?
2. Do the available data warrant a controlled clinical-statistical investigation to evaluate the effectiveness of this treatment-method?
3. Could a sound working hypothesis be offered as a tentative rationale upon which such investigations would be based?

The insulin induced mild hypoglycemic state is defined as one not amounting to a subcoma state, but being terminated shortly after the signs of mild hypoglycemia manifest themselves. Sakel[32, 33] called it borderline insulin treatment. I feel that this term may give rise to confusion and prefer calling it mild hypoglycemia treatment (MHT). This should be clearly differentiated from sub-shock or sub-coma therapy, and obviously, from the insulin coma or insulin shock treatment per se.

The ubiquitous phenomenon of anxiety is looked upon as a manifestation of a slowly and gradually developing pathological condition. The signal aspect of anxiety is disregarded here; only the excess anxiety, disrupting the ego functions and leading to defensive and adaptive countermeasure as they appear in various clinical conditions, will be considered. Basowitz[3] defines anxiety as a "condition of profound organismic arousal with lawfully interrelated somatic, psychological and behavioral events best conceived as a transactional field." I find myself in agreement with this definition.

It is obvious that the only proper objective for the treatment of anxiety should be to modify the etiological factors. Insulin is not considered to be such an agent. It may though control and modify the anxiety syndrome itself. The conclusions of this paper are based on clinical observations. I think that careful clinical observation is an important first step which then must be followed up by controlled experiments and exact statistical evaluations. As Gerard[13] states: "Getting the right hunch is by far the more creative part of the job; but testing the hunch is by far the most important part and the one requiring the greatest expenditure of time and care."

Historical development

In this survey no completeness is attempted. It is hoped that by tracing the historical developments some light might be thrown on the reasons for the almost total abandonment of this treatment method.

There is considerable material published on the non-diabetic use of insulin. It was noted already in 1923[12] that certain depressions cleared in insulin treated diabetics. Soon thereafter insulin was used for the treatment of malnourished infants.[26] In 1924 exophthalmic goiter was treated with insulin.[22] At the 89th meeting of the Swiss Psychiatric Association in Bern in 1937 a film was presented on insulin therapy in psychiatric conditions. On this occasion the work of Steck was discussed. Steck since 1929 used insulin hypoglycemia, but not coma, for the treatment of psychoses and for the mitigation of the withdrawal symptoms of morphine addiction and of delirium tremens.[39, 40] In the same papers Klemperer is named as the originator of the treatment of delirium tremens with insulin. The latter published her results in 1939.[21]

Sakel's original pioneering work on both the borderline insulin treatment and the coma treatment is mentioned here briefly only, because it is well known and is discussed by others at this conference. In his paper given at the same conference in Bern,[32] Sakel stated that he used insulin to check morphine withdrawal symptoms already in 1928: "Insulin abolished the phenomena of irritation during abstinence from morphine . . . starting from this observation . . . I attempted to influence other states of excitation by means of insulin."

American workers[2] used insulin induced hypoglycemia in 1929 for various psychiatric conditions, e.g. melancholia, schizophrenia, psychosis with mental deficiency etc. Their impression was that the treatment shortened the course of these conditions and brought symptomatic relief.

Other important observations were made in 1936 and reported in 1938[5, 6] with using small doses of insulin (10-20 units). These observations jibed with those of Steck's who "long before the advent of insulin-shock therapy praised in a few communications the sedative action of insulin. . . ." These small doses markedly reduced the psychomotor excitement and insomnia and brought about "mental relaxation" of one to several hours' duration. Small doses of insulin in combination with psychotherapy were also tried in a few patients.

From this point on the insulin treatment method took two quite different roads. The first led to the development of coma therapy, the second to the sub-coma treatment. In this paper only the second development will be discussed further.

Sargant and Slater in 1940[37] and Sargant and Craske[35] in 1941 published and advocated the sub-coma insulin treatment in cases of "war-neuroses." According to these authors severe or protracted stress results in acute neurotic symptoms which often get diminished subsequent to the application of this therapy, whereas the long standing neurotic tendencies are not relieved by it. They found rapid improvement of the generalized anxiety; the depression syndrome was less helped. Not all the reports were unanimously favorable though. Insulin was e.g. given by Teitelbaum et al.[42] in sub-shock doses to 50 patients, whereas another 150 men in three groups received group psychotherapy, amytal and placebo respectively. The results of Sargant in producing symptomatic relief were not confirmed in this report. Sargant and Slater[38] criticizing the technique and statistical conclusions felt that the usefulness of the treatment method has been established beyond any doubt. Discussing his seven years of experience with modified insulin treatment in neuroses[36] Sargant states: "We have avoided falling back on crude statistics, which can never assess all the detailed factors involved in the really skilled use of such treatments. Rather we have tried to study as many patients as possible clinically to see how the treatment has affected their individual symptoms. So many factors enter into and influence the results of modified insulin that reliance on broad statistics can be most fallacious." He emphasized in the same paper that it should not be used as a complete treatment in itself, noticing that the persisting tension responds most quickly. The substitution of sterile water for a reasonable period did not bring convincing clinical results disproving the contention that such treatments were largely psychological and abreactive.

Further reports were published in 1944.[34] A mild hypoglycemic state was produced not amounting to light coma. It was found that 60% of the acute anxiety states and anxiety hysterias recovered and much improved, while in the control series (sterile water substituted for insulin) only 15% improvement occurred. According to this report chronic anxiety states rarely benefit from this treatment. The injections were given only for a period of 4-5 weeks. It was felt that the treatment is essentially psychosomatic in type and lasting benefit can be obtained only in conjunction with psychological or even other physical methods.

Numerous, mainly American, workers used it in anxiety tension states,[43] in anxiety states and agitated depressions,[17] and in different mixed psychoneurotic conditions.[11] In a total of 400 cases of psychoneuroses marked clinical improvement was reported in 67% of cases.

Polatin and his co-workers introduced this treatment in America in 1940 for schizophrenic reactions.[27, 28] Their publication was preceded by reports[4] that mild hypoglycemias are of value in controlling those hospital patients who constitute serious management problems. Polatin also treated a group of unselected psychotic cases of organic and functional type as well as a few severe neurotics for an indefinite period of time until the symptoms subsided. He also made the important observation that anxiety as a syndrome diminished and the emotional responsiveness of patients was enhanced, agitated and excited patients were quieted, alertness increased. The rate of improvement was slow and cumulative. He suggested that the therapy must be extended over a period of many months or in schizophrenia indefinitely, in the deteriorating forms for the remainder of the patient's life.

In his discussion of Polatin's paper Bowman[8] shared the opinion that mild hypoglycemia does have a quieting effect, although the manner in which it works is not understood. He suggested that a specific effect of insulin existed and operated. Bowman felt that this treatment had a definite place in our therapeutic armamentarium.

Rennie[31] using sub-coma therapy in cases of depressive, manic and schizophrenic reactions also found that dramatic relief of anxiety could be achieved in various excitement states, wherever "basic anxiety" prevailed. He stressed the specific effect of insulin on anxiety in all of the varieties of the schizophrenic disorder. The alleviation of the anxiety brought about symptomatic improvement in these conditions. He also found it to be the best available method of permitting the patient to utilize psychotherapy. The sedative value was found to be superior to that obtained from chemical sedatives. This paper was published much prior to the discovery of the tranquilizing agents.

Hoch and Kalinowsky[18] believe the subcoma doses of insulin can be used in anxiety states to make the patient more amenable to psychotherapy. They stress the quieting effect on the autonomic nervous system and the improvement of appetite, sleep and increase of weight. They warn against its use as a replacement for insulin coma or electric-convulsive therapy.

Another report also published in the forties[41] dealt with this method used in long standing psychoneuroses of the anxiety-tension type. It ameliorated many of the predominant symptoms rapidly, but no follow up studies were done.

Leo Alexander[1] used this treatment in reactive depressions with anxiety and for the treatment of chronic anxiety states with pronounced epinephrine or nor-epinephrine-triggered anxiety; also in somatization reactions coupled with psychoneurotic symptoms. His Funkenstein graphs show that insulin in subcoma doses markedly reduces epinephrine-precipitable anxiety. He agrees with Hoch and Kalinowsky in advising against its application in schizophrenia. This contention is not shared by all workers.

Polatin and Spotnitz[29] reported on two cases of schizophrenia treated over a period of two and a half years and one and a fourth years respectively. Definite improvement was observed after one year of treatment and both patients maintained it. Both showed a tendency to relapse when insulin was discontinued. These authors recommended treatment for an indefinite period of time in order to obtain and to maintain clinical improvement.

The only worker who used modified sub-coma treatment on office patients was Brickner.[9] He employed the ambulant intravenous insulin method in 18 cases of different types such as anxiety states, schizophrenic reactions and depressions. He found it feasible for office use. He reported that the intense tension could be relieved in whole or in part within a period of weeks.

Summarizing the pertinent findings of the literature: all workers (with the exception of Brickner) agree that sub-coma therapy is a hospital procedure; the target symptoms are anxiety-tension and physically run down condition. With the exception of Polatin, the length of treatment is suggested to be only several weeks or a few months at best. Neither clearcut indications emerged nor has a comprehensive hypothesis of action been formulated which could be usefully integrated into the body of present knowledge about insulin action upon anxiety.

These are some of the reasons which explain why this treatment became obsolescent and got practically forgotten. Another factor was the emergence and somewhat indiscriminate use of the tranquilizers. Reluctance on the part of a great number of therapists to use any other but psychological methods is another cause. It was felt that clarification of some of the concepts and misconceptions surrounding this method may contribute to the re-investigation and revival of the subcoma insulin and of MHT. Should this be successful, the armamentarium of the practicing psychiatrist might be enriched indeed.

Selection of cases

As an associate of Sakel's I have started with the hypoglycemia treatments ten years ago, first on his patients, later on my own ones. About half of the patients were treated by Sakel, but observed and followed up by myself. For the purpose of the present discussion I selected 58 cases, who fulfilled the following criteria:

1. The predominant clinical feature, regardless of the clinical diagnosis, was subacute or chronic, clinically demonstrable anxiety and/or tension.
2. Schizophrenic reactions, with the exception of the pseudoneurotic and residual type, were excluded.
3. All patients had one or more different kind of psychiatric treatments prior to MHT.
4. The duration of the treatment series varied from a minimum of 6 months up to 3 years.
5. In about 60% of all cases a follow up of 1-3 years was possible. The follow up period in the majority of cases ended in 1954. This coincided with the widespread use of tranquilizers in office praxis.

Most of the conclusions drawn in this paper are based on experiences with this group of patients, but some observations were made in connection with the application of this method on other groups of patients as well. The essential findings on the other groups will be published separately.

Some of the vital statistics of the patients, duration of illness and length of treatment are tabulated as follows (Table I):

TABLE I

Age			Sex		Duration of Illness			Length of Treatment			Total
Under 20 years	20-40 years	over 40	male	fe-male	less than 1 year	1-3 years	more than 3 years	6-12 mos.	1 to 2 years	more than 2 years	No. of pa-tients
10	36	12	24	34	7	19	32	13	40	5	58
17%	63%	20%	41%	59%	12%	33%	55%	22%	69%	9%	100%

Although it is emphasized that this treatment is not aimed at altering or "curing" psychopathological conditions underlying the anxiety syndrome per se, it may be of interest to tabulate diagnostically the material presented. The degree of clinical anxiety judged by careful observation of the psychological and physiological concomitants of this syndrome is also estimated and tabulated in Table II.

TABLE II

Clinical diagnosis	No. of cases	light	moderate	severe	Remarks
			Degree of anxiety		
Neurotic anxiety react.	8	1	6	1	
Mixed neurotic reactions	4	2	2		
Conversion reactions	1	1			torticollis
Phobic reactions	3		2	1	
Obsessive compulsive r.	1		1		hand washing
Personality disorders	11	2	8	1	
Alcoholism	7	6	1		without CBS
Drug addiction	2	1	1		barbiturates
Psychosomatic disorders	4	4			
Schizophrenia pseudo-neurotic type	12	3	7	2	
Schizophrenic reaction residual type	3	3			
Chronic brain syndrome after head trauma	1	1			automobile accident
Chronic brain syndrome with Parkinsonism	1	1			20 years after encephalitis
	58	25	28	5	

Technique

The insulin induced MHT has in every case been used as an office procedure. After a thorough psychiatric evaluation is made complete physical and neurological examination, urine analysis and, if possible, blood sugar determination precedes the treatment. It has to be highly individualized. The initial dose of 5 units of plain insulin of the 40 units/cc variety is given subcutaneously at any hour of the day, but on empty stomach. Four hours of fasting precedes the injection. The dose is increased daily unit by unit until signs of mild hypoglycemia occur and the individual pattern of reaction is established. The reaction consists of light sweating, slight trembling, hunger sensation, some tachicardia and mild dizziness. This is usually reached with a dose of 5-20 units. This then becomes the "maintenance dose" which may be readjusted later. The reaction occurs as a rule sometime during the second hour following the injection. The patient is carefully instructed to observe the above signs and after a given period of time he takes carbohydrates in form of sweetened orange juice or a chocolate bar. This terminates the reaction almost immediately. Signs of more severe hypoglycemia such as myoclonic movements, sensory disturbances, faintness, etc. are avoided by immediate termination of the hypoglycemic reaction. After about two hours from the time of the injection a substantial carbohydrate rich meal is consumed, regardless of whether reaction occurred or not, in order to preclude delayed reaction. After the pattern is well established, the patient does not have to stay any more in the office for 1-2 hours, but may leave immediately after the injection. The transportation has to be arranged in such a way that he reaches his home within an hour. Escort is preferable. The number of hypoglycemias per week varies from 3-6. The patients go on with their regular daily activities throughout.

Individual variations of the intensity and duration of reactions, sensitization to insulin as well as diminished sensitivity, allergic reactions, daily fluctuations depending on the blood sugar level and on various other factors, have to be taken into consideration. The intensity of the hypoglycemic reaction can be regulated by manipulating with the following two factors:
1. Dose of insulin
2. Duration of the reaction (which depends on the time of termination)
The duration of the hypoglycemic reaction depending on the clinical picture and on the intensity of the previous reac-

tion is regulated to last from 5-25 minutes. The length of the whole treatment series varies from 6 months to 1-3 years. Agreeing with Sakel's and Polatin's recommendations, in certain selected cases it may last for an indefinite period of time. No formal or analytically oriented psychotherapy was given to this group of patients, only some brief, supportive one. This technique was developed by Sakel and used by him for the last 25 years. I followed his technique with some slight modifications. There were no fatalities. Neither coma, nor any untoward side or after effect of more serious nature took place. There were no severe delayed reactions observed, nonetheless patients were instructed to carry a few chocolate bars with them at all times. Other medication was avoided as much as possible, with the exception of some non-barbiturate sleeping medication. Vitamin, protein, mineral and carbohydrate rich diet was recommended.

The pertinent features of this technique are as follows:

1. It is an office procedure, applied at any hour of the day.
2. The hypoglycemia is kept mild, never reaching even the sub-coma level.
3. The duration of the individual reaction is shorter than in sub-coma treatment.
4. The length of the whole treatment series is prolonged, even indefinite if necessary.

Clinical observations and results

The modifications of the physiological and psychological manifestations of anxiety in the successfully treated patients occur slowly and gradually subsequent to the hypoglycemias. Spectacular sudden changes of lasting nature are rare. The first change takes place in the psychomotor field. The number and intensity of excitement manifestations decrease, a more sedate state of affairs takes place. This results in both lifting of the tense apprehensive feeling of immediate danger, which hangs like a heavy cloud over the patient, and slow diminishing of some of the somatic manifestations, like palpitations, gastrointestinal symptoms and oppressive feeling around the head and chest. This again results in the decrease of the depressive concomitants and the vicious circle loses its grip upon the patient. He is able to engage himself more constructively in his everyday activities. His interpersonal relationships become less ruffled, and his self-confidence increases. Something positive is done for him. His appetite increases; he may gain some weight, gets more sleep. The tonus and turgor of his skin improves. Gradually he is able to utilize his ego defenses better; some of the symptoms resulting from his basic psychopathology diminish. The anxiety being the central theme in neurosis, the lessening of the latter gives rise to a more general improvement of the total picture that can be observed by the therapist and experienced by the patient. Anxiety that caused intense but temporary changes in the organism decreases. He reports longer and more intensive states of relaxation. In those patients who do not react that favorably, only some or none of these changes takes place.

Insulin treatment itself does not terminate an anxiety state, nor does it influence structurally the underlying psychopathology. It does not seem to influence the schizophrenic process, nor does it do much for the endogenously depressed. Shortly after the initiation of treatment a rapid symptomatic improvement is reported in almost every case. This short lasting change is considered to be mainly suggestive-transference improvement. After that a recurrence of symptoms occurs and then a gradual improvement is the rule.

The more acute the anxiety manifestations are, the faster is the response to the treatment; the more chronic states require much longer treatment before improvement occurs, but there are exceptions. The chronic severe cases tend to relapse necessitating re-treatment. As a rule, the improvement becomes definite after 3-6 months. In subacute cases shorter and milder, in chronic cases longer and more intensive hypoglycemic reactions are to be reached. Fluctuations in the anxiety picture should be followed up with modifications of the treatment technique; especially the length and intensity of hypoglycemic reactions should be individually readjusted. There is a tendency to relapse when for any reason the hypoglycemic treatment is discontinued or when no definite hypoglycemic reaction is reached.

In the majority of cases the sedative effect of insulin was more lasting than that of the chemical sedation. These and similar findings were sufficiently regular to be convincing.

Results

TABLE III

Type of anxiety	No. of cases	Recov-ered	Much improved	Improved	Un-changed	Worse
Light	25	5	18	1	1	
Moderate	28	5	13	7	2	1
Severe	5	0	2	1	2	
Total No.	58	10	33	9	5	1

Summarizing the crude, primary treatment results: in 89% of cases favorable modification of anxiety occurred subsequent to the MHT. Out of the 52 patients successfully treated 12 relapsed 3-6 months after the termination of treatment. Eight of these were re-treated and 5 out of the 8 could then be classified under one of the improved categories. Sixty percent of all the cases treated (35 patients) were followed up. After 3 years (in 1954) 24 (68%) out of 35 patients were classified as maintaining their improved clinical status.

The length of treatment series can not be determined in an arbitrary fashion; it depends on numerous factors the main one being the degree and nature of clinical improvement. Every attempt should be made to consolidate the improvement by getting the patient into a constructive psychotherapeutic situation and by wholesome environmental manipulation. This aspect of the management of anxiety states though falls beyond the scope of this paper.

Indications

Rennie called sub-coma treatment "an effective adjunct to the total psychiatric therapy." It is felt that this definition can be equally well applied to the less intensive MHT. The formerly established indications for MHT have been modified since the widespread utilization of the tranquilizers. Since no controlled studies on MHT have yet been made, the indications are tentative and subject to change depending on further investigations.

As a general statement it is suggested that MHT has a limited, but definite place in office treatment. It should be offered to the non-hospitalized patient with marked sub-acute or chronic anxiety and tension manifestations

1. who does not react to psychotherapy or tranquilizers or to a combination of both,
2. who for any reason can not be given psychotherapy,
3. who shows untoward reactions to the tranquilizers, and especially to the patient with chronic anxiety who may develop toxic reactions or severe side-effects on long term tranquilizing regimen.

Although the underlying psychopathology does not play too important a role in setting up the indications a range of diagnostic preference emerges:

1. Neurotic anxiety reactions
2. Anxiety reactions in neurotic character disorders.
3. Anxiety states in psychosomatic conditions.
4. Anxiety with chronic organic mental syndrome, other than vascular in origin.
5. Post-concussion syndrome.

6. Pseudoneurotic and residual forms of schizophrenic reactions.
7. Character disorders with addictions of different kinds.
8. Neurotic-phobic manifestations.

It is felt that in psychoneurotic reactions other than mentioned, in psychotic reactions and in depressions of different kinds, the result do not warrant the application of this method. MHT is not a substitute for insulin coma therapy nor for ECT. It is also felt that in circulatory disturbances with OMS,* in dissociation and in conversion reactions it is contraindicated. Once the indication is made, the treatment must be intense, prolonged and highly individualized; it cannot be given in a routine fashion. In the event of relapse prompt re-treatment is mandatory.

Discussion

In order to evaluate the possible factors responsible for the therapeutic action of mild hypoglycemia, comparison with the insulin coma can not be used. The profound shock effect going way beyond the pharmacological action of insulin itself is not present here. Not even the milder, but still quite intensive effect of the sub-coma treatment is justified to be compared to MHT as an analogous intervention. The mode of action of MHT can be understood only as the end result of the summation of numerous factors: psychopharmacological, psychoendocrinological, metabolic and psychological. The earlier workers looked upon the mode of action as being primarily metabolic, the improvement being secondary to the increased appetite, weight and sleep. The more recent publications emphasize the pronounced anti-anxiety effect as being primary, but with a few notable exceptions, fail to offer any comprehensive explanation that could be used as a rationale for the treatment and for further research. We believe that the effect of insulin as applied in MHT clamps down primarily on the anxiety syndrome,

* Organic Mental Syndrome.

without, unlike some of the tranquilizers, causing secondary depression; the long term somatic changes are secondary to the favorably modified anxiety picture.

Biochemical and psychoendocrinological considerations

Research on stress and on the tranquilizers has shed more light on the biochemical aspect of anxiety. More knowledge about the function of the ascending reticular system gave tremendous momentum to research on this subject. But even so, as Waelsch[44] states, a purely biochemical interpretation of the anxiety state, a state which can be influenced by psychological means and is reversible, somehow impresses one as being too crude.

Glucose is the main fuel of the brain. The energy liberated is utilized for the synthesis of acetylcholine.[23, 24] The other substance utilized by the brain tissue is glutamic acid.[7] Without elaborating here on the intricate intermediate metabolic cycles involved it is safe to state that the rate of these processes influences the amount of useful energy freed for utilization by the brain cells. Numerous abnormal stimuli may interfere with this rate at different points, upsetting its homeostasis. Lack of glucose causes anxiety symptoms by slowing down the energy-yielding metabolic processes.[16, 44] This starts when the blood sugar level is reduced to about 70mg/100. The anxiety-modifying effect of the MHT, the "curative" agent is then of the same variety; anxiety, as a concomitant of hypoglycemia. This aspect of the treatment will be discussed presently.

In considering further the biochemical aspects, it is impossible not to involve what we know today about the action of the tranquilizers. This seems to be a more fruitful endeavor than comparing MHT to the insulin-coma effect on the human organism.

Acetylcholine is probably the only mediator in the nervous system involved in the transmission of excitation at synapses of the autonomic ganglia.[10] It increases the permeability of the nerve membrane for ions. Acetylcholinesterase changes it from a bound to a free form.[25] The energy for this comes from glycophosphate bonds. Tranquilizers probably interfere with this process.

An additional way of interpreting tranquilizer action involves neurophysiological considerations. Without going into details about the role of the Papez circuit and the reticular activating system in the arousal and in the experiencing of anxiety, we may say with Winkler[45] that the action of the phenothiazines on the CNS is predominantly central and is exerted primarily on the reticular system by blocking the excitant actions of epinephrine. Phenothiazines other than chlorprozamine in addition act on the hypothalamus. These two structures are principally concerned with stress and emotional response. Tranquilizers do not cure anxiety, nor does insulin, but both modify it favorably in the majority of cases by their effect on these structures.

A further step is to tie up these data with facts derived from recent psychoendocrinological studies. These studies analyze functional and structural interrelationships of the CNS and the endocrine glands. M. Reiss[30] discusses three elements concerned in the development of psychiatric conditions: Personality pattern, emergency situation and endocrine equilibrium. The endocrine function, the hormone equilibrium and the width of adaptability determines when an existing emergency situation will lead to the precipitation of psychopathological phenomena in an individual of a certain personality pattern. Since anxiety as a stressor can exert its influence via this mechanism and thus produce changes in the peripheral ductless glands, the feed-back initiates a vicious circle. This consideration clearly shows why insulin action is not considered to be specific: since the personality pattern and hormone equilibrium differ from patient to patient, the assumption of such specificity would be untenable.

Deep insulin coma is a form of severe stress, mild hypoglycemic reaction a moderate one. Nevertheless even the

latter breaks into the endocrine and biochemico-neurophys-
iological vicious circle, offering a rational basis for this
treatment. Since there is evidence that the anterior pituitary is at least partly controlled by the hypothalamus, which
is connected to other areas of the brain, and since the
target-hormones can in turn act on the brain as well, the
interrelationship of the CNS and the endocrine system is
clearly established. It was suggested[19, 20] that coma doses of
insulin depress, small doses of the same stimulates adrenocortical functions. The same effect was found by using
tranquilizers. The assumption then is that MHT secondarily
influences the whole endocrine system. Moderate doses of
insulin according to Réiss and his co-workers (unpublished
data 1957) cause changes in weight and function of the thyroid, thymus, testicles, adrenals and pituitary; slight increase
in weight of the pituitary and adrenals and decrease in
weight of the thyroid gland occurs. The pituitary shows an
increase in TSH (thyroid stimulating hormone) content and
first an increase and then a decrease of the ACTH (adreno-
cortico-tropic hormone) content.

Donnelly and Gordon[14] found similarities in the psychosomatic effects of non-coma insulin and chlorpromazine.
Their theoretical formulation involves the hormonal balance question as well. Their contention is similar to ours:
the essence of non-coma insulin effect is neuroendocrinolog-
ical rather than metabolic. Coma dose of insulin was given
by them together with glucose so no coma developed. This
way their method can be compared with ours, although
there is considerable quantitative difference between the
insulin amounts. A 50% decrement of amino acids was found
by them. Large doses of insulin given to rats increased tremendously the proportion of amino-acid—nucleic-acid derivatives in the liver. According to these authors increase in
ribose-nucleic—acid amino-acid derivatives are also stimulated by thyroid, cortisone, testosterone and adrenaline. Insulin encourages the synthesis of nucleic-acid—amino-acid
derivatives and thus causes a drop of circulating amino acid
nitrogen. In a later paper the same authors express their

opinion that the fall of amino acid on phenothiazine medication may be caused by the promotion of the release of adrenaline, which becomes then more available to the tissues, causing an adrenaline deficiency in the blood. This drop of adrenaline, according to these authors, leads to an over-all change in the enzymatic balance and modifies the nutrition for the entire organism including the CNS.

It was also shown that chlorpromazine and promazine induce a fall in amino acid nitrogen similar to the insulin effect. It is possible, according to Donnelly, that the therapeutic effect of the phenothiazines and the non-coma insulin is based on a similar mechanism. This gives a biochemical rationale to our long term insulin treatment. It is obvious that a short term program would permit the return of faulty biochemical conditions with their concomitant behavioral malfunctions.

Two other groups of factors have also to be considered in explaining the mild hypoglycemic action on anxiety.

The metabolic factor can be briefly presented, because it is well known and has been analyzed repeatedly by a multitude of workers. Improved utilization of sugar by the tissues, increased storage of glycogen by the musculature and liver, increase in the general carbohydrate metabolism and a rising respiratory quotient may be mentioned here.

The group of *psychological factors* needs some more elaboration and should not be underestimated. The threat and magic of the "needle" is a powerful psychological factor first, but its impact diminishes later, when the injections are repeated over a long period of time. The authority of the physician representing the "father-healer-medicine man" is another factor to be considered. Frequent personal contact, directive, benevolent, interested, active approach creates a climate, which may be compared in many ways to the "strong positive transference" in the psychotherapeutic situation. It is taken for granted that this transference is analyzed in psychotherapy and is left unanalyzed in MHT. Reassurance and environmental manipulation enhances the psychological effect. The patient feels that something significant is being done for him, his faith and self-confidence grow.

Another psychological factor falls in the realm of the conditioning-deconditioning concept. The unchecked, overwhelming organismic arousal perceived as anxiety is treated with a method causing a rather similar reaction, but the latter is moderate and well in hand, limited in time and repeated at will relieving the patient of his anxious anticipation. It acts as an experimental stress. The correct technique consists of bringing about the right intensity of stimulation, which can yet be tolerated. Using Glover's phrase, the physician plays the role of the "friendly prosecutor" punishing, benevolently relieving guilt and eventually "curing" illness.

There are some puzzling, unsolved questions involved: e.g. differences in the same patient as far as the duration, intensity and start of hypoglycemic reaction is concerned; marked differences among patients getting the same amount of insulin; daily fluctuations; qualitative and quantitative differences in the modification of anxiety syndrome in the same patients after relapse and in re-treatment; and many others.

Sex, age, major endocrinological crises, like puberty, pregnancy and climacterium also make a difference. It is felt that all these factors have to be analyzed individually. Some of the answers can be found in applying the law of initial value[46] to these phenomena, but this goes beyond the scope of this paper.

Hastings and his co-workers[15] presented follow up data on 1638 consecutive psychiatric admissions to a university hospital at the time when organic therapies were not yet utilized (1938-1944). These patients were treated by hospital-nursing care and followed up 6-12 years after discharge. The followed up group constituted 77% of the total group. They found spontaneous remissions judged by social improvement and by adjustment to family and community, in psychoneuroses of all types, as being 47%. The spontaneous recovery rate in these conditions is generally estimated to be 33-50%. Our follow up figures (68% maintained improvement) can be favorably compared with the above ones, being significantly higher.

Conclusions

1. MHT modifies favorably anxiety in 89% of patients with different, non psychotic, subacute and chronic psychiatric conditions.
2. The follow up results are significantly better than the spontaneous recovery rates.
3. MHT can be used as an office procedure; it is harmless and has no side effects of any significance.
4. The target syndrome is anxiety, the somatic-metabolic manifestations are probably secondary.
5. MHT does not cure the anxiety, nor is the underlying pathology influenced by it but it is a useful adjunct in properly selected cases.
6. The mode of action is understood to be based on a summation of psychopharmacological, psychoendocrinological, metabolic and psychogenic factors.
7. Insulin in small doses is considered to be a biologically syntonic psychopharmacological agent.

Summary

A review of the literature covering the history of subcoma insulin treatment is given. The differences and similarities between these previous approaches and the MHT are outlined. Indications, limitations and crude figures on the clinical results are presented. A tentative working hypothesis on the mode of action of this biologically syntonic treatment is offered. Further controlled studies are recommended.

References

1. Alexander, L. Treatment of Mental Disorder. Philadelphia: W. B. Saunders Co., 1953.
2. Appel, K. E., Farr, C. B. Arch. Neurol, and Psychiatry, 21:145-148 (Jan.), 1929.
3. Basowitz, H. The Experimental Induction of Anxiety: Problems, Methods and Theory. Psychiatric Research Reports of A.P.A. No. 8, 1957.
4. Bennett, C. R. and Miller, T. K. Am. J. Psychiat., 96: 961-966 (Jan.), 1940.
5. Beno, N. Observations and Results in the Insulin Treatment. The Amer. J. of Psychiatr., 94 (Suppl.) 213, 1938.
6. Beno, N. Observations and Results Obtained in the Insulin Treatment of 52 Psychotic Patients. The Amer. J. of Psychiatry 94 (Suppl.) 1938.
7. Bessman, S. P. and Schwerin, P. The Function of the System, Glutamic Acid-Glutamine in Brain Metabolism. Federation Proceedings 8, No. 1, 1949.
8. Bowman, K. M. Discussions at the Annual Meeting of the Med. Soc. of the State of New York, NYC, May 8, 1940.
9. Brickner, M. R. The Modified Insulin Technique in the Treatment of Ambulant Psychiatric Patients. J. of the Mount Sinai Hospital, 91-97, 1946.
10. Burgen, A. S. W. and MacIntosh, F. C. The Physiological Significance of Acetylcholine. Elliott K. A. C., Page, I. H. and Quastel, J. H. (editors): Neurochemistry: The Clinical Dynamics of Brain and Nerve. Springfield, Ill. 1955, Charles C. Thomas.
11. Carnet, M., Edwards, F. J. and Fletcher, E. I. Treatment of Certain Psychoneuroses by Modified Insulin Therapy. Canad. M. A. J., 58:22-25, 1948.
12. Cowle, D. M., Parsons, J. P. and Raphael, T. J. Michigan M. Soc. 22:383 (Sept.), 1923.

13. Gerard, R. W. Concluding Remarks. Annals of the New York Academy of Sciences, 67:885-890, 1957.
14. Gordon, M. Zeller, W. and Donnelly, J. A. Biochemical Evaluation of the Activity of Certain Tranquilizers and their Relationship to Hormonal Function. The Amer. J. of Psychiatry 114, No. 3, 1957.
15. Hastings, D. W. et al. Follow up Results in Mental Illness. 113. Annual Meeting of A.P.A., 1957.
16. Hoch, P. and Zubin, J. (ed.) Anxiety. Waelsch, H. Biochemical Aspects of Anxiety, New York, Grune and Stratton, 1950.
17. Hochman, L. B. and Kline, C. L. Subshock Insulin Therapy in Anxiety States and Anxiety Depressions. Dis. Nerv. System, 7:293-298, 1946.
18. Kalinowsky, L. B. and Hoch, P. H. Shock Treatments, Psychosurgery and Other Somatic Treatments. New York, Grune and Stratton, 1952.
19. Kay, W. W. The Endocrinology of Deep Insulin Coma Therapy. Reiss, M. (ed.) Psychoendocrinology. Grune and Stratton (publ.), New York, 1958.
20. Kay, W. W. and Thorley, A. S. Proc. Roy. Soc. Med., 44:973, 1951.
21. Klemperer, E. Die Wirkung des Insulins beim Delirium Tremens. Monatschrift f. Psychiat. und Neurol. 74: 163, 1939.
22. Lawrence, R. D. Four Cases of Exophthalmic Goitre Treated with Insulin. Brit. M. S. 2:753, Oct. 24, 1924.
23. Mann, P. J. G., Tennenbaum, M. and Quastel, J. H. Acetylcholine Metabolism in Central Nervous System. Biochem. J., 33:822-835, 1939.
24. Nachmansohn, D. and Machado, A. L. The Formation of Acetylcholine. A New Enzyme: "Cholin Acetylase." J. Neurophysiol., 6:397-403, 1943.
25. Nachmansohn, D., Cox, R. T., Coates, C. W. and Machado, A. L. Action Potential and Enzyme Activity of the Electric Organ of Electrophorus Electricus II.

Phosphocreatine as Energy Source of the Action Potential. J. Neurophysiol., 6:383, 1943.

26. Pitfield, R. L. Insulin in Infantile Inanition. New York Med. Soc., 118:217, 1923.

27. Polatin, P. and Wiesel, B. Ambulatory Insulin Treatment of Mental Disorders. New York State J. Med. 40:843, 1940.

28. Polatin, P. and Wiesel, B. Effects of Intravenous Injection of Insulin in Treatment of Mental Disease. Schweiz. Arch. f. Neurol. and Psychiat. 43:925, 1940.

29. Polatin, P. and Spotnitz, H. Continuous Ambulatory Insulin Shock Technique in Treatment of Schizophrenia. Archives of Neurology and Psychiatry, 47:53-56, 1942.

30. Reiss, M. Psychoendocrinology. New York, Grune and Stratton, 1958.

31. Rennie, T. A. C. Use of Insulin as Sedative Therapy. Archives of Neurology and Psychiatry, 50, 1943.

32. Sakel, M. The Nature and Origin of the Hypoglycemic Treatment of Psychoses. The Amer. J. of Psychiatry, Vol. 94, May 1938. Orig. Published in Schweizer Archiv. f. Neurology und Psychiatrie. Supplement to Vol. XXXIX.

33. Sakel, M. Classical Sakel Shock Treatment. J. of Clinical and Experimental Psychopathology and Quarterly Review of Psychiatry and Neurology, 15. No. 3, 1954.

34. Sands, D. E. Insulin Treatment in Neurosis. The J. of Mental Science, 90, No. 380, 1944.

35. Sargant, W. and Craske, N. Modified Insulin Therapy in War Neuroses. The Lancet, 2, 1941.

36. Sargant, W. Seven Years of Experience with Modified Insulin Treatment in Neuroses and Early Psychoses. The Amer. J. of Psychiatry, 105: 1948-1949.

37. Sargant, W. and Slater, E. The Lancet, 1940, 2, 1.

38. Sargant, W. and Slater, E. Treatment by Insulin in Sub-shock Doses. The J. of Nervous and Mental Dissease, 105, 1947.

39. Steck, H. Die Behandlung des Delirium Tremens mit

Insulin. Schweiz. Arch. f. Neurol. and Psychiat. 29:173, 1923.

40. Steck, H. and Bovet, H. The Results Obtained by Insulin Therapy from 1929 to 1937. The Amer. J. of Psychiatry, Vol. 94, May 1938. Orig. Published in Schweizer Archiv. f. Neurol. und Psychiat. Supplement to Vol. XXXIX.

41. Sullivan, D. J. Insulin Subshock (Subcoma) Treatment of Psychoses and Psychoneuroses. Sacramento, Calif.: Archives of Neurology and Psychiatry, Vol. 59:185, 1948.

42. Teitelbaum, H. A. et al. The Treatment of Acute Psychiatric Disorders due to Combat by Means of a Group Therapy Program and Insulin in Subshock Doses. J. of Nervous and Mental Disease, 104:123, 1946.

43. Tomlinson, P. J. and Ozarin, L. D. Ambulatory Insulin Treatments. Psychiatric Quarterly, 16:167-173, 1942.

44. Waelsch, H. The Metabolism of Glutamic Acid. The Lancet, July 2, 1949.

45. Winkler, A. The Relation of Psychiatry to Pharmacology. Baltimore, Williams and Wilkins Company, 1957.

46. Wilder, J. Modern Psychophysiology and the Law of Initial Value. Amer. J. of Psychotherapy, 12, No. 2, 1958.

DISCUSSION

DR. BOND: Well, I enjoyed Dr. Bernath's paper as a change from the kind of therapy that we have been speaking of. I am thinking more of the general proposition of what we have to deal with as we get a hundred patients who have been showing some overt symptoms of schizophrenia for 18 months. I think we have a good deal of reason to think that of those hundred patients 15 or 16 are going to get well anyway, sometimes in spite of treatment. Perhaps another 15 or 16 are not going to get well no matter what is done, and probably we are forgetting to some extent the deep psychological and physiological comfort that schizophrenia brings to this group. It was brought forcibly to my mind some twenty years ago when I was in the middle of treatment of a schizophrenic patient who was being roused a little bit toward her normal condition and said to the doctors and nurses, "Who in the hell told you that I wanted to get well anyway." And for the next twenty years, she hadn't made another move toward any kind of improvement. It's in the middle group between the two extremes that any treatment has to look for its value.

DR. SARGANT: I very much enjoyed hearing the paper. I did have considerable experience with it during the development and use of modified insulin in World War II. We found that this treatment greatly helped the anxiety states which were coming back from Dunkirk. And our indications for treatment with insulin subcoma have always been in the treatment of certain anxiety states and anxiety hysterias. We feel it is relatively useless compared to coma in the treatment of schizophrenia. We find that modified insulin therapy is most useful in the treatment of anxiety hysteria where there is pronounced loss of weight. If you try to use it in all cases of anxiety where there is no weight loss, you will inevitably get failures and disappointment.

DR. DONNELLY: I was very much interested in this impressive presentation. I would tend to agree with Dr. Sargant's point about the type of patient, loss of weight and so on. As to the relief of anxiety by insulin, there are several possible factors. One, mechanisms which are involved in insulin coma treatment are presumably active in insulin treatment not producing coma; two, perhaps in modified insulin to relieve anxiety these mechanisms are similar to those in the kind of treatment we are giving, namely, full coma doses but without allowing the patient to become hypoglycemic. We feel there is some evidence that the brain is definitely not dependent altogether on glucose. We feel that amino acid metabolism is going on all the time in the brain and that there is some evidence that this is part of normal brain functioning.

There seems also some evidence that the brain is capable of actually producing amino acids itself; although this has not been fully established this is a possibility that we must keep in mind.

How clinical changes are effected I, of course, don't know but I remember a number of years ago watching Dr. Sargant with a patient coming out of coma treatment; he was talking to the patient trying to elicit memories. I have been very interested in similar experiences with several of my own patients. The patient is placed in a very deep stage of coma and then fed glucose very slowly intravenously or gavaged with small amounts of glucose. As the patient comes out of the coma it is possible by direct questions to elicit some very interesting phenomena. Some patients will talk at first as though they are actually at the age of two years and as the termination continues the patient progresses by years so that if you ask the patient his age at different stages he will actually say that he is two, nine, thirteen, etc. and then shoot right up to the middle teens or to his present age. This is very interesting because one can ask the patients about events in their lives and they speak as though they are at a younger age and as though the events have never happened. A little later they will then talk as though the events have just happened or have happened relatively recently. In this way it is also possible to get some patients to discuss their relationships with their parents when they were young; with the mother, for example, the patient may discuss anxiety which existed in the early age in regard to this parent.

One wonders whether the effect of the insulin is interruption of more recently developed metabolic patterns or whatever constitutes the physical basis of memory; whether the insulin produces changes which in effect disrupt the more recent memories more easily while patterns related to the earliest memories remain the most stable; whether the more persistent patterns are related to more traumatic experiences. I have made observations on about seven or eight patients with this technique over a number of years. Not with all patients, unfortunately, can this "recall" be effected but it is an interesting technique and it certainly is provocation to regress the person to an early age, have him speak as though he were living at that age and to "grow him up" chronologically by the administration of glucose.

DR. KALINOWSKY: I would like to ask an additional question of Dr. Sargant. I take it that this treatment was more successful in the acute neurotic reactions. Was it more effective in war neuroses than in the less acute peacetime neuroses? And my second question would be, now that we use the tranquilizers how do these indications change for this hypoglycemic treatment. I wonder what Dr. Sargant's feeling is about this.

DR. DENBER: Unfortunately, time has prevented Dr. Bernath from expanding on some of the background material of his paper, but it would seem that the effect of subcoma insulin is on anxiety. If he can dampen this feeling, many, if not the majority of his patients, should show improvement. I was not clear on that. From drug studies, it seems that anxiety is affected in an analogous manner. This may be one of the underlying factors in producing improvement with the newer drugs. If this is the case, I would again raise the question regarding specificity of the insulin coma treatment, and point out that the effect may be analogous to that produced with a wide variety of therapeutic techniques.

DR. SARWER-FONER: Our series is similar to those reported. We haven't as yet analyzed some of these groups. We are in the process of doing this now. Our general impressions are very similar.

As to anxiety, there are all sorts of theories about this according to the theoretical framework. It would take too long to go into it here.

DR. GRALNICK: We have had some experience at High Point Hospital in using sub-coma insulin. We have found that it is helpful in the psychotic patient who has anxiety as a prominent symptom. It gives us a better framework in which to work therapeutically with the patient. I'd say further that Dr. Bernath's paper is useful to us in highlighting the fact that various factors are present in the general use of insulin therapy, whether it be on a sub-coma or coma basis. I was particularly interested to hear Dr. Donnelly relate his experiences. It too would certainly suggest that when we subject the patient to these physiological changes, many other things of a highly significant psychodynamic nature are transpiring too. Again I say these demand equal attention. Unless we study psychology as well as physiology, and with equal intensity with individual patients, we are going to continue to lose sight of very significant information.

DR. WAGGONER: I enjoyed the paper very much. It brought out something that I'd just like to mention for a moment, the reverse side of the coin. Often times in psychotherapy if one can mobilize anxiety in the proper way, psychotherapy is very much helped by such a procedure, and I found that in a series of cases, the use of insulin in properly determined doses can help to mobilize anxiety which can be very useful to the patient.

DR. SARGANT: In answer to Dr. Kalinowsky's questions, modified insulin treatment can be useful in both acute and chronic neurotic reactions providing that both anxiety and weight loss are present. So often in adopting a purely psychotherapeutic approach to these problems, people are apt to miss the fact that a patient may be 20-30 pounds below his normal weight. If this weight can be regained with insulin, he is much more likely to resist future stresses which can well get him down if his physical debilitation is not remedied at the same time as his psychological problems are being dealt with.

With regard to the use of tranquilizers and modified insulin treatment, we find that we can combine modified insulin with large doses of tranquilizers such as chlorpromazine in selected cases. My present impression is that combining modified insulin with tranquilizers may accelerate weight gain and diminution in tension. When the weight has been regained, one can often stop the insulin and sometimes keep the patient on a suitable tranquilizer afterwards.

CHAIRMAN RINKEL: Thank you, Dr. Sargant. Time does not permit further discussion. May I ask Dr. Bernath to conclude.

DR. BERNATH: Re Dr. Bond: In my opinion MHT is valueless in the treatment of schizophrenia; only symptomatically helpful. It can not replace more profoundly acting methods.

Re Dr. Sargant: The weight problem was considered but the increase was looked upon as being secondary to the alleviation of anxiety. I feel this is a part only of the total situation. Unlike in your cases, I used MHT for a prolonged period of time and, although I did have some failures and disappointments with my anxiety patients, the successful cases outnumbered them.

Re Dr. Donnelly: I think that the effect of non-coma insulin on the amino-acid metabolism is only one factor, though possibly a very important one. Several other psychopharmacological actions are in operation.

Re Dr. Denber and Dr. Waggoner: I feel that we treat anxiety with anxiety. I don't think that MHT is specific. It ameliorates clinical, excess, disruptive anxiety by the application of measured and controlled anxiety caused by mild hypoglycemic reaction. This is a way of deconditioning. The fact is that the majority of patients did show a great deal of improvement. Nevertheless, MHT is considered to be an adjunctive measure only. As such, it cannot be used justifiably for the treatment of psychoses where more effective treatments may get delayed.

Re Dr. Gralnick: Shortness of time did not permit me to elaborate on the psycho-dynamic factors involved but I did discuss them in the original paper. I certainly agree with what Dr. Gralnick suggested about the significance of these psychodynamic factors. Nevertheless I consider MHT as being essentially psychopharmacological in nature.

Chapter 16

INSULIN COMA THERAPY IN A VETERANS ADMINISTRATION HOSPITAL

DANIEL M. WEISS

The Veterans Administration Hospital is a 1,000-bed general medical and surgical hospital located in Boston, Massachusetts. This hospital was built in 1952 and staffed largely by personnel who had been transferred mainly from the Cushing Veterans Administration Hospital, which had been located in Framingham, Massachusetts, and from the West Roxbury Veterans Administration Hospital. Cushing Veterans Administration Hospital had been organized as a hospital, beginning in January 1947. In effect, then, there has been a continuous hospital for eleven and a half years, despite the change in names, and there has been a continuum of medical staff, thus assuring as much as possible that there has been a progressively-developing, but essentially a continuous, philosophy of therapy. While at Cushing Veterans Administration Hospital 108 beds were on the closed ward section, at the Veterans Administration Hospital in Boston 101 beds are on the closed ward section. Only patients on the closed ward section have received insulin coma therapy. Thus it can be seen that we had a relatively small population from which to draw our patient load.

·

Nevertheless, we were able to maintain a very active insulin coma therapy unit. During the first two years of this unit, Dr. Jack Kneipp was in charge of somatic therapy. Since January, 1949 the author has been in complete charge. Thus there has been no difficulty in terms of frequent changes in attitude or of concept on the part of the doctor in charge, as is all too frequently the case in many hospitals where a staff doctor is "rotated through" this service. Since we have always been a residency training center, we have had residents on the psychiatric service, and these have "rotated through" the insulin therapy unit—but always under the direct direction and supervision of the sole director of the unit. As another means of assuring a continuum of training and of attitude, the nurse to be in charge and the charge aide have always been assigned specifically to the insulin therapy unit, without duties elsewhere within the hospital. In this manner, years of experience were always available within the persons of the three people directly in charge. Assistant nurses and assistant aides were, however, rotated through the unit, so that eventually practically every nurse or aide in the entire psychiatric section became moderately well familiar with insulin treatment, and could be assigned to the unit at any time, and could easily act as part of the team.

During treatment we have had—in addition to the staff doctor in charge, the resident physician, and the nurse in charge—the services of one nurse and one psychiatric aide for each four patients on treatment, in an effort to minimize the dangers of this form of treatment to the patient. I believe that our low mortality and morbidity rates were attributable to the high degree of training and experience of the treatment team, and the fact that we were able to function as an integrated team because of the many hours spent together.

Despite the fact that there had been a maximum of 108 beds on the closed ward section at Cushing Veterans Administration Hospital the insulin treatment unit consisted of 20 beds, and most of the time there were 20 patients being treated simultaneously. At that time about 19% of the patients on the closed ward section at any one time were receiving insulin coma therapy. When the unit was moved to the Veterans Administration Hospital in Boston the room to which the unit was assigned was smaller, and the unit was cut in size to 14 beds. By 1954 the total number of patients who were treated by means of insulin coma was definitely becoming smaller, progressively, and at this time of writing the insulin treatment unit consists of only five beds. At all times we have kept the insulin treatment unit entirely apart from the regular dormitory beds, and this has had the psychological effect of keeping the entire concept of the use of insulin as a form of therapy in the minds of patients and personnel alike, as well as keeping each patient's sleeping quarters entirely dedicated to rest or sleep.

We have given to date 501 completed courses of insulin coma therapy. Included in this total figure are 39 who have had two series of insulin coma therapy, and two who have had three series. 8.2% of our patients have had more than one course of treatment. These figures all concern deep coma therapy, as outlined elsewhere in this paper. Many of those who had a second course of insulin coma therapy had previously had an unsuccessful first course, with the Gradual Increase Procedure, and the second course of the Rapid Increase Procedure was generally much more successful.

In addition to the patients treated by deep coma insulin therapy, we have also treated to date 67 patients with sub-coma insulin therapy mainly for sedative purposes. These have consisted of acute psychoneurotic anxiety reactions. We have considered the optimum level of sub-coma treatment to be at the bottom of Stage ii, after Himwich,[7] where there may be sweating and dulling of the senses, with sleep, but where the patient may be awakened and can respond to questions, and can drink volitionally.

In our experience, insulin coma therapy was prescribed only for patients carrying a diagnosis of schizophrenic reaction, paranoid or mixed type. No patients with serious depressions or manic states, nor with any organic psychotic states, were treated with insulin coma therapy. Our patient population was severely restricted in two senses. Since we were working in a veterans' hospital which was an acute treatment center, the age limits are perhaps more limited than one would find in other hospitals. Thus our youngest treated patient was age 19 at the time of treatment and the oldest patient to have been given deep coma therapy was 55. In addition, neither at Cushing Veterans Administration Hospital nor at the Veterans Administration Hospital in Boston did we treat any female psychotic patients, as other local Veterans Administration mental hospitals were designated as female psychosis treatment centers.

Preparation of Patient and Family

In all cases we have felt that a better end-result might be anticipated if we were able to have the full cooperation of the patient, and of the patient's family. To this end we discussed the projected treatment plan with the patient at length, and we enlisted the aid of our Social Service department to acquaint the family with the plan. We also constructed an information sheet, which was devised to answer many of the common questions about this form of treatment, and gave a copy of the sheet to the patient, and to a responsible member of the family. This simple device has repeatedly been shown to be of value to all concerned.

Before treatment was begun each patient was given a thorough physical examination, pre-treatment x-rays of the spine and a chest film. During a course of treatment, we also took routine chest films at least twice more (usually following the 20th and 40th comas), and following the 60th coma a chest film as well as follow-up x-rays of spine were taken. Routine blood tests were also done. Thus, we were always able to document physiological or osseous changes which might have been attributable to the therapy. We have followed the usual practice of considering a complete course of therapy to be 60 comas. However, if a patient had completed 58 or 59 comas at the end of a week's treatment, we never insisted that he complete the extra one or two comas in the following week.

As to sensitivity testing before insulin therapy was begun, we have given the patient 5, 10, and 25 units of insulin subcutaneously on successive days, and if no untoward reactions have occurred then we have felt that no undue sensitivity was present. In the rare case when we felt that the particular patient was sensitive, a different brand of insulin could be used successfully without any untoward reactions ensuing.

Procedure

For the first two years of our experience we followed the procedure as originally delineated by Dr. Manfred Sakel, in what we now call the Gradual Increase Procedure. In tabulating (Fig. I) our first 108 patients treated with this method, we found that in 7,284 treatment days we were able to achieve coma level 4,848 times. This was a success ratio of 67%. The average number of treatment days which elapsed until the first coma was achieved was 10, and the average number of days lost (where a coma did not ensue) during a course of treatment was 23. Unsuccessful treatments can increase the dangers and discomfort to the patient.

In comparing the total amount of insulin used in a course of coma therapy, we found that this did not seem to vary greatly whether the Gradual or the Rapid Increase Procedures were used, either in building up to the first coma, nor thereafter. A significantly lower number of "missed comas" was seen in those treated with the newer method than with the classical method.

For example, in one patient who was particularly resist-

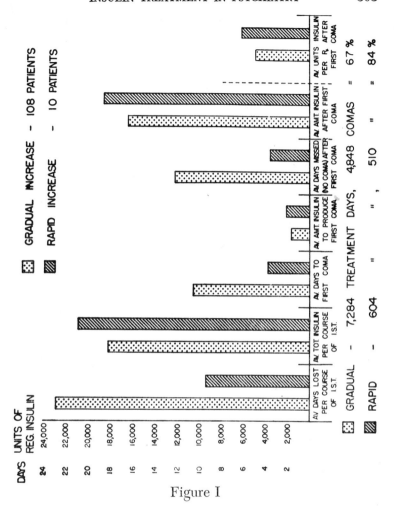

Figure I

ant to insulin (Fig. II) only four comas were achieved in 94 attempts, although both the intravenous and intramuscular modes of injection were employed. We decided that an effort should be made to achieve a more efficient manner of performing this treatment and to that end we attempted the newer method of *Shurley and Bond*[7] called the Rapid Increase Procedure. In order to put it to a real test, our first

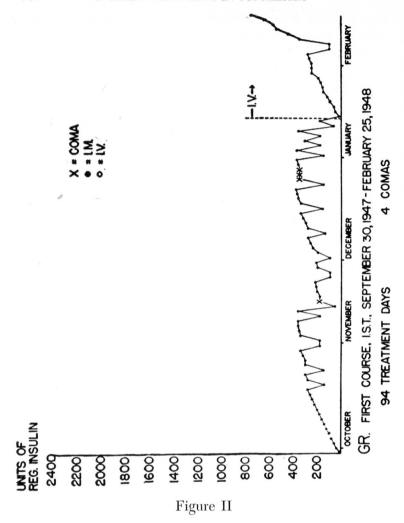

Figure II

patient was the same one with whom we had had such signal failure before. Thus (Fig. III) this patient, who had been considered to have been insulin-resistant, was able to have a · successful course of insulin coma therapy, with 72 treatments and 60 comas. As a result of this experience the Rapid Increase Procedure was adopted as the method of choice.

Using this method, we have had approximately 84% suc-

cess in terms of treatment-coma ratio. The resulting econo-
mies to hospital, personnel, and patients have been very
great. While we have found that most patients were able to
have a successful first coma at the 1600-unit level, we have
given larger doses on many occasions, and in one patient
coma was not achieved until a single dose of 4,200 units was
given. These dosages of insulin may stagger the imagination,
yet our experience indicates that patients can recover from

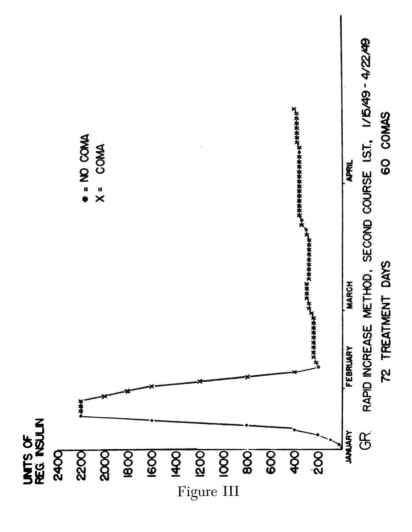

Figure III

these tremendous dosages as easily as from a much smaller dose. As an aid to the attainment of a satisfactory coma, we have stipulated that the patient ingest nothing having food value after 8:00 P.M. on the evening preceding treatment, and to drink no fluids of any kind after midnight. This greatly lessens the dangers of vomiting and of aspiration during the excitement phase of the treatment.

Pre-medication: Each patient was given phenobarbital, grains 1½, before each treatment to minimize the incidence of spontaneous convulsions. To control excessive salivation, and the possibility of aspiration of mucus, Atropine, grains 1/150, was also administered. To insure that vitamin intake is adequate, we have been in the habit also of giving these patients multivitamins daily. During the summer months, when it is hot, perspiration seems to be greatly increased during treatment, and we give the patients salt tablets at that time to replace sodium loss.

The patients were awakened at 6:30 A.M., allowed to complete their toilets, and were then brought to the insulin treatment room by 7:00 A.M. The crystallized regular insulin was then injected intramuscularly and the patients lay down on their beds. The room was kept moderately darkened, and soft music was played via the hospital radio system. Talk among the personnel is kept at a minimum to avoid distractions. The dose of insulin was calculated as far as possible for each patient so that coma would be attained not less than three hours after the administration of the insulin, and not more than four hours.

It is recommended that the patient be in a sturdy bed during this form of treatment, otherwise during the excitement phase the patient might be injured, or the bed damaged. The ordinary Gatch hospital bed is recommended since it is firmly constructed and has good springs and mattress. We have used, however, a modification of the Army-style bunk bed, with a solid bedboard under the mattress. Since these beds are low the possibility of a patient hurting himself by falling is minimized. Another advantage of having firm support for the patient during this treatment is that patients complain of fewer backaches after treatment.

During the excitement phase it is frequently necessary to apply restraints—and these are used basically to prevent the patient from harming himself. By and large, we have ordinarily relied upon a combination of shoulder-and-ankle restraints, and only very rarely was it necessary to use wrist restraints also. A patient who is restricted too severely by means of multiple restraints may struggle even harder, in his confusional state, and becomes severely fatigued. The patients are checked frequently as to pulse, respiration, and signs of Himwich,[7] and we have relied upon three main signs to denote coma level: (1) Absence of pain response to supra-orbital pressure; (2) presence of positive Babinski signs; and (3) absence of corneal reflex. Once coma has been attained the time is noted on a clock-face hanging on the wall behind the patient's bed. This provides for easy checking on the part of the doctor, and serves as a clear visual reminder of the time when coma should be terminated. We allow the first coma to endure for 15 minutes, the second for one half-hour, and the third for 45 minutes. Subsequently comas are allowed to persist for a full hour, unless there is some other reason for an earlier termination. In the event that coma deepens beyond stage 3, and medullary signs are seen, that coma is terminated immediately. If a convulsion occurs, we always terminate the coma immediately, in whatever stage the patient may be. We found that it was not necessary to calculate the amount of glucose which is used for termination of the coma in relation to the dosage of insulin. We chose to use the intra-gastric gavage route for termination of coma routinely and our usual gavage solution consists of 400 cc. of a 50% glucose solution, thus containing 200 grams of glucose. The use of the intra-gastric route as a routine enabled us to preserve the patient's veins for possible emergencies.

After the patient is gavaged, the time is noted on a second clock-face, and careful attention is paid to the awakening period. In most cases the patient has awakened with the gavage only. However, if good signs of awakening are not present by 15 minutes after the gavage, we then administer an intravenous injection of 30 cc. of 50% dextrose solution. Practically always we have found that this will accomplish a successful awakening. The patient is allowed then to rest until he is clear, and then he is urged to have some sort of fruit juice, following which he is brought to the shower room where he is showered, and dressed in warm, clean clothes. Following that he is given a dish of cereal and some hot coffee. Afterwards he is returned to his ward, to resume his daily activities.

In the event that a particular patient could not tolerate the glucose solution, which can irritate the gastric mucosa, the glucose can be dissolved quite easily into chocolate milk, eggnog solution, or protein-enriched solutions of various types. These latter solutions have the value that the protein or fat is absorbed and metabolized more slowly than the glucose itself, and is then continuously available to the patient over a longer period of time. We have noticed that when a coma is terminated by the intravenous route, the patient must be urged strongly to drink something, such as juice or one of the milk or eggnog solutions, preferably fortified with a small amount of glucose, otherwise they usually will soon lapse into a coma again, and the whole process will necessarily be repeated. In addition, we have noticed on occasion that intravenous administration of glucose (which must be accomplished very carefully as it is highly irritating to peri-venous tissue and can cause sclerosis, and loss of the vein) can actually cause the coma to deepen. We have called this the paradoxical effect of intravenous glucose, and we believe that it stems from an endogenous elaboration of insulin, probably by stimulation of the pancreas, although we are unable to substantiate this claim. At any rate, we have found that this deepening of the coma is relatively transient, and we have not felt that an additional injection of glucose was warranted at these times. Recently, we have started to use Glucagon (Lilly) as a means of terminating coma. Glucagon is a naturally-occurring hormone produced by the alpha cells of the pancreatic islets which can cause a temporary rise in the blood sugar level, in the presence of insulin.[6] Generally it is given subcutaneously in 2 cc. doses, and it seems to be very quickly and safely effective in the termination of insulin coma. Again, the patient must drink some sort of fluid which will provide for a more sustained absorption of glucose, to prevent a relapse into coma.

Prolonged and Irreversible Comas

The most serious and dangerous complications of insulin coma therapy are the prolonged and the irreversible comas. These are somewhat confusing conditions because in most cases these can occur even when the circulating blood sugar is within normal limits. Various reasons for their appearances have been proposed: vascular, anoxic, toxic-metabolic, autonomic imbalance, deficiency of tissue essentials, calcium deficiency of the blood, and excessive hydration of the cortical cells.[3] Rivers[5] states that in insulin coma therapy there may be a progressive hydration of the cerebral cells up to a certain point. It is known that a relatively slight oxygen lack in the cerebral cells can produce unconsciousness, and the earliest change in the anoxic brain is intra-cellular edema. If this edema persists then oxygen supplied by external means cannot be utilized by the cells, and a vicious cycle is created, since anoxia in itself leads to further edema. Lucas[3] points out that in hypoglycemia the cortical cells are frequently unable to metabolize efficiently, and so are less resistant to anoxia than normally. Thus, we have felt that the basis of prolonged or irreversible coma is this intra-cellular edema, and we have based our therapeutic efforts towards reduction of the edema. Once the circulating blood sugar has reached normal levels, one needs only to maintain it there, and massive doses of glucose would serve no further useful purpose. There is even some indication that massive doses of glucose then would be harmful because glucose does pass through the blood-spinal fluid barrier, and instead of a reduction in spinal fluid pressure there occurs a delayed or secondary rise in pressure. Since sucrose does not pass through the barrier, it is more effective than dextrose for this purpose, although its osmotic pressure is only one-half that of dextrose in the same strength. Sucrose has some disadvantages in the sense that deposition of sucrose crystals in the renal tubules may cause a nephritis. A number of other materials have been suggested, including Mannitol, magnesium sulfate, and human lyophilized serum. We have found that Sorbitol is the most effective. Sorbitol (an alcoholate of glucose) is as effective a dehydrating agent as is dextrose, and it does not pass through the blood-cerebrospinal fluid barrier. Thus, the secondary rise in pressure is avoided. About 40% of the injected Sorbitol is converted into glycogen by the liver, and thus becomes available to supplement the depleted body reserves. The remainder is recovered from the urine almost unchanged, mostly within the first few hours after injection.[1] There is a positive reduction in cerebro-spinal fluid pressure, and this reduction may endure for 3-4 days. To our knowledge, Rivers[5] was the first to introduce its use in the treatment of prolonged coma. We have felt very strongly that hourly injections of Sorbitol following the onset of prolonged coma have prevented all except three prolonged comas in our series from becoming irreversible. As an aid, we have given these patients, also, injections of Solu-B, a vitamin preparation which has a high content of Vitamin B, because we have felt that the B-fractions have probably become depleted, with resultant malfunction of intra-cellular metabolism. Two of our failures were due to cardiac arrest in prolonged coma. The third was caused by exhaustion of the adrenal glands. Using the Rapid Increase method, we have had a mortality rate of only 3/501 or 0.6% of the total number of patients. This finding compares very favorably with other published figures.

Post-Coma Care

The patients having insulin coma therapy are supervised during the lunch and dinner hours, to ensure that their dietary intake be adequate. We have not, as a rule, given these patients any special diet, since our usual hospital diet is considered to be quite adequate, and is generally over 3,000 calories daily. As a matter of fact, most of our patients have gained between 20 and 30 pounds during a course of treatment. The personnel have all been trained to give special attention to those who eat poorly, and if gently urging does not result in a good food intake, this is reported quickly to the nurse, so that the patient will get special attention during the balance of the day. Supplementary feedings of fruit juices, crackers, or sandwiches are given to these patients during the afternoons, and it has occurred many times that other psychotic patients have reported that one of the treatment patients is perspiring freely, indicating the awareness on the part of all that these patients bear special watching. It would seem that these delayed reactions are due to several causes: Failure to inject the insulin into the muscle may result in a delayed absorption of the insulin, leading to delayed reaction. Another cause is that the dosage might have been too great for a particular day. In addition, we have felt—particularly with high doses—that these patients are probably slightly hypoglycemic for much of the day, and that unusual exertion, especially in the hot weather, may cause another decrease in the circulating blood sugar level which is enough to cause a delayed reaction. In all cases, our first efforts are bent to getting the patient to drink some sort of juice which has been enriched with glucose. If this is not possible, then the next step is to terminate this reaction by either the intragastric or intravenous route, as above. During the night special rounds are made by the personnel to observe the insulin coma patients to prevent a delayed reaction from going unnoticed, and from evolving into an undetected and therefore serious coma. We have been repeatedly struck by the fact that these night rounds may be irritating to the other patients who are not receiving this type of treatment, and yet the morale of the patient group as a whole is such that extremely few complaints have been heard. During the entire course of treatments, we have always been extremely careful to observe ordinary rules of hygiene, and to pay special attention to slight injuries accidentally sustained by the patients during the ordinary daily activities, always having in mind the knowledge that insulin coma therapy is a strenuous form of treatment, and the feeling that the resistance of the patient to infection may be lowered during it.

Results

At this time we have planned a five-year follow-up to determine the actual clinical results. This project is at the point of beginning, and, unfortunately, no results are as yet available from which to quote. We can say, at this time, however, that the number of former patients, who had had a course of insulin coma therapy and who have required re-admission to this hospital, is relatively small, probably not over 15%. It is quite possible that a number may have been admitted to some other veterans' hospital, and this will have to be determined. In addition, a number who have had this form of treatment were not improved, and were subsequently transferred to other veterans' hospitals. Our impression is that at least 70% of our patients have had lasting benefit but we cannot be more definite at this time.

We have made some studies of various aspects of insulin coma therapy, whenever interesting problems arose. One of our first projects was to attempt to determine whether there was a level of circulating blood sugar which would correlate with the onset of insulin coma. Many determinations were done, and examined with the usual laboratory methods. However, we felt that there was too great a spread in the figures. Therefore, we had the blood samples titrated according to the Somogyi method.[8] While this is a more expensive procedure, it seems to be more nearly accurate since it is not distorted by the presence of non-glucose-reducing substances, as is the Folin-Wu test. Using this method, we have found that (Fig. IV) the critical level, in an average of three hourly specimens, is 11 mg. %. Thus it was even possible for the laboratory technicians to state, merely from the laboratory calculations, whether or not a patient had had a coma.

In a recent study which we have made[4] we measured adrenocortical function before, during, and after a complete course of insulin coma therapy in a paranoid schizophrenic

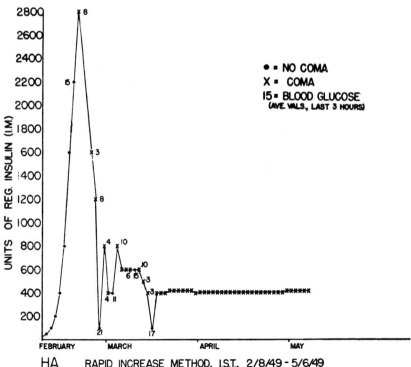

HA.   RAPID INCREASE METHOD, I.S.T., 2/8/49 - 5/6/49

59 TREATMENT DAYS   —   48 COMAS

Figure IV

patient. We observed that on treatment days a moderate increase in urinary corticosteroid excretion was noted. On non-treatment days these levels again decreased. We found that 17 ketosteroid excretion did not parallel the corticosteroid excretion. However, we found that insulin coma therapy did not alter the adrenal responsiveness to intravenous ACTH. Following a course of this therapy, both urinary corticosteroid and 17-ketosteroid excretions remained at a lower level than during the pre-insulin control period, suggesting that adrenocortical functions may be somewhat depressed by a long course of insulin therapy.

Reasons for a Decrease in Numbers of Patients
Being Treated with Insulin Coma

In a number of hospitals which formerly had given this form of treatment, the number of patients now being so treated has been reduced, and in some hospitals the treatment has been discontinued. We still utilize insulin coma therapy in our hospital, but there is no question that there has been a progressive decline in the numbers of patients being treated. There are several probable reasons in our own experience. First, we have come to depend more and more on psychotherapy of the psychotic patient, and on arranging his milieu in a more therapeutic manner. Secondly, for the most part, we have adequate numbers of ward personnel, and of residents, so that it has been possible to see each patient almost daily. With such frequent interviews, and with attention to the milieu, we have found it relatively unnecessary except in a small number of patients to use any somatic therapy. Finally, it has seemed to us that the increasing use of tranquilizers has lessened the necessity in a number of cases to use insulin or other somatic therapy in order to help the patient to become more accessible to verbal therapy. Our accent has been on psychotherapy, and our concept of the use of insulin coma therapy has been that it was very useful as an adjunct, but not as a primary or exclusive form of treatment.

Summary

An account is presented of the history, technique, and results of the insulin therapy unit at the Cushing and Boston Veterans Administration Hospitals, from the inception of the unit to the present time.

Bibliography

1. Browder, J., and Bragdon, F. H. An Evaluation of Sorbitol as a Dehydrating Agent. Am. J. Surg. V. 49. pp. 234-441. 1940.

2. Kalinowsky, L. B., and Hoch, P. H. Shock Treatments, Psychosurgery, and other Somatic Treatments in Psychiatry. Grune and Stratton, N. Y., 2nd ed. 1952. pp. 46-40.

3. Lucas, B. G. B. Some Observations on Anoxia. Anesthesiology. V.12 pp. 762-766. Nov. 1951.

4. Marks, L. J., Weiss, D. M., et al. The Adrenocortical Response to Insulin Coma. I. Effects of an Entire Course of Insulin Coma Therapy on the Urinary Excretion of 17-Hydroxycorticosteroids and 17-Ketosteroids and on Circulating Eosinophils. J. Clin. Endoc. and Metab. V.18 No. 3 March 1958 pp. 235-245.

5. Rivers, T. D. Effect of Vitamin B1, Sucrose, and Sorbitol on Certain Complications of Insulin Hypoglycemia: A Clinical Report. Arch. Psychiat. and Neurol. V.44 pp. 910-912. 1940.

6. Schulman, J. F., and Greben, S. E. The Effect of Glucagon on the Blood Glucose level and the Clinical State in the Presence of Marked Insulin Hypoglycemia. J. Clin. Invest. V.36 No. 1 pp. 74-80 January, 1957.

7. Shurley, J. T., and Bond, E. D. Insulin Shock Therapy in Schizophrenia. Veterans Administration Technical Bulletin #TB10-501 April 16, 1948.

8. Somogyi, M. Determination of Blood Sugar. J. Biol. Chem. V.160 pp. 69-73. September, 1945.

Chapter 17

THE PLACE OF SAKEL'S INSULIN COMA THERAPY IN AN ACTIVE TREATMENT UNIT OF TODAY

KARL THEO DUSSIK

Whatever the place of insulin coma therapy will be ten years hence, there is no doubt that Sakel's initiative had a tremendous impact upon the fate of schizophrenic patients around the world. Figure 1 shows data on three groups of patients in terms of release from the hospital, continued confinement, and mortalities.

The first group consists of 94 patients. From all schizophrenic patients who had passed through the University Clinic of Neurology and Psychiatry in Vienna, Austria, over a period of 15 months immediately prior to the start of Insulin Coma Therapy at this clinic, 100 male cases whose symptoms had not lasted longer than 6 months before admission were first admissions. The data could be established on 94 patients. For six cases sufficient information could not be obtained. Column 1 of figure 1 presents the data on all these 94 cases without selection.[4]

In 1933, when Manfred Sakel had returned from Berlin to Vienna, Professor Poetzl arranged for the introduction of Sakel's method in his clinic. Incidentally, yesterday marked the twenty-fifth anniversary of the day when Sakel and

Figure 1

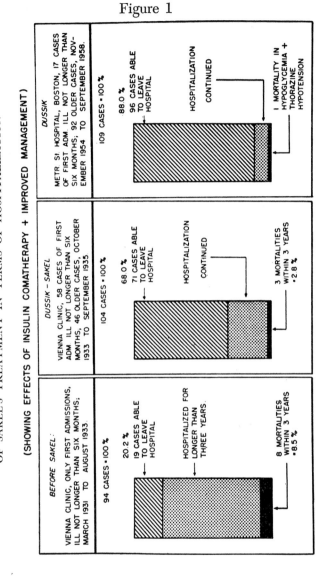

THE COURSE OF SCHIZOPHRENIC PATIENTS BEFORE AND AFTER INTRODUCTION OF SAKEL'S TREATMENT IN TERMS OF HOSPITALIZATION

(SHOWING EFFECTS OF INSULIN COMATHERAPY + IMPROVED MANAGEMENT)

BEFORE SAKEL:
VIENNA CLINIC, ONLY FIRST ADMISSIONS, ILL NOT LONGER THAN SIX MONTHS; MARCH 1931 TO AUGUST 1933.

94 CASES = 100 %

20.2 %
19 CASES ABLE TO LEAVE HOSPITAL

HOSPITALIZED FOR LONGER THAN THREE YEARS.

8 MORTALITIES WITHIN 3 YEARS = 8.5 %

DUSSIK – SAKEL
VIENNA CLINIC, 58 CASES OF FIRST ADM. ILL NOT LONGER THAN SIX MONTHS, 46 OLDER CASES, OCTOBER 1933 TO SEPTEMBER 1935

104 CASES = 100 %

68.0 %
71 CASES ABLE TO LEAVE HOSPITAL

HOSPITALIZATION CONTINUED

3 MORTALITIES WITHIN 3 YEARS = 2.8 %

DUSSIK
METR. ST. HOSPITAL, BOSTON, 17 CASES OF FIRST ADM. ILL NOT LONGER THAN SIX MONTHS, 92 OLDER CASES, NOVEMBER 1954 TO SEPTEMBER 1958.

109 CASES = 100 %

88.0 %
96 CASES ABLE TO LEAVE HOSPITAL

HOSPITALIZATION CONTINUED

1 MORTALITY IN HYPOGLYCEMIA + THORAZINE HYPOTENSION

myself started Insulin Coma Therapy for the first patient (R.H., case 41 of the report on the first series of 104 patients).[5] The respective data of this first Vienna series are presented in the second column of figure 1. The third column of figure 1 concerns the 109 patients who have been completely treated by Sakel's method in Boston since 1954.*

These data illustrate the great progress since Sakel's method was used. While the pharmacological effect of hypoglycemic coma should not be claimed as the only factor which is responsible for this development, it hardly can be denied that it is by far the most deciding one. Psychological milieu factors and improved management alone, important as they may be, could not have brought about a statistical trend showing changes of such a dimension.

These data are simple and unquestionable. More details of the case histories of schizophrenic patients than the ones which are presented in figure 1 have to be known, and they are known for these patients: (a) The duration of the disease before the treatment had started, (b) the type of symptomatology, (c) the duration of the hospitalization required to obtain the results, (d) the degree and nature of the improvement, (e) the further course, especially in terms of relapses. So far as the cases of the untreated group in column 1 are concerned, all but one of these patients had to be rehospitalized within three years. The first hospitalization was in average three times as long as the one for the insulin treated cases of the series which are presented in the second column.

The problems of the quality of results and of the interrelation of the pharmacological or neuro-humoral factors and the psychological factors were subjects of many investigations and controversies. These problems are so complicated that it is difficult to discuss them here. One can refer to several excellent reviews such as the ones contained in the books of Sargant and Slater,[12] Kalinowsky and Hoch,[6] Alexander,[1] and Mueller.[8] To these authors who thoroughly and

* Since 1954, the treatments and investigations have taken place at the Active Treatment Unit of the Metropolitan State Hospital in Waltham, Massachusetts, William McLaughlin, M.D., Superintendent. A grant of the Manfred Sakel Foundation made it possible that in April 1958 an Insulin Treatment Research and Teaching Division was added to this Active Treatment Unit (Karl Theo Dussik, M.D., Director).

with avoidance of bias analyzed the evidence which was available until 1951, Insulin Coma Therapy appears to be well established as an effective and preferable therapy for schizophrenia, with certain limitations of the indication in terms of the pre-treatment period of the symptoms and the type. Alexander compiled data in 1951 from world literature,

Figure 2

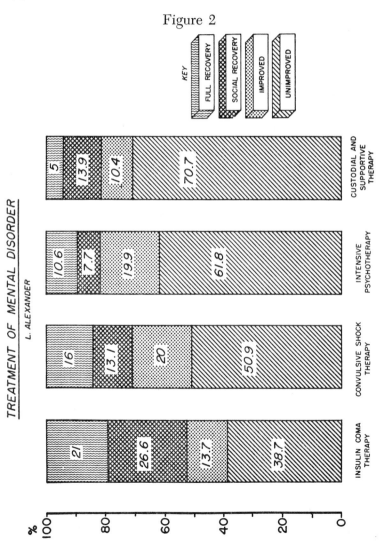

on the outcome of 30,000 schizophrenic patients, and in this way compared various therapies. From his exhaustive statistical studies, figure 2 presents the over-all breakdown. Psychotropic drugs did not come into wide use before the release of these publications.

In spite of this, psychiatrists have not agreed upon the therapeutic significance of ICT. There are several reasons for this. The evaluation of any therapy for schizophrenia poses tremendous difficulties. Lacking any unequivocal knowledge as to the etiology, and with courses as variable as they are in this condition, one can never be certain in an individual patient if occurring changes are spontaneous or are brought about by a therapeutic measure. We are dependent upon the impressions of the interviewer who is appraising the results obtained, since objective laboratory methods are not yet available. A valid evaluation of treatment requires a great number of patients who are treated and observed for many years according to the same principles. In the report on the 104 patients treated by Sakel and myself between 1933 and 1935, we did not fail to point out these problems.

Evidence was only circumstantial. This allows for the opinion of the medical reader to be more influenced by the subjective element than if he were presented with data which would be more comparable to a mathematical equation. The single facts were correctly reported. However, I have to admit that our presentation occasionally failed by not describing clearly enough the reasons for our conclusions. Furthermore, Sakel's classical technique includes many details which have not been sufficiently investigated.

Their didactic presentation did not carry enough weight. It remained unclear as to which technical details have to be emphasized as deciding. Therefore, one must say that the classical technique had little real chance to be applied and to be evaluated. A few authors have consciously or unknowingly modified the classical technique. Some of them have concluded that ICT is not effective. Their disappointment may have been due to their modifications of the Sakel technique. The percentage of success, the quality and stability of the obtained results may greatly depend upon technical factors which are difficult to define.

In 1954, I was given the opportunity to organize a 20-bed insulin unit at the Metropolitan State Hospital in Waltham, using the classical method. Our results closely resemble those which were reported by Sakel and myself in 1936.

The results obtained in the later cases of the insulin treated series were better than in the initial period of each series, due to increasing experience. The same trend continued in regard to results as well as to safety. Among the 109 patients, we had one serious prolonged coma two years ago. Now the patient is at home leading a useful life. Her schizophrenic symptoms have subsided and clinical evidence of the organic brain syndrome has nearly disappeared. One of our patients succumbed following a convulsion during the awakening period. It was later learned that this patient had been given 150 mg thorazine on his ward that morning prior to coming to the unit for insulin. A severe hypoglycemic seizure with marked hypertension due to thorazine combined in the fatal effect.

In order to comment on several controversial questions we present in Figure 3 data in terms of the type of psychosis, duration of manifest symptoms before the treatment, quality of outcome, and relapses.

The cases are arranged according to the time elapsed between the onset of the first symptoms and the start of ICT. The degree of obtained results are expressed in four grades referring to an evaluation made four weeks after the treatment was completed. Grade I means that all psychotic symptoms have disappeared. The patient returns to his previous function and adjustment in the family and in the community. He recognizes the unrealistic nature of his past psychotic experiences and behavior. Grade II means that the patient has left the hospital to lead a reasonably adjusted life, but shows either residual symptoms which he

Figure 3

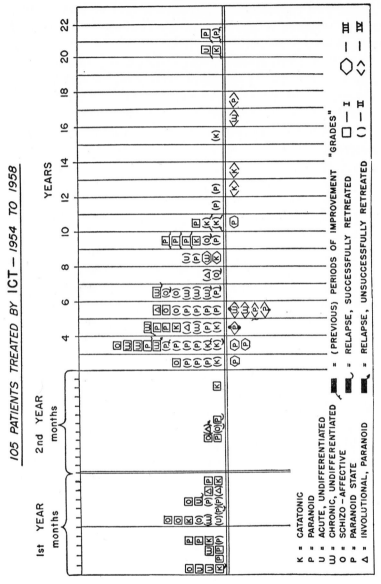

is able to control well, and/or still clings to an unrealistic attitude in regard to his previous psychotic experiences and behavior. Patients whose hospitalization has to be continued are listed as Grade III or Grade IV, depending upon whether adjustment is significantly improved or not. Two patients lived outside of the hospital for years after treatment, but are dependent upon the protective care of their families, and therefore are indicated as Grade III (but above the horizontal line dividing the cases who are living outside the hospital and those who are still in the hospital).

Many controversies have arisen over the terms "full remission" or "social recovery" and "cure." In his recent book on schizophrenia, Arieti[2] claims that the remissions of patients released as "cured" from hospitals after somatic treatment without intensive psychotherapy are only fragile and incomplete. Others have found that these allegedly "cured" patients still show so-called schizophrenic features in the Rorschach test. However, if it could be possible to free all schizophrenics of these symptoms which made their confinement necessary so that they could return to their families and live a satisfactory life, this alone would be a tremendous achievement even if they could not pass a probing psychodynamic interview or a Rorschach test. Most of our Grade I results do not warrant Arieti's doubts. As long as we do not know more about the schizophrenic process, one is not able to decide the theoretical question of whether a patient is "cured" or not. However, it is generally agreed upon that if a person remains well five years after a schizophrenic episode has subsided, he is practically safe, since later relapses occur very rarely (Langfeldt).[7] In 1944 Poetzl[9] mentions that 50% of the treated patients were found completely well after 10 years. The relapse rate in the Boston series is small up to now, about 17% for Grade I results within three years, but only 4% had to be rehospitalized. The other relapses could be treated successfully with tranquilizers on an outpatient basis. The percentage of cases whose manifest symptoms had lasted not longer than six months before treatment is much smaller in this series than in the Vienna series 1933-1935. All seventeen cases of a pre-treatment duration of not more than six months, which are contained in our last series were able to leave the hospital. Six of them had been treated three years ago and they are still well; the others were treated later. One patient of this group had a relapse after the delivery of a baby one year after treatment. Two other women had children after treatment, one of them had two, without any recurrence of psychotic symptoms. Relapses in the first year are very rare. Perhaps we have been favored by the law of averages. The number of our cases is still small. The present series does not date back more than four years. The continued follow-up observations become more valuable with additional time. Five year periods of observation will allow the prediction that the respective patients who reach Grade I results will remain free of psychotic symptoms in their future life.

So far, the patients with a pre-treatment period of not longer than six months do not fit with the rule which was recently expressed by Langfeldt, that 25% of schizophrenics fail to respond to any treatment even if treated as early as possible. Also, this sub-group does not fit Manfred Bleuler's[3] concept that only those schizophrenics respond to ICT who have a good prognosis anyway. It seems improbable that one could select seventeen schizophrenics anticipating correctly an unexceptionally benign prognosis. Furthermore, in the whole series three fourths of our patients who obtained Grade I or Grade II results after ICT had a series of ECT first during which they failed to reach an optimum remission. If Manfred Bleuler's concept would be valid for these cases, at least some of them should have shown their relative benign prognosis during the weeks that they were treated by ECT exclusively. I believe that the graphic presentation of the cases of our last series gives a clue as to how this apparent contradiction perhaps could be explained. Both Manfred Bleuler's and our conclusions are based on observations. Differences in the techniques of treatment can probably explain this contradiction to some degree only. It would be very difficult to establish exactly what these differences may be.[8] However, if one would consider only those cases in our series who are ill for a longer time than two years, and do not reach more than Grade II results, such a selection from our material could also possibly lead one to the interpretation that only cases respond to treatment who have a more benign prognosis. If one would only consider the cases of our series who are ill longer than two years and do not reach Grade I results, one would find the following: the majority of the cases of such a selected group who respond is composed of patients who had previously shown periods of improvement. It is much rarer that cases respond who had previously a straight down-hill course or had been stationary for several years. But it does not seem to be justified to extrapolate this observation on older cases with poorer response to cases which were treated in an earlier period of their disease and obtained Grade I results.

It is my contention that these and other contradictions in the evaluation of statistical trends are explained by the enormous difficulties of arriving at valid conclusions on the limited number of cases which are available to one observer. Factors beyond the control of the investigator as well as his interpretation of statistics enter into the formation of opinions. Every effort must be made to evaluate statistically larger series of cases treated and recorded according to the outlined principles. This has not yet been done sufficiently. This poses a great challenge to a combined effort in the future. Only in this way the difficulties of the evaluation of the treatment of schizophrenia can be overcome. Also, in a similar sense the controversy in regard to the frequency of relapses may be explained. There are differences in technique. In addition statistical analysis helps us to understand the reasons for this type of controversy.

If one isolates those cases of our series who are ill longer than two years and reach only Grade II results, one would also arrive at a relapse rate of 50%.

It might be true for certain patients that one can not obtain more than a limited remission. One is, however, obliged to exhaust all available efforts before one considers it the unavoidable fate of an individual not to reach a Grade I result.

In this respect the need for individualization especially becomes apparent. No standardization can lead to optimal results. If a patient fails to improve towards Grade I, one must not blame either the incurability of the schizophrenic process or the ineffectiveness of ICT in general. One must attempt to adjust the coma depth and duration, add convulsive treatment during hypoglycemia, try to modify the period of awakening, and other factors. This individualization depends upon the observance of subtle and gross changes in the pathological picture during each treatment day. In taking these changes as leads for the further steps of individualized application of treatment, one learns to modify the manifest picture of the psychosis and can work step by step toward an optimum end result.[11] Insulin, as a tool of psychiatric therapy, has a unique characteristic. One can tranquilize and/or activate the reactions of a psychotic patient. Insulin is a unique factor in two physiological respects. First, it is the only substance produced by the organism itself which is capable of bringing about a reversible state of extreme relaxation comparable to hibernation (Sakel—1937).[10] No other hormone is known to have this function. Second, insulin is a hormone and is constantly functioning to a lesser or greater extent in the organism. This may be the reason that one can give larger amounts, within established limits, than those the organism spontaneously utilizes, and can produce a deep coma which is reversible at will and has no untoward aftereffects. The nature of this reaction is comparable to sleep or hibernation rather than to intoxication by a drug which is foreign to the organism.

From the beginning of his work, Sakel combined insulin with the then available respective pharmaca, such as atropin, adrenalin, gynergen, thyroxin, and metrazol. The arrival of the tranquilizers has opened a new avenue. They can control pathological behavior. In a percentage of cases they can also condition recovery in a deeper sense, from psychosis. Tranquilizers are in common use for four years only. This is still too short a period as a final assessment for a treatment of schizophrenia. Thus far our experiences suggest that even if one tries to keep the other factors of the therapeutic situation, such as attention on special treatment wards, group meetings with the patients and with the relatives, an activity program, liberal weekend permits, planning for the period following release from the hospital from the beginning of treatment, on a similar level for both insulin and tranquilizer cases, the classical ICT technique still gives better results. The ratio for our insulin patients of mixed pretreatment duration between Grade I and Grade II results is about 1:1. For comparable tranquilizer cases, this ratio is estimated as being only 1:4. This may herald a greater tendency for relapses in cases that are treated by tranquilizers alone. However, it is possible to treat relapses with tranquilizers on an out-patient basis if the patients are willing to come for follow-up visits. In this respect, it is probably significant that the insulin patients usually have a better attitude toward the hospital and the physician after being released. We use meprobamate if again-arising difficulties are characterized only by tension, self-consciousness, or anxious uneasiness. We give or add thorazine if autonomic symptoms appear, such as sleep disturbance or weight loss. If delusional ideas, e.g. ideas of reference, or hallucinations reappear, we prefer compazine or trilafon. If paranoid hostility dominates the picture, stelazine is our choice. In order to obtain satisfactory results these drugs must be given in relatively large doses. In some of the rare Grade II results, where lack of initiative still hampers the readjustment, although all delusional or hallucinatory symptoms have subsided, iproniazid may give good effects. We give it in daily doses of 50 to 100 mg. In corroboration with Nathan

Kline's observation, we rarely see an effect before four weeks. We perform liver function tests every other week and from the beginning add sufficient Vitamin B. No liver damage was seen in our cases.

A judicious combination of ICT with the above mentioned drugs is in line with Sakel's program. With tranquilizers, activation during hypoglycemia and the behavior during free week-ends in the first phase of ICT may be controlled. We avoided the simultaneous use of serpasil or iproniazid with ICT, because of assumed risks. We do not consider doses larger than 50 mg of thorazine as safe during hypoglycemia.

The use of psychotropic drugs certainly holds promise. But the responsibilities for treatment in the case of an incipient schizophrenic is so great, especially since mistakes may only show after years, that I believe it would be a great loss to our schizophrenic patients if ICT would be abandoned. ICT still gives a schizophrenic patient who is in the first years of his disease the greatest chance of recovery especially in regard to a long term result. In Figure III the common impression is illustrated that the percentage of success diminishes the longer ICT is delayed after the onset of symptoms. During the years 1933 to 1935, we were under the impression that the critical turning point in most cases is the period of six months. Therefore, we classified the patients of our report in 1936 in two groups, consisting of those who were ill no longer than six months and of those who have a longer pretreatment duration respectively. Later experiences as discussed, among others, by Mueller[8] showed that the pretreatment periods with relatively satisfactory chances are probably longer. Once in a while a case whose symptoms had dated back many more years responds to ICT to a surprising degree. However, it has been impossible so far to predict which case of longer duration would exceptionally so respond.

Figure III shows that all cases of the Boston series which could be treated by the classical ICT during the first two years of their manifest symptoms, could be brought at least to a Grade II result. The ratio between Grade I and Grade II results gradually becomes less favorable. Although it still seems best to treat schizophrenics as early as possible, it is our present impression that the critical turning point in respect to responsiveness to ICT is for the majority of patients not in the proximity of six months, but rather at the beginning of the third year. I do not feel that the statistical trend can be interpreted only in terms of decreased responsiveness to treatment with the increased pretreatment periods since the start of symptoms, although this factor is probably the most significant one. That good results are obtained more readily in cases with relatively short pretreatment histories, is partly related to the fact that these patients represent a selection of cases whose resistance to the schizophrenic process is comparably greater and may have a better potential to resist deterioration. The cases coming to treatment later are likely those with a more insidious onset and may have less potential to defend themselves against the disease. Furthermore, I feel that one should not overlook the following: The gradual diminished responsiveness with duration of pretreatment history became apparent to us at an early period of this work. The concept of decreasing responsiveness in older patients may have influenced our emphasis in the technique. It may be that we have not yet learned more effective ways for cases of longer standing. Studies would be warranted in this sense.

As mentioned in various respects, the collection of appropriately detailed material is very important. We were fortunate that six months ago, a research and teaching division could be added to our unit by a grant of the Manfred Sakel Foundation, Inc. In this way, a facility for controlled therapeutic investigations became available. Details of Sakel's classical insulin technique in their objective relevance, and interviews of treated patients by psychiatrists who otherwise are not connected with the individual treatment situation, are among our program.

Furthermore, we have had the opportunity to do coordinated research with Dr. Samuel Bogoch of the Massachusetts Mental Health Center, Boston. This investigation deals mainly with the longitudinal follow-up of the neuraminic acid content in the spinal fluid during treatment. Sakel's ICT has a very definite place in an active treatment program of today. It can and should be integrated in a good therapeutic community and in an active treatment program. Sakel's ICT ranks foremost under the weapons which are available at present in the fight against schizophrenia.

References

1. Alexander, Leo. Treatment of Mental Disorder. Philadelphia and London: W. B. Saunders Co., 1953.
2. Arieti, Silvano. Interpretation of Schizophrenia. New York: Robert Brunner, 1955.
3. Bleuler, Manfred. "Forschungen zur Schizophreniefrage." Wien. Zschr. f. Nervenheilkunde u. Grenzgebiete, Bd 1, Heft 2/3, 1947.
4. Dussik, Karl Theo. "Les résultats du traîtement da la schizophrenie par les chocs insuliniques d'après la méthode du docteur Sakel en comparison avec les évolutions spontanèes de la schizophrenie." Pol. Jb. f. Psychiatry 28, 1936.
5. Dussik, Karl Theo and Sakel, Manfred. "Ergebnisse der Hypoglykaemie—Schock behandlung der Schizophrenie." Z. neur. 155:351, 1936.
6. Kalinowsky, Lothar B. and Hoch, Paul H. Shock Treatments, Psychosurgery, and Other Somatic Treatments in Psychiatry. New York: Grune and Stratton, 1952.
7. Langfeldt, G. Prognosis in Schizophrenia. Scandinav: Acta psychiat. et neurol. Supp. 110, 1956.
8. Mueller, Max. Die Koerperlichen Behandlungsverfahren in der Psychiatrie. Stuttgart: Georg Thieme Verlag, 1952.

9. Poetzl, Otto. "Uber die Erfolge der Schocktherapie bei Geisteskrankheiten." Wien: Wien Med. Wochschr. 94, 1944.
10. Sakel, Manfred. The Pharmacological Shock Treatment of Schizophrenia. New York and Washington: Nervous and Mental Disease Publishing Co., 1938.
11. Sakel, Manfred. Schizophrenia. New York: Philosophical Library, 1958.
12. Sargant, William and Slater, Eliot. An Introduction to Physical Methods of Treatment in Psychiatry. Baltimore: The Williams and Wilkins Company, 1954.

DISCUSSION

DR. GOTTLIEB: I certainly want to compliment the presenters of the last two papers. They gave a very full and detailed description of their activity and the extent of their operations.

In this discussion I would like to expand a little bit beyond the point of their papers, if you will permit. As I look at the problem of treatment of the patient with schizophrenia, I see two fundamentally different approaches. On the one hand is the psychological method of therapy, psychotherapy. The essence of this treatment is to established emotional support for the patient by means of the patient-physician relationship, which has for its purpose the reduction of the effects of all those factors, both conscious and unconscious, which were disturbing to the patient. Essentially, through the techniques available by this method, one is attempting to either remove or minimize the personalized stresses under which the patient has been living, and thus improve his adaptability by making him more flexible and better able to cope with emotional stress. The means by which this type of therapy is applied and its implications on stress mechanisms, however, is not a subject of discussion for this conference. On the other hand, through the use of the somatic treatments, we are doing just the opposite. We are using stress to overwhelm the patient. Historically, as was pointed out by Dr. Hoff, it has been observed that trials by water, by fire, by physical illness—overwhelming stressors—have been noted from time to time to lead to therapeutic benefit.

We have heard at this conference several theories as to how the insulin procedure may bring about the desired results. Dr. Arnold presented a theory to the effect that those cells which were already partially damaged would be the first to be lost, and hence restore the organism's equilibrium. In contrast the presentations on the physiology, the biochemistry, and the electrical potentials of the brain certainly gave us a comprehensive picture of the tremendous metabolic changes that were brought about through insulin, through electric shock, and more recently, through the new drugs.

Yet, in spite of the knowledge of the metabolic changes produced by these therapeutic agents, we do not know which changes are the important ones related to the therapeutic benefit that the patient receives, and which ones are epiphenomenal. We really don't know whether the sequence of experiences through these stressors is to abolish some metabolic or cellular systems, or to produce a rebound effect on some metabolic system that is disturbed so that it assumes a more normal pattern, hence allowing the person with illness to return to a better adaptive framework. Certainly some of the comments that were given suggesting combining insulin with convulsive treatment and with the tranquilizers as producing the better results, suggest that the specificity depends upon the totality of the stress in order to achieve the necessary physiological responsiveness and therapeutic goals.

It seems to me that from this conference there are several very basic problems that deserve investigation. Can we in some way develop indicators that will give us some idea of the mechanisms that are involved in these various therapeutic approaches? What are the mechanisms that are really defective, a cellular distortion, a metabolic system crippled by a defective enzyme, or a pattern ascribable to disturbances in psychological learning?

Although the presentations that have just been given indicate the importance of this method of treatment on an empirical basis, I wish to beg that we extend our observations in order to be able to understand just what are the important and what are the unimportant variables that are involved.

DR. NATHAN KLINE: Both of the authors made what I believe is an extremely important point, that the patient to be counted has to be 100 per cent cured by all psychological, physiological and outer space tests is a highly questionable requirement.

Gruenberg in an article last year made this point rather tellingly, pointing out that in the rest of medicine relief of disabilities constitutes about 80 per cent of the activity. For some reason in psychiatry no one is satisfied unless the patient has been completely relieved or completely "cured" of his illness.

It is certainly a very appropriate and proper function to relieve disability so that the patient can return to society and in most branches of medicine this is regarded as a satisfactory therapeutic result.

One of the claims made not too overtly is that the insulin and the drugs only relieve symptoms. I would state in my own opinion, we don't know the cause of schizophrenia and therefore we cannot talk about a cure. We don't know by what criteria we can judge cure, and I think until we know the etiology of the disease, the best we can speak of is the degree of relief of symptoms including the fact that they are all gone. Now this does not necessarily constitute a cure in the sense that we know the etiological pathology has disappeared.

My feeling about the relationship of the drug to insulin is rather definite at the moment. I think there are a number of specialized techniques of therapy in psychiatry which are by and large expensive and prolonged and require highly skilled personnel to administer. These would include psychoanalysis, deep sleep treatment which has been, I gather, not referred to, and insulin therapy.

In medicine one does not do a gastric resection if Gelusil

will work. The principle of good medicine is to use the most rapid, least expensive treatment if it will do the job. Now my feeling would be in those cases where pharmaceuticals can be used they should be used first. In the ordinary course of administering the drugs probably no longer than three or four months is needed before you know whether you are going to have a good therapeutic result or not.

I think that patients who then do not respond after having been given an adequate quota of pharmaceuticals should be considered for a series of expensive prolonged highly skilled therapies, and I feel that this is the time at which the three treatments, psychoanalysis, deep sleep and insulin should be taken into consideration.

I would further say that because of the limitations of personnel and space for this type of treatment, that even if this is done we will need a hundred times the number of beds available for insulin treatment that we presently have. I think it is a great mistake to try out and treat every patient with a single technique. Even with this screening there is a great need for expansion of insulin therapy. I have no question that there are patients who respond to insulin who fail to respond to the drugs but I feel rather strongly that the drugs should be used first and that to talk about the fact that drugs merely repress symptoms is leaving yourself open to the dubious position that the same can be said and is said about insulin therapy.

I feel that there is nothing incompatible in the use of the various treatments we have available but they should be used with the appropriate patient.

CHAIRMAN DR. RINKEL: Thank you, Dr. Kline.

May I call to your attention that Dr. Hoch made the remark that the introduction of the drugs did not obviate insulin treatment, although most State Hospitals in the state of New York use pharmaceuticals for treatment instead of insulin.

With regard to your remark as to the cure, I fully agree with you. We often have discussed this matter in our hospital. It is a matter of semantics. What do we consider cure? What do we consider a cure in a heart condition? What do we consider a cure of tuberculosis and so on. You are quite right in bring up this question.

DR. JOSEPH WORTIS: Dr. Hoch yesterday and Dr. Kline today brought up a very important point which simply amounts to this: If you have a schizophrenic patient who is brought to you, say a young person in his twenties, with an acute onset a few weeks previously, do you start by giving him one of the tranquilizing drugs or do you start by giving him insulin shock treatment?

Dr. Hoch said very clearly that when you deal with large numbers of patients in the State Hospital system, which is his present responsibility, you don't use expensive elaborate treatments when you can use simple and inexpensive treatments which lend themselves to use with large numbers of patients.

Dr. Kline said something similar. Those of us who have worked in the field know that an acute schizophrenic case presents very promising material for successful treatment, that in a matter of months the likelihood of success diminishes very rapidly.

I make a plea for clarification of one simple question. Do we have any data to justify the use of a method of treatment that is cheap, on the assumption that the results are just as good as the more expensive and elaborate methods?

DR. KLINE: We have such data.

DR. WORTIS: Well, I say the risks involved are great because months are very valuable, and I think most of us are obligated to operate according to our clinical experience as described in the literature and so on. This is an unfortunate state of affairs where the stakes are so high.

We should have some very clear data to justify which of the treatments deserve to be used, and the argument of cheapness is very unconvincing particularly to the families of the patients who may have non-recoverable illnesses after valuable time has been lost.

DR. KENNEDY (Central Islip State Hospital): Some years ago, before the advent of tranquilizing drugs, I caused a study to be made of patients that made spontaneous improvement and had been released, then returned to the hospital and on the advent of the second admission were treated with insulin. I can't quote now the exact number but it was sizable. As we get relapses we expect the patient to become more chronic. But of this entire series only one patient did not do as well following his second release as he did the first time. Two others did just about the same and all other patients in the series made a better adjustment. This was based on a series of tests, as employability, adjustment to the family, duration of their capacity to stay away from the hospital and so on.

From that time on I have felt strongly that there is something in the insulin treatment that the other treatments and drugs have not had. This was before, as I say, any tranquilizers came up.

DR. DENBER: Dr. Dussik has made an excellent presentation, and it should be commended for its clarity and technique. There are, however, several points open to question. He seemed to convey the idea that it was possible to convert most, if not all patients, to a Grade I result with the Sakel technique.

DR. DUSSIK: I'm sorry I gave this impression. I did not say that. I wanted to convey my conviction that we must not think it the inevitable fate of an individual schizophrenic patient not to reach a Grade I result before exhausting all therapeutic possibilities, including ICT.

DR. DENBER: You indicated to me that with this method one should be able to convert—

DR. DUSSIK: We showed a lot of cases who don't.

DR. DENBER: It would appear to me that there are many patients who will never be able to achieve Grade I and always rest in Grade V. On the research service at Manhattan State Hospital, I have observed such individuals who can be considered as chronic, and in whom the prognosis is almost hopeless—at least, with the techniques available today.

Dr. Wortis has brought up a very potent question. It can be answered with some of the New York State statistics concerning admission, discharge, relapse and readmission during many years in the past. It is fairly well known that most new treatments have a beneficial effect at the outset. As time goes on, this beneficial action seems to diminish or disappear. The relapse and readmission rate until 1954 has been fairly constant around 30%.

It is a matter of general knowledge, that since 1954 drugs have been introduced on a large scale into the state hospitals. This is the first time that there has been a consistent decrease in the population of these hospitals, as well as the readmission rate. In some places, this has fallen as low as 12%.

As Dr. Gottlieb has pointed out, there is no question that insulin coma treatment has been of great value. However, it is questionable whether or not it has the absolute value as claimed by Dr. Dussik.

CHAIRMAN RINKEL: I believe that nobody would disagree with Dr. Joseph Wortis' statement that no patient should be denied treatment because it is expensive.

(Applause)

DR. KALINOWSKY: I think we have to stress this once more. If a patient needs a treatment he should get it and the financial situation should not enter at all.

The answer which I have to give to Dr. Kline is the same I gave him once before in a lively discussion we had: it is that insulin and electroshock are effective only during the first year of illness. It is for this reason that I think that after three or four months of pharmacotherapy we should discontinue and give the patient the benefit of the other treatments if he relapses.

DR. CONRAN (Metropolitan State Hospital, Waltham, Massachusetts): I have been able to show that it may take about nine months before you can see whether the tranquilizing drugs are going to have any effect or not. There are certain patients that do not respond for nine months. Therefore I think what we've got to do is to establish the best possible treatment in each case as early as possible.

DR. O. H. ARNOLD: We have developed a new method to produce coma. The dose of insulin is not important, but there is a contra-regulation against the insulin. We have to interrupt this tendency of contra-regulation against insulin. Therefore, we use the ganglion blocker, hexamethonium. The patient should have 100-400 mg of hexamethonium. Using this method, we obtain coma with 40 to 80 units of insulin, beginning with about 10 or 20 units. In most cases, coma is achieved on the third or fourth day.

CHAIRMAN DR. RINKEL: May I ask Dr. Arnold a question: Hexamethonium is a quaternary ammonium base with a chain of six carbons. It has the effect of lowering the blood pressure. How does this effect combine with that of insulin? Is there any danger involved?

DR. O. H. ARNOLD: The method is without danger. Hexamethonium blocks the synapses for the hormonal regulation.

DR. KLINE: The crucial question is how does insulin treatment compare with the other types of treatment, and in all fairness one must give both sides of the case. The clinical impressions of people using insulin is strongly that it is superior. The very few studies which have an adequate experimental design, such as those of Fink et al.,[1] Boardman et al.,[2] Ackner et al.,[3] Scherer and Trehub[4] and a number of others, have shown that the clinical results are approximately the same when chlorpromazine is compared with

1. Fink, M., Shaw, R., Gross, G. E. and Coleman, F. S. Comparative Study of Chlorpromazine and Insulin Coma in Therapy of Psychotics. J.A.M.A. *166:* 1846-1850, April 12, 1958.

2. Boardman, R. H., Lomas, J. and Markowe, M. Insulin and Chlorpromazine in Schizophrenia; a comparative study in previously untreated cases. Lancet 2; 487-494, Sept. 8, 1956.

3. Ackner, B., Harris, A. and Oldham, A. J. Insulin Treatment of Schizophrenia: control study, Lancet 2; 607-611, March 23, 1957.

4. Scherer, I. W. and Trehub, R. Effects of physiodynamic treatments in a hospital over a ten year period. Dis. Nerv. System *18:* 55-58, Feb., 1957.

insulin. There are relatively few follow-up studies so that long-term effects cannot be adequately compared.

The advantages as shown in the studies I know of are that chlorpromazine treatment is more rapid, requires less personnel and also does not require such skill, plus the fact that it is consequently less expensive. Assume for the moment that we have cured 100 of the cases with insulin and the drugs cured only five per cent—having just returned from India where there are 11 million patients per psychiatrist, the impossibility of treating any proportion of the psychotics there with insulin is rather staggering.

In the meantime even if the drugs were only five per cent effective, if you had a choice of treating a thousand schizophrenics with drugs of whom only five per cent would recover (i.e., 50) or of treating 25 patients with insulin, the drugs should prevail. Since current statistics give about the same percentage of response for the drugs and the insulin, I do not see how one can seriously advocate using insulin first and to the exclusion of the other treatments.

I don't think that the enthusiasm, rightly or incorrectly, for one method of treatment should outweigh our moral responsibility to treat as many people as adequately as we can.

DR. WEISS: I am very gratified at the comments that were given. They allow a lot of food for thought.

I'm glad that Dr. Wortis brought up the subject of acute schizophrenic reactions and I offer this in the interests of clarification more than anything else because I ran up against this question myself in our own hospital, and I culled out of the records all those who had what I would call an acute schizophrenic reaction meaning that there were no antecedent qualities of schizophrenia that we can determine, that the patient was hospitalized once and was not hospitalized since that time. This was 1953. It is not yet ready for publication. However, I have 40 cases, most of which are at least five years old. Using these criteria and going into the manner of treatment, ten were treated with insulin, ten without insulin. None of them stayed in the hospital more than six months. If that is statistically significant, so be it.

I am afraid that we have been in the habit of lumping all schizophrenic reactions together. I believe that acute schizophrenics will recover quite nicely and the question is up to the individual therapist whether to use insulin or not.

DR. DUSSIK: The time is too advanced to go into the details so excellently brought up in the discussion, for which I would like to express my sincere appreciation. Many of the points concern important problems brought up and not solved for decades. Their formulation was helpful for further progress.

However, I should like to point out one practical point. I believe that the issue of the expenses is not as significant as it is sometimes said but most of the time a "red herring" which is occasionally used as an excuse for lack of activity and courage.

You are completely right, Dr. Denber, I feel strong emotions in view of the present situation in regard to the treatment of schizophrenic patients. Those of us who believe in the merit of ICT feel on the defensive because of the present trend in this country. Out of the 26 mental hospitals in Massachusetts, 11 never used ICT, 7 gave it up in recent years. It is dangerous now to give up a proven weapon in the fight against such a disastrous condition as schizophrenia which is responsible for the hospitalization of over one-fourth of all people who are hospitalized for any reason, before one knows that one can reach at least the same benefits for the patients with other means. If one holds my enthusiasm against me, I have to admit it. But I feel that as a physician one has to be enthusiastic, which should not be identified with lack of critical judgment. I am enthusiastic about every way to treat successfully schizophrenic patients, but not uncritical in favor or against a particular technique. The respective merits of various techniques have to be critically evaluated in regard to long-term results. I am interested in the new drugs but they have not been in use for a sufficient length of time. So far, we estimate that the ratio between grade I and grade II results is much less favorable for drugs than for ICT. The active treatment of a schizophrenic psychosis is more expensive when one uses drugs alone than when using ICT alone, so far as the expenses for pharmaca is concerned. I estimated that the drugs in the first technique cost about $1,200, but those which are used in ICT (Insulin, Glucose, etc.) about $100. The additional personnel of our unit consisting of only one nurse and two attendants costs about $10,300 a year or 0.25% of the budget of the hospital of about $4,000,000. This is, of course, only valid for a hospital which is very active and would not be the same for a hospital which either has first to provide building facilities or for a private hospital. It is much easier to close an insulin unit than to set up a new one. I believe it is indicated to express a strong warning against the abandonment of insulin units.

Besides the problem of the long-term results, another factor to be considered is the duration of the hospitalization. One must not forget what it means for a patient to be four months, six months, or one year out of his routine life. If the hospitalization lasts longer, the chances that the patient loses his standing in his community increase, the husband has to get a housekeeper and sometimes he gets more, the job is gone, in younger people the education is interrupted for good, life has to be started anew. I believe that also in this respect ICT is still superior in statistical terms. Therefore, I believe that it is unfounded to adopt the opinion that ICT can be substituted for all patients today. We cannot be sure how it will be in 10 or 30 years. I think this conference helped us to take a good look at very important problems, or at least to understand where to look. I do not want to advertise for sentimental reasons a specific technique but to contribute within the limitations we have. I try to be as modest and humble as appropriate with the formidable difficulty of the problem toward progress in the field of the treatment of schizophrenic patients.

Chapter 18

NEURAMINIC ACID IN THE CEREBROSPINAL FLUID OF SCHIZOPHRENIC PATIENTS

SAMUEL BOGOCH

When the definitive physicochemical disturbances which occur in the nervous system in the schizophrenic psychoses are elucidated, it may then be possible to determine the specific effects of insulin and other therapies upon these disturbances.

The reality of recurrent, persistent and crippling schizophrenic illness demonstrates that there is much to be learned. The required knowledge is lacking not only with reference to pathological phenomena, but also with regard to the normal structure and function of brain constituents.

My work is directed towards basic studies of the chemistry and physiology of the central nervous system, with a constant effort to relate structure and function—not as individual coexistent entities, but as a single unitary phenomenon. Both the methodology of the clinic and of the laboratory are used in these studies. I shall briefly summarize my recent investigations on the chemical structure and function of several complex macromolecular substances of the central nervous system. These substances contain lipid, protein and carbohydrate constituents, of which neuraminic acid forms only a small part. I shall, in addition, describe some studies which have only just begun, on the effects of treatment upon the clinical status and the state of neuraminic acid in the cerebrospinal fluid of individual patients.

The Determination of Neuraminic Acid in the CSF

Neuraminic acid is a hexosaminouronic acid which occurs in gray matter of the brain in association with nerve cell bodies. In the brain it forms part of a macromolecular glycolipid called brain ganglioside, whose structure has been the subject of recent work in this laboratory.[6] The structure of brain ganglioside suggested the possibility[6] that this material was involved in membrane receptor and transport functions in the central nervous system, and studies on the interaction of viruses with brain ganglioside[7] have provided evidence in support of this concept. The hypothesis was advanced[1,2] that both fixed (cellular) and free (fluid) neuraminic acid-containing components ('Barrier-Antibody System') consisting of gangliosides, glycoproteins and other substances are present in the central nervous system, which are concerned with the maintenance of a constant biochemical environment for inter-neuronal function in the brain, and that breakdown of this function would permit entry to the brain by many body metabolites which ordinarily do not gain access. The disorganization of function which might result could account for the observed characteristics of the psychotic state. In order to obtain evidence relevant to the above hypothesis, much more would have to be known about the chemistry and metabolism of the neuraminic acid-containing substances of the nervous system.

It thus became of interest to study the presence of neuraminic acid in the more accessible fluid component of the central nervous system, the cerebrospinal fluid (CSF) and to define its mode of chemical association in that fluid. A micromethod was developed[1,2] which was a modification of the classical Klenk-Bohm-Bial's reaction[11] for neuraminic acid in blood serum. Using this method the normal range of concentration of neuraminic acid in the CSF was demonstrated in what is now 475 patients with a variety of psychiatric disorders, neurological disorders, and no disorders of the nervous system. It was shown that the concentration of neuraminic acid tends to increase in the CSF with age. Thus, children under 7 years of age had values of neuraminic acid between 20 and 65 micrograms per cc., whereas over 7 years of age and throughout the adult years, the nonschizophrenic subjects examined had values above 41 micrograms per cc. Schizophrenic adults, on the other hand, had values below 41 micrograms per cc., values comparable in range only to those observed in about half of the nonschizophrenic children examined under seven years of age. The possibility that the increase in concentration of neuraminic acid in the CSF represents a maturation phenomenon was suggested, and the corollary that the low values observed in schizophrenic adults represented a form of chemical immaturity also presented itself as a possibility.[1,2]

Since the Bial's reaction for neuraminic acid may be influenced by very high concentrations of glucose[11] it became important to eliminate any possible interference by the usual glucose present in CSF in the determination of neuraminic acid. Simultaneous glucose and neuraminic acid determinations were done on all CSF samples, and it was observed that there was no consistent correlation between the total amount of neuraminic acid present and the total glucose present, and, in fact, the two were not infrequently inversely correlated. That is, high concentrations of neuraminic acid (or total Bial-positive substances) were frequently associated with low concentrations of glucose, and vice versa. Therefore it did not appear that the normal concentrations of glucose in CSF interfered appreciably with the Bial's reaction in CSF. At any rate, whatever interference might exist was clearly non-linear, so that no simple correction factor could be applied.

It remained necessary however to account for all of the Bial-positive material quantitatively. To this end recent studies in this laboratory[3,4] have been concerned with the development of methods for the separation of micro- and macromolecular species in CSF with reference to neuraminic acid. The distribution of neuraminic acid between dialyzable and non-dialyzable fractions of CSF was studied in 104 cases. In addition to obtaining a large amount of previously unavailable quantitative data on the protein and carbohydrate constituents of the CSF, a water-soluble glycoprotein fraction was isolated,[3,9] whose composition distinguishes it chemically from previously described glycoproteins of blood serum. This glycoprotein fraction (Fraction G) was shown to differ in the amount of neuraminic acid which it contained in schizophrenic and non-schizophrenic subjects, while the 'total protein' fraction did not show these differences. Fraction G accounts for between 0.6 and 22 micrograms per cc. of the 'total' neuraminic acid of the CSF, and appears to be the fraction which is primarily responsible for the differences observed between children under 7 and adults, and between schizophrenic and non-schizophrenic subjects. Further studies are in progress to further define the physical and chemical properties of the components of Fraction G.

Repeated Determinations of Neuraminic Acid in Individual Subjects

Perhaps one of the first questions which comes to mind regarding the significance of the above observations with regard to individual patients concerns the constancy of the value for 'total neuraminic acid' in a given patient over a period of time. If the concentration of neuraminic acid is indeed of significance in the schizophrenic process, several possibilities present themselves. The concentration might be a constant characteristic for a given individual, like a fingerprint, a biological landmark. On the other hand, the concentration might vary slightly with certain functional states, but vary over a relatively narrow range which is itself in some way characteristic of the individual.

To obtain information relevant to these possibilities individual patients were followed in various circumstances of hospitalization, with and without insulin and other therapies, by careful clinical evaluation and repeated determination of the concentration of neuraminic acid in the CSF over a period of several weeks and months.[10]

A 'double blind' method was employed, whereby the investigators evaluating the clinical state of the patient had completed and recorded their observations before the laboratory findings were made known to them, and, similarly, the clinical information was not available to those performing the laboratory determinations. The clinical observations were recorded on a standard form, which included all of the pertinent clinical and psychological data, with special attention to such parameters as evidence of withdrawal, vagueness, fantasy activity and dissociative phenomena, as well as the presence of hallucinations, delusions, extremes of affect, manifest anxiety, speech and motor activity.

A total of 41 schizophrenic and 18 non-schizophrenic patients were examined. A total of 163 neuraminic acid determinations were performed on 59 patients, with between two and five determinations per patient. A thorough clinical evaluation accompanied each determination. 21 of the patients studied received coma insulin therapy, 13 received drug therapy, 3 received EST, and the remainder received no specific therapy. While all of the observations made cannot be discussed at this time, some of the results will be briefly summarized.

Despite active treatment in 33 schizophrenic patients 80 out of the 94 neuraminic acid determinations showed a concentration of neuraminic acid at or below 41 micrograms/cc. of CSF. This demonstrates that, on the one hand, the low values previously reported for schizophrenic patients[1,2] are reasonably 'group consistent' even despite active treatment. On the other hand, only one out of 18 determinations on 8 untreated schizophrenic patients (5.5%) was above 41.0 micrograms/cc. (7.9% in the previous larger series)[2] so that the percent of schizophrenic patients showing higher neuraminic acid values may be slightly greater with active therapy. Especially in those cases where three or more determinations were done is it possible to state with some assurance that these low values are in some way a characteristic phenomenon. It may also be noted that variation does indeed occur in the concentration of neuraminic acid in the CSF of most of these patients, but that it is not large, representing only a change of 1-4 micrograms/cc. in most. Thus, variation occurred about the mean for the schizophrenic group, but values seldom reached into the range of the non-schizophrenic adult values (42.0 to 70.0 micrograms/cc.). Similarly, variation in the values of the 18 non-schizophrenic patients occurred, but these variations seldom led to values which fell into the range of the schizophrenic group.

The question of whether the variations which occur are in any way significantly related to changes in the clinical status of the patients is examined in the following individual studies which are very briefly summarized.

Figures 1 through 12 show the concentration of total neuraminic acid in the CSF plotted against time, with determinations made approximately once a month for four months. The shaded area represents the range of normal adult values.

Case No. 184 (Fig. 1) is a 30-year-old schizophrenic patient who had demonstrated increasing seclusiveness and withdrawal since 1946, and who since 1957 had suffered delusions of persecution and auditory hallucinations. She had two previous mental hospital admissions. On her present admission she was given a course of coma insulin therapy, from November 27, 1957 to March 6, 1958, with 66 treatments, 49 comas, and a maximum dose of 360 units of insulin. She was clinically improved, with disappearance of hallucinations and delusions, the attainment of a 'social remission' permitting her to leave hospital. It may be seen that the concentration of neuraminic acid increased slightly

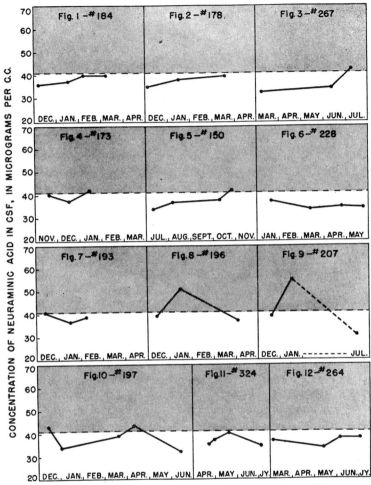

FIGURES 1-12: CONCENTRATION OF NEURAMINIC ACID IN CSF ON REPEATED DETERMINATIONS OVER SEVERAL MONTHS. (SEE TEXT FOR LEGENDS)

(Reproduced from AMA Archives of Neurology and Psychiatry 1959)

over the period of therapy, reaching a final concentration of 40.0 micrograms/cc., but not higher.

Case No. 178 (Fig. 2) is a 30-year-old paranoic schizophrenic admitted for the first time on November 15, 1957 because of increasing withdrawal with lack of activity and spontaneity over the past two years. She feared that someone would enter her room and that she was being persecuted by outside forces. She received a course of insulin therapy between December 2, 1957 and March 20, 1958 with 65 treatments, 51 comas, maximum dose 180 units. She was discharged improved, with diminished paranoid ideation and able to live at home and work, although this was not a full remission. The neuraminic acid levels increased over the four month period up to 40.0 micrograms/cc.

Case No. 267 (Fig. 3) is a 50-year-old schizophrenic patient who had been ill for at least 20 years. He was quiet, withdrawn, with lack of spontaniety and paranoid delusions. He was observed between March and July, 1958. He received no drug or insulin therapy and no formal psychotherapy. During the last two months he appeared more spontaneous, began to speak to many people, played chess with various ward personnel, joined the baseball team, and generally seemed considerably improved. The neuraminic acid concentration rose from 33.5 micrograms/cc. in March to 34.7 micrograms/cc. in June, to 42.5 micrograms/cc. in July.

Case No. 173 (Fig. 4) is a 33-year-old schizophrenic patient, who showed symptoms since the age of 20 associated with loss of interest in life, withdrawal, and what appeared to her family as depression. She had a previous mental hospital admission following a suicidal attempt. On this occasion she was admitted in a state of catatonic stupor, speaking only an occasional word. She was treated with compazine beginning October 23, 1957 to discharge. She was discharged in June, 1958 as a full remission, superficially happy, and able to take care of her children and the home, but lacking in insight. Her neuraminic acid concentration showed an initial depression, followed by an elevation to 42.0 micrograms/cc.

Case No. 150 (Fig. 5) is a 40-year-old woman who had been in a mental hospital for 10 years, withdrawn, uncoordinated and incoherent in her thinking, with the delusion that her mother was still alive. She received insulin therapy from

August 7, 1957 to November 12, 1957 with 64 treatments, 55 comas, maximum dose 110 units. She was discharged considerably less withdrawn, and more coherent, maintaining her delusions, although with considerably less intensity. The neuraminic acid concentration rose from 34.0 micrograms/cc. to 42.2 micrograms/cc.

Case No. 228 (Fig. 6) is a 29-year-old pseudoneurotic schizophrenic woman with two maternal aunts, mother and a cousin who suffer the same disorder, who was hospitalized for the fourth time in January 1958 for symptoms of vagueness and 'depression.' She was treated with marsilid, 50 mg daily, beginning February, 1958. She showed no improvement but rather demonstrated worsening of her symptoms with more clear-cut schizophrenic ideation coming to the fore. During this period her neuraminic acid concentration fell from 37.5 micrograms/cc. with repeat determinations during the stationary phase of her illness in April and May showing values of 35.0 micrograms/cc. and 34.5 micrograms/cc.

Case No. 193 (Fig. 7) is a 29-year-old schizophrenic patient who had shown symptoms including paranoid ideas and fears that she suffered from various venereal and other infectious diseases as well as a brain tumor, and who was admitted in December, 1957. She received a course of coma insulin therapy beginning December 17, with 38 treatments, 36 comas, and a maximum dose of 120 units. She had a full remission with complete disappearance of symptoms and is working at home taking care of four children, although she has not returned to her previous work as a nurse. The preinsulin neuraminic acid concentration was 41.0 micrograms/cc., followed by values of 37.0 micrograms/cc. and 39.0 micrograms/cc.

Case No. 196 (Fig. 8) is a 28-year-old schizophrenic woman who was admitted in 1956, anxious, confused, incoherent, giggling, with marked paranoid ideation. After a period of psychotherapy she was given a course of coma insulin therapy between December 1957 and May 1958, with 108 treatments, 83 comas, maximum dose 220 units. She improved markedly in December and January with almost complete loss of symptomatology. However, towards the end of January and throughout the next three months she demonstrated a marked deterioration with return of anxiety, confusion, and delusions. The neuraminic acid concentration increased markedly, coincident with the clinical improvement, reaching a value of 51.0 micrograms/cc., then showed a decline coincident with the clinical relapse, to a value of 37.5 micrograms/cc.

Case No. 207 (Fig. 9) is a 30-year-old schizophrenic woman who was hallucinated and suffered paranoid delusions on admission to hospital in December 1957. She received 75 mg of vesprin per day from admission through July 1958. She improved markedly during the first month of hospitalization, with disappearance of hallucinations and almost complete absence of paranoid ideation. However, in February and March 1958 she began to show some return of symptoms, being somewhat more anxious again and more paranoid in her thinking. The neuraminic acid concentration rose markedly in the first month of her hospitalization, from 40.0 micrograms/cc. to 55.0 micrograms/cc. temporally coincident with her improvement, but in July 1958 showed a new low of 36.0 micrograms/cc. temporally coincident with her relapse.

Case No. 197 (Fig. 10) is a 25-year-old schizophrenic woman who had a previous hospital admission in 1955 for paranoid illness following the birth of her first child. She recovered from this, but was admitted in December 1957 after several months of neglecting herself, and being preoccupied with over-religious ideas, sexual delusions, visual and auditory hallucinations. On admission she was paranoid, aggressive, assaultive, and very excited. She improved quickly in the first weeks of hospitalization in terms of her excitement and aggressivity, but remained grossly delusional. She received a course of thorazine and trilafon therapy from January through March, 1958, with some slight improvement. In April 1958 she was placed on insulin therapy and improved further, so that she was able to go home on weekends. Towards the end of April she became pregnant and insulin therapy was withdrawn. She remained moderately improved through June 1958, but was still quite deluded. The neuraminic acid concentration was 42.5 micrograms/cc. on admission (coincident with her excited behavior), dropped to 34.0 micrograms/cc. when she was outwardly calm but grossly psychotic, rose to 43.5 micrograms/cc. as she improved with thorazine and insulin therapy, and then showed a new low value of 32.0 micrograms/cc. temporally coincident with her second month of pregnancy.

Case No. 324 (Fig. 11) is a 61-year-old schizophrenic patient who had two previous admissions to a mental hospital and who was admitted on this occasion on April 19, 1958 because of withdrawal, vagueness, inability to work, and auditory hallucinations. During the first month of hospital stay he received no definitive therapy, but improved somewhat, spending more time with other patients and ward personnel. At the end of May he was placed on pacatal, 150 mg per day. The neuraminic acid concentration increased during the first month to a level of 40 micrograms/cc. coincident with his clinical improvement. His last value dropped to 34.5 micrograms/cc. coincident with the administration of pacatal, but with no observed change in his clinical status.

Case No. 264 (Fig. 12) is an 18-year-old schizophrenic boy who had been ill for at least 5 years and had two previous mental hospital admissions. His recent admission on January 28, 1958 was because of illness characterized by inappropriate smiling, flattened affect and threatening behavior. He was placed on trilafon therapy from February through July, 1958, showing no significant clinical change. His neuraminic acid values showed no major fluctuation.

Discussion

The above cases illustrate that 1) repeated neuraminic acid values tend to fall within the range of 30-40 micrograms/cc. in schizophrenic patients, and 2) the direction of change in the concentration of total neuraminic acid in the cases so far examined appears to frequently parallel closely the direction of change in the clinical status. In a few cases, such as No. 196 and No. 207 the parallel holds in quantitative terms as well, that is, in these cases a marked clinical improvement was accompanied by a marked increase in the concentration of total neuraminic acid in the CSF, and, similarly, a marked deterioration in clinical condition was accompanied by a marked drop in the concentration of neuraminic acid. In three of the 42 schizophrenic patients so far studied by repeated determinations, the direction of change in concentration of neuraminic acid was opposite to the direction of the change in clinical status. Eleven patients who received no definitive therapy showed no essential change in their clinical status and no marked change in their neuraminic acid values. Eleven of 12 determinations on 5 non-schizophrenic mental hospital patients showed non-schizophrenic values for neuraminic acid consistent with their diagnoses. Two schizophrenic patients demonstrated high values of total neuraminic acid temporally associated with convulsive activity of the nervous system.

Of the 21 cases treated with insulin five demonstrated a significant increase in concentration of neuraminic acid which accompanied a similarly significant clinical improvement. The moderate clinical improvement which was present in 10 of the 21 cases was unaccompanied by a significant change in the concentration of neuraminic acid in the CSF. In one case only was an apparent clinical improvement associated with a drop in the concentration of neuraminic acid. This small group of cases serves only to suggest certain questions for future work with reference to the effect of insulin therapy on the neuraminic acid concentration and the relationship of this effect to clinical changes in the patients. Thus, for instance, is a clinical improvement which is accompanied by a marked increase in the neuraminic acid in the cerebrospinal fluid more lasting than one which is accompanied by no change in the concentration of neuraminic acid? Are there some patients who demonstrate a degree of modifiability as indicated by the change in the concentration of neuraminic acid, in contrast to other patients who show a more fixed, and perhaps more serious type of schizophrenic illness related to neuraminic acid concentrations which do not change?

An important finding indirectly derived from the study of schizophrenic patients treated with insulin is the following: In the 21 cases who received insulin therapy over a period of several months, the adequacy of the diet consumed and the weight gain which resulted in all cases were in only five cases associated with an increase in neuraminic acid concentration sufficient to bring it over 41.0 micrograms/cc. Thus, the difference in neuraminic acid concentration which has been observed between the schizophrenic and non-schizophrenic groups is apparently unrelated to the diet consumed by the patients.

Conclusions

While the chemical determination of total neuraminic acid, when carefully done, has proved to be extremely useful, the assignment of a great deal of significance to a single determination in a given patient is as unwarranted as it is in any other laboratory determination in clinical medicine. On the other hand the finding of 'group consistent' values in a given individual over 2-5 repeated determinations makes the possibility that a low value is due to chance diminish to an insignificant level.

Despite these promising results the diagnostic value of the determination must remain an open question until many more cases in various diagnostic categories and at various stages in the clinical course of their psychiatric illness have been examined.

The data so far available suggest by the constancy of the values obtained that what is being measured is, in fact, in some way characteristic of the individual, and that the variation which occurs is in many cases temporally coincidental with and qualitatively related to the manifest clinical changes which occur both spontaneously and with treatment. Whether this finding for CSF is paralleled by changes in the state of neuraminic acid in the brain itself and by changes in its function in the central nervous system[5,6,7] is yet to be determined.

Whether the repeated determinations of the neuraminic acid concentration in individual patients will provide an objective index which may be of use in following the clinical course and determining the efficacy of a particular treatment in individual schizophrenic patients, has yet to be determined.

Perhaps most important is the possibility that detailed chemical studies of the structure of these complex constituents of the nervous system and of their interaction will provide new information which will permit a better understanding of the unity of structure and function.

Acknowledgments

These studies have been supported in part by grants from the United States Public Health Service (B-1221 and M-1491) and from the Supreme Council 33° Scottish Rite Northern Masonic Jurisdiction, USA.

References

1. Bogoch, S.: Cerebrospinal Fluid Neuraminic Acid Deficiency in Schizophrenia. Am. J. Psychiat., *114*, 172, 1957.

2. Bogoch, S.: Cerebrospinal Fluid Neuraminic Acid Deficiency in Schizophrenia. A.M.A. Arch. Neurol. & Psychiat., *80*, 221, 1958.

3. Bogoch, S.: Fractionation and Quantitative Analysis of Cerebrospinal Fluid Constituents with Reference to Neuropsychiatric Disorders. Am. J. Psychiat., *114*, 108, 1958.

4. Bogoch, S.: Protein and Carbohydrate Constituents of Cerebrospinal Fluid in Neuropsychiatric Disorders. In press.

5. Bogoch, S.: Neuraminic Acid in the Central Nervous System. In Rinkel, M. (ed.) *Chemical Concepts of Psychosis.* New York: McDowell, Obolensky & Co., 1958.

6. Bogoch, S.: Studies on the Structure of Brain Ganglioside. Biochem. J., *68*, 319, 1958.

7. Bogoch, S.: Inhibition of Viral Hemagglutination by Brain Ganglioside. Virology, *4*, 458, 1957.

8. Bogoch, S.: Neuraminic Acid in the Central Nervous System. Symposium on the Central Nervous System. Proceedings IV International Congress of Biochemistry, Vienna, 1958.

9. Bogoch, S.: Isolation of Neuraminic Acid-containing Proteins from Cerebrospinal Fluid. IV International Congress of Biochemistry, Supplement to International Abstracts of Biological Sciences. Pergamon Press Ltd., London. 1958. Page 217.

10. Bogoch, S., Dussik, K. T. and Lever, P. G.: Repeated Observations on the Clinical Status and on the Concentration of Neuraminic Acid in the Cerebrospinal Fluid of Individual Schizophrenic Patients. In preparation for publication.

11. Bohm, P., Dauber, St., and Baumeister, L.: Neuraminic Acid: Its Occurrence and Estimation in Serum. Klin. Wchschr., *32*, 289, 1954.

DISCUSSION

DR. W. HIMWICH: I'd like to compliment the speaker upon the very nice piece of work which he has presented here. We have been very much interested in what he has been doing on neuraminic acid. We first heard rumors about it. Unfortunately we have not had any opportunity to do it ourselves, to work with this substance. I am very interested in the developmental curve of neuraminic acid in the cerebrospinal fluid.

If I understood your hypothesis correctly, this may be one of the many substances which regulate the exchange between blood and brain. If that is true then this developmental curve takes a form which we would expect from our very limited data on what does happen to blood and brain exchange in the human and in the young of other animals.

BERNARD BRODIE: I would like to congratulate Dr. Bogoch for having skilfully sidestepped the trap which might well have led him to spend all his efforts looking for abnormalities in levels of neuraminic acid in mental disease. While not ignoring the possibility that, despite the immature state of our knowledge, it might be possible to formulate a unitary chemical theory of schizophrenia, he is focusing his attention on the structure and properties of neuraminic acid containing substances and on the role of these large molecules in normal brain function. The presence of neuraminic containing ganglioside material, in brain only, suggests that it may well be an important link between biochemistry and brain function.

DR. BOGOCH: I would like to thank the discussants for

their comments. With reference to Dr. W. Himwich's comments, as you know, the maturation of the brain is a complex phenomenon that is not complete at birth. The first four or five years show great changes with reference to myelinization and the development of synaptic connections, much of which we know almost nothing about. The excellent chemical findings of Dr. Himwich's group with regard to the exchange of substances in the developing central nervous system indicate an important area of investigation which will be of interest for some time to come.

I would like to thank Dr. Brodie for his comments. Certainly brain ganglioside is a fascinating material. I did not have time to show you some of its chemical relatives which occur in other parts of the body, which differ slightly in their structural components and are less complex, yet very closely related. I believe that this family of glycolipid substances will be shown to be important wherever they occur in terms of membrane function.

This general problem of the membrane and transport function of these materials throughout the body is the one that is closest to our interest and is the one with which we shall be most concerned in the next few years.

Chapter 19

SUMMARY

MAX RINKEL

The concept of schizophrenia as an organic disease (although environmental, hereditary and developmental factors are important in its etiology) provides the basic theory justifying research in organic treatments of this disease. Hoff has presented an historical survey of such treatments with a clarification of the diagnoses and prognosis of the disease process. Most of the organic treatments have been on a trial-and-error basis; even insulin shock therapy was primarily introduced by Sakel as a result of astute clinical observations rather than from a theory based on knowledge of chemical changes occurring during psychosis. Hoff states emphatically that "Insulin treatment is the only successful treatment of our time."

Wortis reviewed very carefully the history of insulin shock treatment, which originally was used to accomplish gain in weight in psychotic patients, a use yielding the subordinate observations that in many of these patients their psychotic condition improved. It is amazing that so many scientists had observed this fact without investigating its implications. Sakel approached this problem from an entirely different direction; his rationale for insulin therapy in psychoses was based on his use of insulin as a vagotonic antagonist to the sympathotonic overactivity observed during the withdrawal symptoms in abstinence cures of morphine addiction. In reference to the early use of insulin shock therapy, the chairman was struck by one point of Sargant's remarks to the effect that the value of the therapy can largely be judged by the gain in weight of the patients.

Sargant has emphasized the need for combined treatments of insulin sub-coma or coma, electric shock, and tranquilizers as the best hope for curing early schizophrenics and preventing lapses into chronicity. One of his most cogent remarks was that "we must continue searching for much of our information at the bedside, rather than in the statistician's office, or from the high-powered advertising of the drug houses."

This particular theme of the necessity for carefully controlled clinical observation recurred throughout the meeting, more often in negative aspects, pointing out the inadequacies of statistical evaluations. Differences in diagnosis (even though it was stressed that a schizophrenic is a schizophrenic regardless of where he lives or his cultural background) and differences in the methods of treatment used prevent logical statistical interpretation.

Some of Hoff's remarks in the discussion should be mentioned. He said, "We believe in a many-sided cause of schizophrenia because we believe both in organic and functional origins." "We believe that a combination of insulin treatment with organic and psychological measures represents the most effective weapon against schizophrenia." "Schizophrenia to us is a serious disease, and we thus feel justified in using any and every method of treatment which offers promise of improvement."

Bermann's report contains one specific warning that should be reiterated: "The existence of fatal cases due to the simultaneous use of the Sakel method and reserpine makes it necessary to avoid the administration of reserpine under all circumstances while hypoglycemia shocks are being given."

The global view of insulin treatment in psychiatry was neatly and comprehensively presented by the most traveled contributor to this conference. Bowman reported on the use of such treatment in the Orient, giving as a side remark that medical supplies left in China by the armed forces had not only provided the material but had stimulated extensive use of it in the treatment of schizophrenia. One statement that particularly interested me compared the new "miracle drugs" with insulin. The drug therapy "is no curative treatment. It is primarily drugging a person to make him more comfortable and make him able to adjust outside of a hospital whereas he required hospitalization before such therapy. This is very different from the technique of giving insulin therapy, wherein after a certain period the patient is completely taken off the treatment and it is hoped that insulin per se will have had a certain curative value." Another remark from Bowman; in his conclusion he states, "I feel that we are on the verge of working out the physiological bases of schizophrenia and with a better understanding of them, newer and improved methods of treatment will quickly follow."

Hoch emphasized the major theme of the meeting: the need for research. He stressed the question of differences in treatment of acute and sub-acute schizophrenics as contrasted with the treatment of chronic schizophrenics and the development of differential treatment of the various sub-groups of schizophrenia. Both insulin shock and drug therapy seem to be successful in cases of catatonic and paranoid schizophrenia, but result in little success in cases categorized as hebephrenia or simple schizophrenia. An almost precise quotation of his views on insulin and drug therapy is: While I personally feel there are patients who respond better to insulin than to drugs, I am interested in applying some form of treatment to many unfortunate and helpless individuals who otherwise would receive nothing.

The discussion following these papers was begun by Ewalt who took exception to the statement that schizophrenia is schizophrenia wherever it occurs. He remembered that "the incidence of schizophrenia was much higher in Philadelphia than it was in Baltimore, during the time that Bond and Strecker were interested in schizophrenia in Philadelphia, and Dr. Adolph Meyer had a very conservative attitude toward schizophrenia over in Baltimore." His remark that "For a westerner these places are pretty close together" is painful, in that I remember that in a single hospital at about the same period diagnoses shifted easily between schizophrenia and affective psychoses. Ewalt spoke about the process of cure, saying that "no treatment ever cured a patient of anything"—"we can only provide conditions that will enable the natural curative processes of nature to cure the patient."

Greenblatt brought into sharp focus the many factors involved in insulin treatment, such as the special regimen and added attention, the patients' role in the hospital community, the attitude of the staff towards this method of therapy. His last point deserves further emphasis (many of the contributors and discussants have referred to this idea directly and indirectly), the enthusiasm of the doctor for any type or method of therapy is one of the most essential elements in successful treatment.

Cameron elaborated on Ewalt's discussion of cure by saying, "When we think about recovery, one of the things which we must take into consideration is that the human organism is an emergent phenomenon."

Mann interpreted schizophrenia as the example par excellence of psychophysiological disease so inclusive that it involves all biochemistry, all physiology and all of society. There are trends in the direction that the treatment or investigation of schizophrenia is going far beyond the chemical, the neurophysiological, the psychological, into the wider field of society itself.

Gralnick indicated research potentialities in studying doctor-patient relationships which have as yet not been adequately observed in the course of insulin therapy.

Hoff reemphasized his views that no one treatment by itself will produce satisfactory results. We must combine biological treatment with psychotherapy. It is possible that drug treatment, in selected cases, will substitute effectively for insulin shock treatment.

Conran concurred with the previous discussion and added, on the basis of his many years of experience with insulin treatment, that a "therapeutic milieu structured on dynamic principles quite specifically is an aid to insulin therapy."

The next paper, presented by Arnold, produced some of the most vehement scientific discussion. It offered the theory that disturbance of the performance metabolism in the singular ganglion cells leads to a process which successively decreases the differentiation stage of the common function. This forms the basis of a schizophrenic process or defective state. Insulin is a drug which causes a tight stranglehold on the life function of a ganglion cell. One may expect that those cells will successively be destroyed which have an heredito-genetical disturbance of the organization of their carbohydrate metabolism and which are in an actual state of injury, meaning that they are supporting the psychotic process. The ganglion cells without actual dysfunction, but having a potential trend to it, have more resistance to this destructive stranglehold. Healthy ganglion cells are practically never affected. Arnold sums up his observations "that I.S.T. by Sakel after it was developed according to the described technique has become, in our day, the standard treatment for all cases of schizophrenia."

In discussion of this paper, Hoff strongly supported Arnold's theory, saying that "we must go back to the original treatment of Sakel. That means it must be a treatment with the destruction of cells." He also gave his opinion that in all cases psychotherapy and occupational therapy should be used and that he believes that insulin in combination with electroshock treatment and psychotherapy is the right means of treatment.

Denber raised the question whether the anatomical

changes are the result of anoxia due to insulin coma, or may these changes be the result of a non-specific action produced by any type of coma. There is a considerable amount of evidence to show that, in E.E.G. findings, the presence of high voltage slow waves can be produced not only by insulin coma, but by many other types of treatment in psychiatry.

Kalinowsky commented, "I think it is important for us to realize that we can get twice as many patients well with treatment as get well without treatment."

Hoff added some further remarks to the effect that: "We believe that in the first stage (of schizophrenia) there are only functional disturbances; that later on there is a true organic disruption of cell function, apparent not only clinically but visible in histological pictures as well."

Himwich questioned the evidence for the suggestion that cells concerned with schizophrenia patterns are the ones most sensitive to hypoglycemia. He suggested the use of the expression "deprivation of energy" to distinguish between glucose lack and oxygen lack.

Kline suggested a controlled experiment of making a brain cell count of schizophrenic patients treated by I.S.T. whose deaths had no connection with insulin therapy, contrasting patients who had recovered with those who had failed to recover. On spontaneous remissions, he presumed that defective brain cells somehow recover through some physiological metabolic process.

Dussik commented, "I feel it is necessary to point out that their theory concerns the assumed mechanism of the curative insulin effect but that no symptoms of defect whatsoever result from this treatment after it has been successfully terminated."

Arnold in closing the discussion agreed with Dussik that following insulin shock treatment the patient shows Bleuler's syndrome during some months, but in control examinations after five years no signs of an organic brain lesion can be observed.

Pacheco e Silva referred to several articles on modification of insulin treatment in reaching the conclusion that, "In our opinion the modifications introduced into the original technique of Sakel, on the one hand had the advantage of not requiring such an exacting technique and not carrying so many risks, on the other hand brought the drawbacks of not causing such complete remission in schizophrenia cases."

One really disturbing paragraph in Sal y Rosas' article contributes to the arguments concerning the difficulty in obtaining adequate and comparable statistics: "The insulin treatment is carried out independently in each building under the supervision of a female or male nurse who is assisted by several non-skilled employees. The personnel receive no special instruction in insulin therapy beyond that given in the nursing school. Moreover, due to a system of rotating the nursing staffs of the different departments, the insulin stations have no permanent staff."

Greenblatt reported on a pertinent study made at the Massachusetts Mental Health Center, "We attempted to assess the comparative value of deep and light comas. We found to our amazement that deep coma shows no marked peculiarities over light coma. However, we had the impression that in severe cases deep coma treatments were more successful, even though our results did not attain statistical significance."

Delgado analyzed the results of various methods of insulin treatment of 540 cases of schizophrenia on the bases of age, sex, heredity, diagnosis and duration of illness. He concluded that, "among the four methods used, the one that gives the best result is the combination of insulin, electroshock and chlorpromazine."

Bernath early in his paper made a statement with which I am sure the conference is in complete agreement: "I think that careful clinical observation is an important first step which then must be followed up by controlled experiments and exact statistical evaluations." It is not necessary to repeat his concise and thorough presentation of historical material on mild hypoglycemia treatment and the use of such treatment in alleviating anxiety. I would like to call your attention to two of the conclusions derived from his own research: M.H.T. (modified hypoglycemia treatment) favorably modifies anxiety in 89 per cent of patients with various non-psychotic, subacute and chronic psychiatric conditions, and, a very practicable observation, that M.H.T. can be used as an office procedure since it is harmless and has no side effects of any significance.

Sargant, in discussing this paper, said while mild insulin therapy is relatively useless in the treatment of schizophrenia, his experience has been that it is most useful in the treatment of anxiety hysteria where there is pronounced loss of weight.

Donnelly agreed as to the importance of loss of weight as a prognostic sign and went on to speculate as to whether the effect of insulin is interruption of more recently developed metabolic patterns or whatever constitutes the physical basis of memory.

Denber again raised the question regarding specificity of insulin coma treatment and pointed out that the effect may be analogous to that produced with a wide variety of therapeutic techniques.

Gralnick found that subcoma insulin is helpful in treating psychotic patients who have a prominent symptom of anxiety. However, he stressed the fact that general use of insulin therapy has shown that in addition to the physiological changes there are others of a highly significant dynamic nature.

Sargant in answering questions from Kalinowsky said that: "My present impression is that combining modified insulin with tranquilizers may accelerate weight gain and diminution in tension. When the weight has been restored, one can often stop the insulin and sometimes keep the patient on a suitable tranquilizer afterwards."

Bernath clarified his views in his response to the discussion. One new statement was, "I feel that we treat anxiety with anxiety. I do not think that M.H.T. is specific. It ameliorates clinical, excess, disruptive anxiety by the application of measured and controlled anxiety caused by mild hypoglycemic reaction."

Weiss gave a precise account of insulin therapy in a V. A. Hospital, specifying the rationale for changing from Sakel's original technique to Rapid Increase Procedure. He explained the decline in the number of patients being treated by insulin on the basis that "increasing use of tranquilizers has lessened the necessity in a number of cases to use insulin or other somatic therapy in order to help the patient to become more accessible to verbal therapy. Our accent has been on psychotherapy, and our concept of the use of insulin coma has been that it was very useful as an adjunct, but not as a primary or exclusive form of treatment."

Dussik discussed his results from insulin treatment and reviewed a considerable portion of the literature. He stated that a judicious combination of I. C. T. with the various tranquilizers is in line with Sakel's program. He concluded that "Sakel's I. C. T. has a very definite place in an active treatment program of today."

Gottlieb, in his comments on various of the papers, pointed out two fundamentally different approaches: psychotherapy which attempts to remove or minimize the personalized stresses under which the patient has been living; somatic treatment in which stress is being used to overwhelm the patient. He brought up some basic problems that deserve investigation: "Can we in some way develop indicators that will give us some idea of the mechanisms that are involved in these various therapeutic approaches? What are the mechanisms that are really defective, a cellular distortion, a metabolic system crippled by a defective enzyme, or a pattern ascribable to disturbances in psychological learning?"

Kline in referring to cures said that, "It is certainly a very appropriate and proper function to relieve disability so that the patient can return to society, and in most branches of medicine that is regarded as a satisfactory therapeutic result." Another point he emphasized was, "The principle of good medicine is to use the most rapid, least expensive treatment if it will do the job."

Wortis asked Kline, "Do we have any data to justify the use of a method that is cheap, on the assumption that the results are just as good as the more expensive and elaborate methods?"—"the argument of cheapness is very unconvincing particularly to the families of patients who may have non-recoverable illnesses after valuable time has been lost."

Denber answered Wortis on the basis of New York State statistics covering many years. "It is fairly well known that most new treatments have a beneficial effect at the outset. As time goes on, this beneficial action seems to diminish or disappear. The relapse and readmission rate until 1954 has been fairly constant, around 30 per cent." Since 1954, drugs have been introduced and there has been a consistent decrease in hospital population as well as in the readmission rate. "There is no question that insulin coma treatment has been of great value. However, it is questionable whether or not it has the absolute value as claimed by Dr. Dussik."

Kalinowsky expressed the view that after three or four months of unsuccessful pharmacotherapy we should discontinue and give the patient the benefit of the other treatments.

Conran reported that, "there are certain patients that do not respond for nine months to drug therapy."

Kline replied, "Since current statistics give about the same percentage of response for the drugs and the insulin, I do not see how one can seriously advocate using insulin first and to the exclusion of other treatments."

Dussik responded, "I believe that the issue of the expense is not so significant as it is sometimes said, but most of the time a 'red herring' which is occasionally used as an excuse for lack of activity and courage."—"It is dangerous now to give up a proven weapon in the fight against such a disastrous condition as schizophrenia." "I think this conference helped us to take a good look at very important problems, or at least to understand where to look."

Bogoch pointed out the possibility that the increase in the concentration of neuraminic acid in the cerebrospinal fluid with age, which he observed, represents a maturation phenomenon, and indicated the corollary that the low values, observed in 92 per cent of untreated chronic schizophrenic adults, represents a form of chemical immaturity of the nervous system. Investigation with repeated neuraminic acid determinations on patients being actively treated with I. S. T. showed a low concentration of neuraminic acid in 84 per cent of the patients, a finding which demonstrates that the low values previously reported for schizophrenic patients are reasonably "group consistent" even despite active treatment.

Williamina Himwich suggested that neuraminic acid may be one of the many substances which regulate the exchange between blood and brain, and that the developmental curve takes the expected form of what happens to blood and brain exchange in young humans and animals.

Brodie commented that, "The presence of neuraminic containing ganglioside material, in brain only, suggests that it may well be an important link between biochemistry and brain function."

In concluding this summary, I would like to remind you of some pertinent comments by Himwich in his opening address as chairman of the first session of this conference. He said, this treatment is most important from a practical point of view for it returns patients to society; but it has done more than that, it has changed our ideas about the prognosis of schizophrenia. With the advent of Sakel's treatment, our ideas of an invariably bad prognosis have had to change to a more optimistic outlook and to increased efforts in treatment. I also wish to quote Joseph Wortis who, in his discussion of Physiological Treatment in the Review of

Psychiatric Progress, 1958, answered the question, raised by the Second International Conference on Insulin Treatment, whether insulin treatment has been outmoded, as follows: "The critical consensus was that it was not."

In my opinion, this conference has succeeded in providing a comprehensive review of the progress of insulin therapy in psychiatry throughout the world, and has stimulated further research in the important relationship between biochemistry, physiology, psychology, and psychiatry.

Part Four ·

A P P E N D I X

APPENDIX

EDITORS' NOTE

The publishers have presented us with a copy of Manfred Sakel's speech at the ceremony in his honor, in Vienna, accepting a citation from the Psychiatrisch-Neurologische Klinik of the University of Vienna in September, 1957. We are grateful to Dr. Runes for his careful and conscientious work in putting the rough translation of Dr. Sakel's address into smoother English. Dr. Runes states: "I really am convinced that, from the point of view of medical history, this is a significant address, as it was delivered by the discoverer after thirty years of practical experience."

The editors feel impelled to include this speech, and the citation, as an appendix because of its historical interest.

Ed.

SAKEL'S ADDRESS AT THE UNIVERSITY OF VIENNA AT THE THIRTY-YEAR CELEBRATION OF HIS DISCOVERY

September 12-14, 1957

I am very happy to be present at this anniversary of the important discovery made in 1927 at the University of Vienna Clinic regarding the treatment of nervous and mental diseases. As it happens, the Medical School has chosen this occasion to honor me as author of this discovery. For my part, I do not believe that discoverers should be honored. They do what they do because they are compelled to, either by some higher plan or by the endowment of their genes, which make them tools in the uncovering of knowledge and the providing of ways and means for advancing the progress of mankind. In other words, their deeds are not the consequence of their own volition. Acts of discovery should, rather, be considered deeds of "mission" or compulsion.

I consider it far more appropriate that homage and honor should be paid those who, seeking no glory for themselves and at the risk that the discovery may be a fiasco, throw behind it the whole weight of their position and authority—powers which I, in my youth, did not possess—to make possible its general acceptance and its availability to the unfortunate patients for whom it is intended. I am of course referring, in this instance, to Professor Otto Poetzl, that great master of psychiatry, and to Professor Hans Hoff, at that time his able assistant, at present his worthy successor. As is always the case with new ideas and discoveries, however valid they may be, they must first overcome the inevitable opposition of the deeply ingrained thought habits of the past, however invalid these may eventually prove to be. Taking into account, furthermore, the facts of my barely having come of age in psychiatry, and my complete lack of experience in the indirect approach, which arouses, as everyone knows, even more concentrated resistance, the discovery would certainly have remained a theory only, and have never reached the stage of general application, had it not been for the selfless and dedicated struggle of Professor Poetzl, and his associate, Professor Hans Hoff, to force upon the reluctant profession this long-awaited, new approach to nervous and mental diseases. Or, at least, force them to try it, and prove or disprove its efficacy, rather than dismiss it out of hand.

The Medical School of Vienna has been lucky—and I

hope its luck will continue—in having had at the head of its Psychiatric Department a man of Professor Poetzl's vision, with the capacity to understand and entertain unconfirmed concepts, unorthodox ideas, and afford them an opportunity to prove their usefulness to mankind. I hope that this attitude will continue, not only in Vienna, and that ideas which are accepted habits of thought in medical science will not be clung to once their ineffectiveness has been shown.

To come back to my discovery—and I suppose that is what is expected of me—I would like to say that it was simply inevitable. Being of a critical temperament, and trying to be as objective about myself as anyone can be, I realized that my use of orthodox psychiatric procedures was not yielding results that justified my efforts. Naturally, I realized my ineffectiveness, and I began to search the whole psychiatric literature for evidences of the success of others. To my surprise and sorrow, ineffectiveness proved to be general. Having been trained to be logical, the only conclusion I could reach was that we were all stuck with a wrong approach, which we were pursuing only out of inertia and out of the momentum of our beliefs. I realized suddenly that psychiatry, the newest branch of modern medicine, was, and is, working from a basis of faith and belief rather than achievement. For me, this was unacceptable as a scientific discipline. Postulates and theories, however eloquently and elegantly expressed, should have no place in a scientific discipline, and can be of no use therapeutically. So I fell back upon the approach of empirical science. That is, if we want to uncover some unknown law of cause and effect in nature, we must first formulate precisely the question for which we seek an answer. If properly formulated, the question will already contain half the answer, and lead to a complete one. Hazily formulated definitions, common enough in psychiatry, lead in a vicious circle to parochial beliefs. Therefore, I had first to decide what psychiatry was meant to be. For me as a doctor and scientist, it meant simply a discipline to cure a *sickness*, which needed to be cured rather than talked about. It could not possibly serve the doctor as a diving board from which to take off on flights of literary dexterity, or as a starting point for philosophical, or even worse for mystical, speculations. That is not to say that the doctor can ignore or neglect the human attitude. It must be used as a therapeutic tool in every sickness, even physical ones, and particularly in psychiatric cases, which differ from other sicknesses in one major particular—that their main symptoms appear in the dysfunction not, say, of the intestines, but of the mental faculties. In treating cholera, even after Koch, a doctor knew that he had not only to combat the infection, but also to take careful consideration of the diet so as not to aggravate the infected intestines. A similar approach, which according to my line of thought might prove successful, had to be sought to psychiatric sickness. I emphasize the word "sickness" because I do not want to leave the impression that I am ignoring other disturbances in human beings, which may be just as upsetting but which cannot be considered sickness. No one can deny that doctors are frequently called upon to deal with unhappiness caused by psychological, mental, educational, economic or other circumstantial factors; or even by a nervous system not sufficiently robust to cope with the normal hardships and adversities of life without guidance and spiritual support. But then we should differentiate sharply and strictly between medical psychiatry and so-called psychiatry. One deals with sickness, the other calls for an abundance of emotional and psychological strength on the part of the doctor with which he can succor those who lack it.

If, as doctors, we confine ourselves to the purely medical, we will see that this celebration is among the few such in history; for among the thousands of "new" treatments devised in centuries past, fewer than can be counted on the fingers of one hand could continue to claim effectiveness after thirty years.

The reason must be that in this case the treatment went to the very fundamentals of the sickness. I am especially happy, not merely to have opened a new avenue to the treatment of nervous and mental diseases, but to have been apparently correct in recognizing the basic causes of these disturbances. Devised as an over-all grand strategy, the treatment supplied, at the same time, tactical means of modifying its application to suit the individual patient and his illness. This seems to be borne out particularly in the literature of the past few months. The metabolic-biochemical treatment by means of endogenous insulin (the Sakel technique) not only has survived, but is reconquering the ground it lost to its (to be sure, flattering) imitators, who selected part factors and devised short cuts through the use of physical or chemical exogenous agents. It now appears certain that the best that can be achieved by these imitations of the main factors in the treatment—that is, convulsion and hibernation—is amelioration but not cure. Ameliorations achieved by exogenous agents have proved in psychiatry, as in other branches of medicine, not capable of permanently correcting distorted metabolic-biochemical functions. As in other branches of medicine, it becomes clearer and clearer that cures can be achieved only by imitating the natural, corrective, biological capacity of the body. It will likewise become clearer and clearer that the doctor has his own human limitations which he cannot exceed. He can stimulate the body's innate, self-regulatory, defense mechanisms to achieve enduring health, but he cannot invent and add to nature anything that nature has not already provided for its protection.

That is the reason why, in spite of the similar nerve effects which other synthetic or foreign body agents may have, these agents cannot intrude themselves as insulin can into the established biochemical life processes, fixed for millions of years. That is why, however astounding the effects of "miracle" drugs upon nervous disease, their working mechanism is not a biological one, and therefore not permanently acceptable to the body cells.

Insulin, on the other hand, is a bodily product, which

properly used seems to achieve—as I originally claimed it achieved—improvement and recovery in the nerve cells because it works biologically. Thus the "unscholarly," but still indisputable, discovery by Jenner of immunization against smallpox, which has saved hundreds upon hundreds of millions of lives, and the "unscholarly" and furiously resisted lay discovery by Pasteur of infections, diseases and immunization against rabies by an attenuated toxin, are still effective because fundamentally true. It should be recalled in this connection that if it had rested with the prevailing medical thinking of his time, Pasteur would not have survived his first publication. But fortunately for mankind, Pasteur was a genius even if he was not a doctor. Even that would have done him little good had not nature further equipped him with the special skills of a good popular writer. So he succeeded in selling the truth to the medical profession via the readers of the daily press. But that is how life is; and these human factors not only repeat themselves, but remain eternal.

When I announced my biochemical-metabolic discovery for the treatment of nervous and mental diseases, it might still—in spite of Poetzl's support, into which he threw all he could give—have remained only a parochial affair or a local fight within the Vienna Medical School, because I lacked utterly the gift of writing. But the very fact that opposition to my discovery was so vociferous and turbulent made the headlines of the daily press in Europe. Therefore, I must give my opposition credit for having spread my findings, however unwillingly, by making front-page headlines, with the result that all the scientific centers of Europe were informed, aroused and alarmed, so that they could not ignore the issue. Thus, the daily press not only discharged its proper function, but served the ultimate good of humanity.

Award from the Psychiatrisch-Neurologische Klinik of the University of Vienna.

Die

Psychiatrisch-Neurologische Klinik

der

Universität Wien

gratuliert dem Erfinder der
Insulin-Schocktherapie

Herrn Prof. Dr. Manfred Sakel

anläßlich des 30. Jahrestages
vom ganzen Herzen.
Sie empfindet diese Erfindung als
einen Markstein in der Entwicklung
der Therapie der Psychosen.

Wien, 12. 9. 1957

Prof. Dr. Hans Hoff

INDEX

A

Ackner, viii, 152, 339
Adey, 112
Alexander, 46, 47, 63, 318, 319
Appel, 21
Arduini, 110, 112
Arieti, 323
Arnold, O. H., 134, 164, 168, 196, 222, 223, 224, 225, 226, 227, 228, 229, 333, 339, 364, 365

B

Babinski, 307
Bahr, 23
Banting, 50, 179
Barcroft, Sir Joseph, 139
Basowitz, 267
Batt, 61, 67
Becker, 19
Bennett, 23, 139, 140, 192
Berger, 106
Bermann, G., 163, 235, 361
Berkowitz, 110, 112, 114, 116, 117, 119
Bernath, 292, 294, 295, 296, 366, 367
Berson, 140
Berze, 5, 25
Berson, 56
Best, 62, 179
Beyer, 21
Bial, 344, 345
Billig, 59
Bini, 12, 147
Binswanger, 163
Birnbaum, 67
Bleuler, Eugen, 5, 6, 165, 324, 365
Bleuler, Manfred, 324
Bliss, 59, 67, 69

Boardman, 339
Bogoch, Samuel, 329, 358, 370
Bohm, 344
Bond, Earl, 52, 73, 166, 168, 169, 171, 188, 225, 235, 292, 296, 304, 363
Bone, 58
Borelli, Nelson, 162
Borenz, 48, 50
Boschi, 235
Bourne, viii
Bowes, ix
Bowman, Karl, xix, 26, 60, 270, 271, 362
Bremer, 109
Brenman, 110
Brevais-Pearson, 201
Brickner, 272
Brodie, Bernard B., 127, 128, 135, 136, 141, 358, 359, 370
Brodman, 14
Bumke, 29

C

Campbell, McFie, 29, 128
Cameron, Ewen D., 26, 48, 106, 191, 195, 363
Cerletti, 12, 147, 232
Chesler, 87
Chicata, Miguel A., 264
Colfer, 94
Conn, 51
Conran, 197, 338, 364, 369
Cori, 213
Corwin, 56
Costa, 92
Cotton, 168
Cowie, 19
Craske, 147, 269

Cravioto, 89, 91
Crossland, 93
Cunza, Jose L., 264

D

Daley, 235
Dawson, 89, 90
Dax, 232, 235
de Gourmont, Remy, 33
Delgado, Honorio, xviii, 244, 366
Denber, 223, 229, 294, 297, 337, 341, 364, 367, 369
DeWesselow, 55
Dohan, 63, 69
Donnelly, John, 131, 132, 135, 136, 137, 284, 285, 293, 295, 297, 367
Doussinet, Pierre, 22
Dunning, Henry, 128, 129
Dunkirk, 292
Dussik, 11, 25, 229, 230, 337, 338, 341, 365, 368, 369

E

Ehrlich, Paul, 179
Elkes, 17
Elliot, 93
Engel, 106
Ewalt, Jack R., 187, 362, 363

F

Farr, 21
Fazekas, 93, 94
Fernandez, 110
Ferris, 87
Feuerlein, 262
Fink, 121, 135, 339
Folin-Wu, 313
Fraser, Russell, 146
Freeman, 49, 63, 128
Friedman, 57
Freud, 18
Freudenberg, 146, 149
Funkenstein, 46, 271
Furtado, Diogo, 235

G

Gallinek, 21
Geiger, 91, 136, 138

Gelhorn, 47, 52, 126
Gerard, Ralph W., 126, 136, 138, 139, 267
Gerty, 54
Ghantus, 86
Glueck, 26
Glover, 286
Gold, 46
Goldner, 55
Goldwater, S. S., 172
Goncharova, 88
Goodwin, 107
Gordon, Malcolm, 131, 284
Gottlieb, 332, 338, 368
Gralnick, Alexander, 195, 295, 363, 367
Gray, 59
Greenblatt, Milton, 189, 191, 192, 251, 363, 366
Green, 112
Grenell, 110
Griffiths, 55
Gruenberg, 334
Grundler, 22

H

Haack, 19, 23
Haavaldsen, 140
Harris, 50, 55
Hartmann, 16
Hastings, 286
Haugaard, 55
Heath, 140
Hellbrunn, 60, 89
Hesser, 59
Heuyer, 244
Hewitt, 51
Himwich, Harold, 17, 86, 87, 92, 93, 94, 107, 110, 114, 120, 121, 134, 136, 192, 227, 230, 300, 307, 359, 365, 370
Himwich, Williamina A., 89, 90, 91, 126, 127, 128, 129, 130, 132, 358, 370
Hinkle, 49
Hippocrates, 198
Hoagland, 106, 107
Hoch, 15, 187, 189, 191, 195, 271, 318, 335, 336, 362
Hoff, Hans, x, 164, 166, 168, 171, 182, 184, 185, 187, 191, 193, 196,

222, 225, 226, 229, 332, 360, 361, 364, 365, 376
Hoffman, 55
Hokfelt, 58
Holmes, 167
Holzbauer, 58
Horvath, 57
Hoskins, 26
Hough, Heloise, 128, 129
Houssay, 262

I

Ibor, Lopes, 232
Imache, 19

J

Jackson, Hughlings, 107, 139
Jacob, France E., 22
Jacobowsky, 235
Jaschke, 21
Jaspers, 163
Jenner, 380
Jones, 235

K

Kalinowsky, 12, 164, 224, 226, 233, 271, 294, 296, 318, 338, 365, 367, 369
Keele, 130
Kennedy, Foster, 163, 337
Kerr, 86, 87
Killam, K. F., 121, 141
Killam, E. K., 121, 141
Klasi, 8
Klein, 87
Klemperer, 268
Klenk, 344
Kline, Nathan S., 227, 230, 328, 334, 335, 336, 338, 339, 365, 368, 369
Kneipp, Jack, 299
Kolle, 262
Kraepelin, xxii, 6, 29
Kraines, 55
Kretschmer, 7
Kuppers, 22

L

Lamache, 21
Langfeldt, 323, 324
Lehmann, 62, 63
Lerman, J., 55, 81

Lestani, Hector, 161
Liebert, 60, 89, 213
Lingjaerde, 140
Livingston, 109
Looney, 48
Luft, 59

M

Machado, Mario, 161
Magoun, 109
Maher, 48
Malzberg, 248
Mann, 62, 63, 193, 363
Mansalet, Delman, 233
Mansour, 51
Margolis, Lester, 176
Marks, 68
Marsh, 55
Marshall, 21
May, 187
Mayer-Gross, 232, 235
McGhee, 91
McLaughlin, William, 318
Mebel, 22
Meduna, 11, 12, 27, 33, 54, 143
Meyer, 29, 30, 188, 235, 363
Millar, 59
Miskolczy, 19
Moniz, 14, 145
Morgan, 55
Morris, 46
Moruzzi, 107, 109
Moya, 55
Mueller, 25, 26, 248, 318, 328
Munn, Charlotte, 23, 24
Munson, 59

N

Naatanen, 56
Nadeau, 50
Nahum, 86
Nathan, 327
Nauta, 112
Neander, 63
Neutzel, 48, 51
Neveu, 232

O

Olsen, 48, 51, 87
Okizane, 113
Owens, 110, 114, 120

P

Paasonen, 93
Pacheco e Silva, 235, 365
Palisa, 11
Pamboukis, 235
Papez, 16, 112, 141, 283
Pappins, 93
Parfitt, 23
Parsons, Frederic, 19, 172, 173
Pasteur, 380
Patterson, 53, 262
Patton, ix
Petersen, 90
Pfister, 49, 257
Pilgrim, 55
Plattner, 248
Pogorinski, 162
Polatin, 270, 271, 277
Polonio, 150
Poetzl, Otto, 9, 10, 11, 14, 25, 212, 323, 376, 377, 380
Preston, 121
Prince, Morton, 29
Proctor, 48
Puca, 19, 21
Pullar-Strecker, 146

R

Randall, 91
Raphael, 19
Reiner, 53
Reiss, M., 283
Rennie, 271, 280
Revoredo, Leonor, 249
Richter, 17
Ricketts, 55
Rinkel, 168
Rivers, 309, 310
Roberti, 21
Rorschach, 257
Rosa, Sal y, 366
Rosenthal, 21
Rouleau, 50, 235
Rubin, 106
Rumke, 171
Runes, 375
Russell, 146

S

Saavedra, Alfredo, 264
Sakel, Manfred, vii, ix, x, xiv, xv, xx, xxi, xxii, xxiii, 10, 11, 13, 18, 19, 24, 25, 26, 27, 29, 30, 32, 33, 41, 75, 85, 86, 106, 107, 139, 142, 143, 147, 148, 152, 154, 158, 159, 160, 161, 162, 163, 165, 166, 167, 169, 170, 172, 173, 179, 180, 182, 183, 185, 189, 191, 193, 195, 219, 231, 232, 233, 234, 235, 236, 242, 243, 244, 248, 253, 255, 267, 277, 304, 320, 321, 326, 328, 337, 360, 361, 364, 366, 368, 370, 375, 379
Samson, 91
Sargant, William, 164, 166, 167, 170, 187, 189, 197, 223, 232, 235, 269, 292, 293, 294, 296, 318, 361, 367
Sarwer-Foner, 191, 295
Sawyer, 114, 120, 226, 131, 136, 141
Scheflen, 53
Sherer, 339
Schilder, 8, 172
Schmidt, Paul, 20, 21, 22
Schultz-Henke, Harold, 163
Seggiaro, Juan, 161
Semrad, 23
Selye, 232
Sharp, 23
Shurley, T., 46, 52, 73, 304
Slater, 269, 318
Slein, 213
Slotopolsky, 21, 22
Somogyi, 48, 313
Sorin, Miguel, 162
Southard, 187
Speidel, 126
Spiegel, 14
Spotnitz, 271
Stanesco, 21
Steck, 22, 24, 268
Steinfeld, 26
Stewart, 121
Stone, 87, 94
Stransky, 5, 8
Strecker, 188, 363
Strehl, 22
Sullivan, Harry Stack, 89, 90, 91, 94, 191
Sundsten, 110, 114

T

Targowa, 19, 21
Teitelbaum, 269
Tietz, 58, 67

Titeca, 235
Tokizane, 120
Torp, 24
Trehub, 339
Trelles, J. O., 253
Tsau, 62

U

Urse, 54

V

Vaichulis, 54
Vanderkamp, 46
Van Meter, 92, 110, 114, 120
Vogt, 58, 93, 226
Von Braunmühl, 51, 262, 224, 253
Von Euler, 59

W

Waelsch, 282
Waggoner, Raymond, 165, 295, 297
Warner-Jauregg, 5, 10
Walaas, 140
Walter, Allan, 232
Wartegg, 257
Weil-Malherbe, 58, 59
Weiss, 340, 368
West, F. H., 235, 262
Whitehorn, ix
Wilson, Isabel, 24, 146
Winkler, 283
Wolf, 49
Wolff, Harold G., 128, 130
Wortis, Joseph, xxi, 126, 172, 173, 336, 338, 340, 360, 369, 370
Wycis, 14

Y

Yalow, 56
Yannet, 88, 89, 90